The *PREVENTION* How-To Dictionary of HEALING REMEDIES AND TECHNIQUES

The *PREVENTION* How-To Dictionary of HEALING REMEDIES AND TECHNIQUES

From Acupressure and Aspirin
to Yoga and Yogurt
Over 350 Curative Options

By the Editors of *PREVENTION*
Magazine Health Books

Edited by John Feltman

Rodale Press, Emmaus, Pennsylvania

If you have any questions or comments concerning this book, please write:

Rodale Press
Book Readers' Service
33 East Minor Street
Emmaus, PA 18098

Library of Congress Cataloging-in-Publication Data

The Prevention how-to dictionary of healing remedies
    and techniques.

        1. Therapeutics—Dictionaries.   I. Feltman, John.
II. Prevention Magazine Health Books.
RM36.P74   1992   615.5'03   92–9053
ISBN 0–87596–114–2   hardcover

Distributed in the book trade by St. Martin's Press

2   4   6   8   10   9   7   5   3   1   hardcover

NOTICE

This book is intended as a reference volume only, not as a medical manual. The information here is designed to help you make informed decisions about your health. It is not a substitute for any treatment that may have been prescribed by your doctor. If you suspect that you have a medical problem, we urge you to seek competent medical help.

CONTRIBUTORS

Editor: John Feltman

Contributing Writers: Douglas Dollemore, Sharon Faelten, Deborah Grandinetti, Matthew Hoffman, Marcia Holman, Anne Remondi Imhoff, Sid Kirchheimer, Gale Maleskey, Ellen Michaud, Hank Nuwer, Hollis Paschen, Jean Rogers, Richard Schorske, Porter Shimer, Lyn Votava, Joe Wargo, Russell Wild

Book Designer: Acey Lee

Cover Designer: Lisa Nawaz

Illustrators: Maryanne Buschini, John Carlance, Susan Rosenberger

Research Chief: Ann Gossy

Research/Fact-Checking Staff: Christine Dreisbach, Sharon Stocker, Jewel Flegal, Anne Remondi Imhoff, Cemela London, Melissa Meyers, Paris Mihely-Muchanic, Linda Miller, Cynthia Nickerson, Deborah Pedron, Bernadette Sukley, Michele Toth

Production Editor: Jane Sherman

Copy Editor: Ellen Pahl

Office Staff: Roberta Mulliner, Karen Earl-Braymer, Julie Kehs, Mary Lou Stephen

Managing Editor, *Prevention* Magazine Health Books: Alice Feinstein
Executive Editor, *Prevention* Magazine Health Books: Debora Tkac
Vice President and Editor in Chief, *Prevention* Magazine Health Books: William Gottlieb
Group Vice President, Health: Mark Bricklin

CONTENTS

• corrective lenses • cortisone • cotton swabs • cough medicines • CPR • cranberry juice • crying • cryosurgery

INTRODUCTION

Read any good dictionaries lately? In an age of spy novels, romances, and whodunits, the prospect of actually reading (or even browsing through) a large book that calls itself a dictionary might seem like an exercise in tedium. But for *The Prevention How-To Dictionary of Healing Remedies and Techniques,* you just might want to make an exception.

In fact, please don't even think of this book as a dictionary in the usual sense. It's definitely not the kind of volume you turn to once every four or five months to look up the definition of *onomatopoeic,* to check on the spelling of *somnambulate,* or to find a synonym for *ebullient.*

What you *will* be consulting this dictionary for regularly is something far more important: helpful, easy-to-understand information on hundreds of available healing options—from the latest prescription drugs and surgical techniques to the most traditional herbal and dietary home remedies. From balm of Gilead to biofeedback, from gamma globulin to gotu kola, from low-fat diet to liposuction, you'll be able to find out what works and why. And you'll learn from medical experts what practical steps you can take to make these remedies most effective.

If you have a particular health problem or concern, the Master Chart of Complaints and Remedies at the beginning of the book can help you zero in on dictionary entries you may want to consult first. Or you may want to simply turn directly to items of interest to find answers to questions you may have. In either case, "see also" suggestions at the end of many entries will direct you to additional headings that can supply more useful information.

So welcome to a dictionary with a difference, a unique guidebook to the myriad healing agents at your disposal. Use it in good health!

John Feltman

John Feltman
Senior Editor
Prevention Magazine Health Books

MASTER CHART OF COMPLAINTS AND REMEDIES

The following comprehensive listing of health problems and treatments is designed to help you quickly locate the information you need. For each problem at the left, dictionary entries that discuss aspects of treatment or prevention are provided to the right. If you are concerned about *allergies*, for example, you might want to turn to *affirmations, air cleaners, allergy shots, antihistamines, behavior therapy, decongestants, elimination diet,* and *eyedrops* to get a good overview of the problem and potential solutions. Check for additional "see also" notes at the end of many entries for suggested further reading.

Health Problem	See These Entries . . .
Abnormal menstrual bleeding	D & C hysterectomy
Abrasions	witch hazel
Acid indigestion	heat therapy
Acidosis	baking soda
Acne	acne remedies alcohol, rubbing imagery retinoids stress management tetracycline
Addictive habits	behavior therapy computer therapy group therapy
Addison's disease	hydrocortisone steroids
Age spots	bleaching cream chemical peels
Agoraphobia	group therapy self-help audiotapes
AIDS	art therapy AZT

Health Problem	See These Entries
Alcoholism	art therapy
	aversion therapy
	group therapy
	self-help groups
Allergies	affirmations
	air cleaners
	allergy shots
	antihistamines
	behavior therapy
	decongestants
	elimination diet
	eyedrops
Altitude sickness	hyperbaric oxygen
Anal fissures	petroleum jelly
Anaphylaxis	epinephrine
Anemia	nutritional therapy (folate)
Angina	angioplasty
	atherectomy
	beta blockers
	calcium channel blockers
	coronary bypass
	nitroglycerin
Anorexia nervosa	self-help audiotapes
Anxiety	acupuncture
	antianxiety drugs
	barbiturates
	beta blockers
	breathing techniques
	cognitive therapy
	color therapy
	dream therapy
	Gestalt therapy
	hypnosis

Health Problem	See These Entries
Anxiety—*continued*	imagery
	meditation
	music therapy
	phenobarbital
	plant therapy
	psychoanalysis
	sedatives
	therapeutic touch
	tranquilizers
	yoga
Arrhythmias	beta blockers
	calcium channel blockers
	nutritional therapy (magnesium)
Arthritis	acupuncture
	Alexander Technique
	anti-inflammatories
	aspirin
	balm of Gilead
	cold therapy
	cortisone
	exercise therapy
	ginger
	gold
	heat therapy
	hydrocortisone
	hydrotherapy
	imagery
	mattresses and beds
	music therapy
	oil of wintergreen
	painkillers
	physiatry
	poultices

Health Problem	See These Entries
	shoes, therapeutic
	stretching
Asthma	air cleaners
	anticholinergics
	atropine
	behavior therapy
	breathing techniques
	bronchodilators
	caffeine
	coffee
	cortisone
	cough medicines
	epinephrine
	fish oil
	hydrocortisone
	inhalers
	onions
	prednisone
	steroids
	stress management
	tea
	therapeutic touch
Astigmatism	corrective lenses
Athlete's foot	alum
	athlete's foot remedies
	cotton swabs
	deodorants
	hair dryer
Athletic injuries	hydrotherapy
Back pain	acupuncture
	Alexander Technique
	bed rest
	chiropractic

Master Chart of Complaints and Remedies

Health Problem	See These Entries
Back pain—*continued*	cold therapy electrotherapy flotation tanks gravity inversion hydrotherapy mattresses and beds mustard plasters oil of wintergreen orthoses physiatry physical therapy pillows posture therapy Relaxation Response weight loss yoga
Baldness	minoxidil
Bedsores	imagery mattresses and beds sugar
Birthmarks	laser surgery
Bite problems	mouth guards posture therapy
Blisters	pads and plasters petroleum jelly
Blood clots	anticoagulants aspirin ibuprofen leeches onions
Body odor	chlorophyll deodorants electrotherapy

Health Problem	See These Entries
Boils	heat therapy poultices
Breast cancer	lumpectomy mastectomy
Breast pain	evening primrose oil
Broken tooth	dentistry, restorative
Bronchitis	atropine breathing techniques cough medicines eucalyptus physical therapy slippery elm tetracycline
Brown skin patches	bleaching cream chemical peels
Bruises	alum cold therapy comfrey heat therapy plantain witch hazel
Bruxism	apple mouth guard
Bulimia	interpersonal psychotherapy
Bunions	orthoses pads and plasters shoes, therapeutic
Burns	aloe bandages cold therapy growth factors hyperbaric oxygen

Master Chart of Complaints and Remedies

Health Problem	See These Entries
Burns—*continued*	nutritional therapy (vitamin A) physical therapy skin grafts
Bursitis	ultrasound
Calluses	castor oil orthoses pads and plasters
Cancer	affirmations art therapy chemotherapy heat therapy imagery interferon laser surgery light therapy low-fat diet macrobiotic diet nutritional therapy (vitamin A) (vitamin C) onions radiation therapy retinoids self-help groups weight loss
Candidiasis	gentian violet
Canker sores	baking soda chamomile imagery lysine tea
Carpal tunnel syndrome	banana nutritional therapy (vitamin B_6) physiatry

Health Problem	See These Entries
Cataracts	imagery
Cerebral palsy	Feldenkrais Method
Cervical cancer	hysterectomy retinoids
Cervical dysplasia	cryosurgery
Chapped lips	petroleum jelly
Chickenpox	acyclovir calamine lotion oatmeal, colloidal
Childbirth problems	nutritional therapy (magnesium)
Chlamydia	tetracycline
Choking	Heimlich maneuver
Cirrhosis of the liver	dandelion
Cluster headaches	oxygen therapy
Colds	acetaminophen aspirin bed rest chicken soup cold remedies dandelion decongestants echinacea heat therapy humidifiers hydrotherapy ibuprofen imagery interferon lozenges menthol mustard plasters nutritional therapy (vitamin C)

Health Problem	See These Entries
Colds—*continued*	peppers, hot
	slippery elm
	thyme
	vaporizers
Cold sores	acyclovir
	aloe
Colitis	progressive relaxation
	yoga
Congestion	balm of Gilead
	cold remedies
	decongestants
Congestive heart failure	digitalis
	diuretics
Conjunctivitis	eyedrops
Constipation	bran
	castor oil
	fiber
	kelp
	laxatives
	mineral oil
	prunes
	psyllium
	vegetarian diet
Convulsions	anticonvulsants
	barbiturates
	phenobarbital
	sedatives
Corneal ulcers	eyedrops
Corns	castor oil
	orthoses
	pads and plasters
Coughs	cold remedies
	cough medicines

Health Problem	See These Entries
	eucalyptus
	horehound
	menthol
	slippery elm
	thyme
Cracked nipples	plantain
Crooked teeth	dentistry, restorative
Cross-eye (strabismus)	corrective lenses
	vision therapy
Cuts	alum
	plantain
Cystitis	baking soda
	penicillin
Cysts	cryosurgery
Cytomegalovirus	acyclovir
Dandruff	thyme
Decompression sickness	hyperbaric oxygen
Dehydration	fluids
	sugar
	water
Dental plaque	dental floss
	ultrasound
Depression	antidepressants
	assertiveness training
	cognitive therapy
	computer therapy
	electroconvulsive therapy
	exercise therapy
	Gestalt therapy
	interpersonal psychotherapy
	laughter
	light therapy
	lithium

Health Problem	See These Entries
Depression—*continued*	nutritional therapy (folate)
	pet therapy
	plant therapy
	psychoanalysis
	Relaxation Response
Dermatitis	cold therapy
	hydrocortisone
	oatmeal, colloidal
Diabetes	bran
	dandelion
	diabetic diet
	exercise therapy
	fiber
	imagery
	low-fat diet
	music therapy
	nutritional therapy (chromium)
	shoes, therapeutic
	weight loss
Diabetic coma	sugar
Diabetic neuropathy	peppers, hot
Diabetic retinopathy	laser surgery
Diaper rash	hair dryer
	petroleum jelly
Diarrhea	banana
	bismuth
	clay
	electrolytes
	Imodium (loperamide hydrochloride)
	Kaopectate
	lactase
	sugar
	yogurt

Health Problem	See These Entries
Dishpan hands	petroleum jelly
Diverticulitis	fiber
Drowning	CPR
Drug abuse	art therapy aversion therapy group therapy
Drug overdose	charcoal, activated emetics
Dry eyes	eyedrops tears, artificial
Dry skin	castor oil humidifiers mineral oil moisturizers oatmeal, colloidal petroleum jelly
Eczema	group therapy hydrocortisone light therapy moisturizers oatmeal, colloidal
Edema	diuretics mattresses and beds
Emotional problems	art therapy assertiveness training behavior therapy cognitive therapy crying dream therapy Gestalt therapy group therapy interpersonal psychotherapy journal writing

Health Problem	See These Entries
Emotional problems—*continued*	laughter lithium meditation pet therapy poetry therapy psychoanalysis self-help groups therapeutic touch touch therapy
Emotional trauma	prayer
Emphysema	breathing techniques oxygen therapy physical therapy therapeutic touch
Endometriosis	endoscopy hysterectomy
Epilepsy	anticonvulsants barbiturates phenobarbital
Excess stomach acid	antacids
Eye infections	eyedrops
Eyelid dysfunction	gold
Fat deposits	liposuction
Fatigue	coffee electrolytes yoga
Fever	acetaminophen alcohol, rubbing aspirin balm of Gilead ibuprofen
Fever blisters	acyclovir

Health Problem	See These Entries
Fibroids	hysterectomy
Fibromyalgia	yoga
Flatulence	caraway fennel thyme
Flu	acetaminophen aspirin bed rest eucalyptus heat therapy hydrotherapy peppers, hot
Food allergies	elimination diet
Foot odor	charcoal, activated tea
Foot pain	orthoses shoes, therapeutic
Functional halluxlimitus	orthoses
Fungal infections	hair dryer
Gallbladder disease	laser surgery
Gallstones	endoscopy lithotripsy low-fat diet weight loss
Gangrene	hyperbaric oxygen
Gas	anise antacids fennel lactase peppermint
Gas pains	charcoal, activated
Gastric reflux	mattresses and beds

Master Chart of Complaints and Remedies

Health Problem	See These Entries
Genital herpes	lysine
Genital warts	interferon
Glaucoma	beta blockers
	eyedrops
	ultrasound
Glucose intolerance	nutritional therapy (chromium)
Goiter	kelp
Gonorrhea	antibiotics
	penicillin
Gout	cherries
Growth retardation	touch therapy
Gum inflammation	hydrogen peroxide
	salt
Hairy cell leukemia	interferon
Hairy cell leukoplakia	acyclovir
Hamstring injuries	cold therapy
Hay fever	air cleaners
	allergy shots
	antihistamines
Headache	acetaminophen
	acupressure
	art therapy
	aspirin
	behavior therapy
	biofeedback
	caffeine
	cold therapy
	electrotherapy
	elimination diet
	ergot
	flotation tanks
	ibuprofen

Health Problem	See These Entries
	oxygen therapy
	painkillers
	pillows
	progressive relaxation
	Relaxation Response
	therapeutic touch
	yoga
Hearing loss	hearing aids
Heart arrhythmias	atropine
	digitalis
Heart attack	anticoagulants
	CPR
	epinephrine
Heartburn	antacids
	baking soda
	ginger
	weight loss
Heart disease	alcohol, drinking
	angioplasty
	aspirin
	atherectomy
	bran
	chelation therapy
	cholesterol-lowering drugs
	coffee
	coronary bypass
	digitalis
	estrogen replacement therapy
	fish
	fish oil
	garlic
	laser surgery
	low-fat diet
	low-sodium diet

Health Problem	See These Entries

Heart disease—*continued*	macrobiotic diet
	monounsaturated oils
	nutritional therapy
	   (magnesium)
	   (niacin)
	onions
	pet therapy
	polyunsaturated oils
	prayer
	vegetarian diet
	weight loss

Heat rash	slippery elm
Heel pain	orthoses
Hemorrhoids	bran cortisone cryosurgery electrotherapy fiber hydrotherapy witch hazel
Hepatitis	gamma globulin interferon
Herniated disk	chymopapain laser surgery physiatry stress management
Herpes infections	acyclovir lysine
Hiatal hernia	antacids mattresses and beds
High blood pressure	affirmations antihypertensives banana beta blockers

Health Problem	See These Entries
	biofeedback
	blood pressure monitors
	calcium channel blockers
	diuretics
	dream therapy
	exercise therapy
	flotation tanks
	imagery
	low-fat diet
	low-sodium diet
	macrobiotic diet
	meditation
	monounsaturated oils
	nutritional therapy
	(calcium)
	(magnesium)
	(potassium)
	(vitamin C)
	pet therapy
	progressive relaxation
	Relaxation Response
	stress management
	therapeutic touch
	vegetarian diet
	weight loss
	yoga
High cholesterol	apple
	banana
	bran
	cholesterol-lowering drugs
	exercise therapy
	fiber
	fish oil
	garlic
	ileal bypass

Health Problem	See These Entries

High cholesterol—*continued*	macrobiotic diet
	milk
	nutritional therapy
	  (niacin)
	  (potassium)
	pectin
	polyunsaturated oils
	progressive relaxation
	prunes
	psyllium

Hives	antihistamines elimination diet hydrotherapy
Hoarseness	horehound
Hot flashes	estrogen replacement therapy
Hyperactivity	amphetamines
Hyperopia	corrective lenses
Hyperthyroidism	beta blockers
Impaired concentration	ergot
Impotence	papaverine penile implants
Incontinence	anticholinergics behavior therapy estrogen replacement therapy Kegel exercises
Indigestion	antacids baking soda bitters caraway charcoal, activated fennel ginger peppermint

Health Problem	See These Entries
	soda crackers
	thyme
Infections	affirmations
	antibiotics
	echinacea
	garlic
	growth factors
	heat therapy
	hydrotherapy
	iodine
	lavender
	penicillin
	peppers, hot
	sugar
	tea tree oil
	tetracycline
Infertility	nutritional therapy (vitamin C)
Inflammation	aloe
	anti-inflammatories
	aspirin
	balm of Gilead
	cold therapy
	comfrey
	cortisone
	hydrocortisone
	ibuprofen
	peppers, hot
	poultices
	prednisone
	steroids
Ingrown toenails	laser surgery
Injuries	cold therapy
	physiatry
	physical therapy
	posture therapy

Master Chart of Complaints and Remedies

Health Problem	See These Entries
Inner ear infections	antibiotics
Insect bites and stings	alcohol, rubbing allergy shots alum aspirin baking soda calamine lotion charcoal, activated cold therapy cryosurgery epinephrine meat tenderizers poultices witch hazel
Insomnia	acupuncture behavior therapy biofeedback hydrotherapy mattresses and beds Relaxation Response sedatives sex tranquilizers valerian
Interstitial cystitis	DMSO Kegel exercises
Intestinal cramps	anticholinergics
Intestinal polyps	endoscopy proctosigmoidoscopy
Irregular heartbeat	pacemaker
Irritable bowel syndrome	bran Kegel exercises peppermint

Health Problem	See These Entries
Itching	calamine lotion cold therapy hair dryer humidifiers menthol oatmeal, colloidal steroids
Itchy eyes	elimination diet
Jaundice	color therapy
Jaw pain	arthroscopy orthoses posture therapy
Jellyfish stings	meat tenderizers
Jet lag	sunlight
Jock itch	hair dryer
Joint injuries	arthroscopy aspirin exercise therapy RICE
Joint stiffness	cold therapy Epsom salts heat therapy hydrotherapy physical therapy poultices
Kaposi's sarcoma	interferon
Kidney failure	diuretics water
Kidney problems	low-sodium diet
Kidney stones	baking soda banana fluids

Health Problem	See These Entries
Kidney stones—*continued*	lithotripsy nutritional therapy 　(magnesium) 　(vitamin B_6)
Knee pain	arthroscopy cold therapy Feldenkrais Method orthoses pillows weight loss
Lack of concentration	flotation tanks
Lactose intolerance	lactase
Lead poisoning	chelation therapy
Learning disabilities	amphetamines art therapy music therapy
Leg pain	pillows
Leg ulcers	skin grafts
Leukemia	light therapy retinoids
Leukoplakia	nutritional therapy (vitamin A) retinoids
Liver spots	bleaching creams cryosurgery
Loneliness	pet therapy prayer
Low blood pressure	salt
Low self-esteem	affirmations exercise therapy plant therapy
Lung disease	oxygen therapy
Lupus	music therapy

Health Problem	See These Entries
Lyme disease	tetracycline
Mania	electroconvulsive therapy
	lithium
Manic-depression	lithium
Measles	gamma globulin
	nutritional therapy (vitamin A)
Memory impairment	ergot
	music therapy
Meningitis	penicillin
Menorrhagia	D & C
Menstrual cramps	acetaminophen
	chamomile
	heat therapy
	ibuprofen
	nutritional therapy
	(magnesium)
	painkillers
	sex
Migraine headaches	acupuncture
	art therapy
	aspirin
	beta blockers
	biofeedback
	calcium channel blockers
	coffee
	color therapy
	ergot
	feverfew
	hydrotherapy
Mood disorders	lithium
Morning sickness	antiemetics
	ginger
	soda crackers

Master Chart of Complaints and Remedies

Health Problem	See These Entries
Motion sickness	antiemetics
	ginger
	motion sickness remedies
Multiple sclerosis	physiatry
Muscle atrophy	electrotherapy
Muscle pain	acupuncture
	baking soda
	balm of Gilead
	elimination diet
	Epsom salts
	eucalyptus
	heat therapy
	hydrotherapy
	mattresses and beds
	menthol
	oil of wintergreen
	physical therapy
	posture therapy
Muscle spasms and tremors	anticholinergics
	cold therapy
	electrotherapy
	massage
	nutritional therapy
	(magnesium)
Muscle stiffness	exercise therapy
Muscle tension	acupressure
	massage
	Relaxation Response
	sedatives
	yoga
Musculoskeletal problems	chiropractic
Myopia	corrective lenses
	vision therapy

Health Problem	See These Entries
Narcolepsy	amphetamines
Nausea	antiemetics
	Coke syrup
	ginger
	motion sickness remedies
	soda crackers
Neck pain	acupuncture
	Alexander Technique
	imagery
	oil of wintergreen
	physiatry
	pillows
	posture therapy
	Relaxation Response
	yoga
Negative thinking	affirmations
Nervousness	hydrotherapy
Neuromuscular disorders	Feldenkrais Method
Nicotine withdrawal	baking soda
Night sweats	estrogen replacement therapy
Nosebleeds	cauterization
	epinephrine
Obsessive-compulsive disorder	antianxiety drugs
Osteoporosis	antacids
	estrogen replacement therapy
	exercise therapy
	milk
	nutritional therapy (calcium)
Overeating	behavior therapy
	color therapy
	self-help groups
Overweight	affirmations
	aversion therapy

Health Problem	See These Entries
Overweight—*continued*	apple
	caffeine
	color therapy
	exercise therapy
	fasting
	fiber
	flotation tanks
	hypnosis
	kelp
	liposuction
	low-fat diet
	pectin
	self-help audiotapes
	vegetarian diet
	weight loss
Pain	acetaminophen
	acupressure
	acupuncture
	aloe
	anti-inflammatories
	aspirin
	behavior therapy
	caffeine
	cold therapy
	cortisone
	electrotherapy
	Feldenkrais Method
	flotation tanks
	heat therapy
	hydrotherapy
	hypnosis
	ibuprofen
	imagery
	massage
	meditation
	menthol

Health Problem	See These Entries
	music therapy
	painkillers
	peppermint
	peppers, hot
	physiatry
	physical therapy
	placebo
	posture therapy
	sex
	therapeutic touch
	willow bark
Palsy	electrotherapy
Panic attacks	antianxiety drugs
	biofeedback
	cognitive therapy
	sedatives
	tranquilizers
Parkinson's disease .	levodopa
	nutritional therapy
	(vitamin E)
Pelvic pain	posture therapy
Pemphigus	gold
Periodontal disease	dental floss
	hydrogen peroxide
Phobias	antianxiety drugs
	behavior therapy
	cognitive therapy
	flotation tanks
	Gestalt therapy
	psychoanalysis
	self-help audiotapes
Pimples	acne remedies
	calamine lotion

Health Problem	See These Entries
Pinched nerves	Alexander Technique physiatry
Pneumonia	antibiotics penicillin physical therapy tetracycline
Poisoning	charcoal, activated emetics
Poison ivy	alum baking soda calamine lotion clay cold therapy cortisone deodorants oatmeal, colloidal
Posttraumatic stress disorder	art therapy
Posture problems	Alexander Technique orthoses yoga
Pregnancy-induced hypertension	aspirin
Premature ejaculation	Kegel exercises
Premenstrual syndrome	imagery nutritional therapy (calcium) (vitamin E)
Presbyopia	corrective lenses
Pressure sores	aloe
Prickly heat	oatmeal, colloidal
Prolapsed uterus	hysterectomy Kegel exercises
Prostate cancer	radiation therapy ultrasound

Health Problem	See These Entries
Psoriasis	cotton swabs
	fish
	fish oil
	light therapy
	mineral oil
	moisturizers
	sunlight
Psychosis	lithium
Pulled hamstring	hydrotherapy
Rabies	gamma globulin
Rashes	calamine lotion
Raynaud's disease	fish oil
Red eyes	eyedrops
Respiratory disease	breathing techniques
Respiratory infections	antibiotics
Rheumatic pains	thyme
Rheumatoid arthritis	anti-inflammatories
	cortisone
	evening primrose oil
	fish
	fish oil
	flotation tanks
	gold
	hydrocortisone
	ibuprofen
	light therapy
	physiatry
	physical therapy
	prednisone
	salt
	steroids
	vegetarian diet
Rickets	sunlight

Master Chart of Complaints and Remedies

Health Problem	See These Entries
Rocky Mountain spotted fever	tetracycline
Runny nose	antihistamines
Schizophrenia	nutritional therapy (folate) psychoanalysis
Sciatica	acupuncture
Scleroderma	light therapy
Scoliosis	Alexander Technique
Scratches	witch hazel
Seasonal affective disorder (SAD)	light therapy
Seizures	anticonvulsants barbiturates phenobarbital
Shingles	acyclovir calamine lotion electrotherapy lysine peppers, hot
Shoulder pain	arthroscopy electrotherapy Feldenkrais Method pillows posture therapy yoga
Shyness	group therapy
Sinus problems	endoscopy heat therapy humidifiers hydrotherapy peppers, hot
Skin cancer	chemical peels cryosurgery retinoids

Health Problem	See These Entries
Skin growths	cauterization
Skin problems	aloe antibiotics chamomile cortisone moisturizers oatmeal, colloidal petroleum jelly slippery elm steroids
Smoking	aversion therapy behavior therapy computer therapy flotation tanks hypnosis nicotine gum
Snoring	mattresses and beds
Solar keratoses	cryosurgery
Sore feet	Epsom salts
Sore throat	eucalyptus gargling heat therapy horehound humidifiers lozenges menthol poultices salt slippery elm sore throat remedies vaporizers
Speech disorders	poetry therapy
Spinal cord injuries	art therapy physiatry

Master Chart of Complaints and Remedies

Health Problem	See These Entries
Spinal cord injuries—*continued*	prednisone steroids
Splinters	poultices
Sprains	anti-inflammatories bandages cold therapy cortisone electrotherapy hydrotherapy menthol prednisone RICE ultrasound yoga
Stained teeth	dentistry, restorative hydrogen peroxide
Stomachache	heat therapy
Stomach cramps	chamomile
Strains	bandages cold therapy electrotherapy RICE yoga
Strep throat	penicillin
Stress	acupressure affirmations autogenic training behavior therapy biofeedback breathing techniques color therapy crying dream therapy exercise therapy

Health Problem	See These Entries
	flotation tanks
	group therapy
	hydrotherapy
	imagery
	journal writing
	laughter
	massage
	meditation
	plant therapy
	progressive relaxation
	reflexology
	Relaxation Response
	sedatives
	self-help audiotapes
	stress management
	stretching
	therapeutic touch
	valerian
	yoga
Stretch marks	retinoids
Stroke	antihypertensives
	art therapy
	diuretics
	Feldenkrais Method
	low-fat diet
	nutritional therapy (potassium)
	physiatry
	physical therapy
Stuffy nose	decongestants
	hydrotherapy
Suffocation	CPR
Sunburn	aloe
	baking soda
	witch hazel

Master Chart of Complaints and Remedies

Health Problem	See These Entries
Sweaty feet	salt
	tea
Sweaty palms	electrotherapy
Swelling	aspirin
	cold therapy
	comfrey
	ibuprofen
Swimmer's ear	alum
Syphilis	tetracycline
Tardive dyskinesia	nutritional therapy (vitamin E)
Tattoos	laser surgery
Tendinitis	cold therapy
	ultrasound
Tendon injuries	acupuncture
Tennis elbow	acupuncture
	physiatry
Tetanus	gamma globulin
Thinning hair	minoxidil
TM disorder	mouth guard
Toothache	cloves
	cold therapy
	dentistry, restorative
	painkillers
Tooth decay	dentistry, restorative
	fluoride
	tea
Trigger finger	prednisone
Turista	bismuth
Ulcerative colitis	prednisone
	steroids

Health Problem	See These Entries
Ulcers	antacids
	bismuth
	endoscopy
	progressive relaxation
	stress management
	therapeutic touch
	ulcer drugs
Urinary tract infections	antibiotics
	cranberry juice
	fluids
	tetracycline
	water
Uterine cancer	hysterectomy
Vaginal atrophy	sex
Vaginal dryness	estrogen replacement therapy
Vaginal infections	estrogen replacement therapy
Vaginal itching	douching
Vaginal odor	douching
Varicose veins	mattresses and beds
	sclerotherapy
Violent behavior	color therapy
Viral infections	heat therapy
Vision problems	color therapy
	vision therapy
Vitiligo	light therapy
Vomiting	antiemetics
	ginger
	motion sickness remedies
	sugar
Warts	cauterization
	cryosurgery

Health Problem	See These Entries
Warts—*continued*	imagery
	laser surgery
Whiplash	chiropractic
Windburn	witch hazel
Wounds	aloe
	bandages
	cauterization
	chlorophyll
	cotton swabs
	echinacea
	growth factors
	heat therapy
	honey
	hydrotherapy
	imagery
	kelp
	nutritional therapy
	(vitamin A)
	(vitamin C)
	plantain
	poultices
	skin grafts
	slippery elm
	sugar
	tea tree oil
	therapeutic touch
	ultrasound
Wrinkles	chemical peels
Yeast infections	acidophilus
	douching
	echinacea
	estrogen replacement therapy
	gentian violet
	tea tree oil

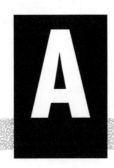

Accutane. *See* **acne remedies**

acetaminophen (ah-seet-ah-MIN-ah-fen *or* ah-set-ah-MEE-na-fen) Even if you've never heard of acetaminophen, the chances are good you've *taken* some. Do any of these brands—Tylenol, Anacin-3, Dristan Decongestant, or Sine-Aid Maximum Strength—sound familiar? Along with more than 100 other products listed in the *Physicians' Desk Reference,* they all contain this safe, hard-working painkiller that for most people produces fewer side effects than aspirin.

By all accounts, acetaminophen is every bit as strong a painkiller as aspirin, the time-honored gold standard for analgesics. Aspirin and acetaminophen have a lot in common. Both lower fevers, relieve headaches, and ease the aches of colds and flu. Both relieve menstrual cramps, and both are available without prescription.

"If they're so much alike," many people ask, "why not stick with aspirin? It's cheaper."

Aspirin and acetaminophen don't do *quite* the same jobs; there are small but significant differences.

Acetaminophen, for example, has no effect on inflammation. It won't reduce the swelling in a banged-up elbow or ease the inflammation of arthritis. If it's swelling you want to control, stay away from acetaminophen.

You also should stay away from acetaminophen if you're looking for an antiplatelet drug—that is, a drug that inhibits clots from forming in your bloodstream. Unlike aspirin, acetaminophen won't "thin" your blood.

On the other hand, doctors sometimes ask people to switch from aspirin to acetaminophen before some kinds of surgeries or dental procedures, the better to control excessive bleeding.

Both acetaminophen and aspirin inhibit your body's production of prostaglandins, compounds that are believed to trigger inflammation and send pain sensations to your brain. However, aspirin affects prostaglandin production everywhere in your body; acetaminophen affects only your brain's supply. That's why acetaminophen will stop pain but not inflammation.

EASIER ON THE STOMACH

Acetaminophen rarely causes the stomach upset regular aspirin users may be plagued with, and pediatricians generally feel it's a lot safer than aspirin for children.

Long-term aspirin use, to put it simply, is tough on your gut. People who can't tolerate aspirin because of stomach irritation, however, *can* take acetaminophen. Acetaminophen is also a welcome substitute for those people who are allergic to aspirin.

For many pediatricians, acetaminophen now is the analgesic of choice. One reason is that in recent years, aspirin has been linked with Reye syndrome, a sometimes-fatal liver and neurological condition that can strike children with little warning.

Acetaminophen appears to work as well for kids as it does for adults. In one study, Los Angeles researchers monitored 282 children who received diphtheria, tetanus toxoids, and pertussis (the DTP series) vaccinations. Children who took acetaminophen had considerably less pain and fever than children who didn't.

Even though acetaminophen is remarkably free of short-term side effects, it isn't meant for long-term use. So you may want to talk with your doctor before taking acetaminophen for pain that persists more than a few days. Hepatotoxicity (liver damage) may result from acetaminophen overdosing.

In one study, researchers investigated 554 adults—all with newly diagnosed kidney disease—to discover what analgesics they had been taking. The researchers found "an increased risk associated with daily use of acetaminophen." Acetaminophen-related fatalities, however, are rare.

Taken as directed, acetaminophen does an excellent job of relieving the aches and pains we all experience from time to time. Apparently safer for children than aspirin or ibuprofen—and better tolerated by adults—acetaminophen is a popular player in the painkiller game. *See also* **painkillers**

acidophilus (ass-ih-DOF-ih-lus) Eating live bacteria may not sound like the healthiest thing to do, but people who seek out acidophilus-containing products do it all the time. You'll find this type of bacteria (full name: *Lactobacillus acidophilus*) in milk labeled acidophilus milk, in certain brands of yogurt, and in tablets, powders, capsules, and liquids sold in health food stores. If the product contains live or "viable" acidophilus strains, the label will say so.

There is one key difference between acidophilus and the two principal bacteria used in most yogurts. Acidophilus is similar to beneficial bacteria normally present in the human body. Yogurt bacteria can't claim that resemblance, giving acidophilus its edge.

These naturally occurring bacteria play a beneficial role in the vagina, for example, where they protect against yeast infections. That may account for the fact that dietary supplementation with acidophilus appears to reduce recurrent yeast infections. At least that's what a doctor at Long Island Jewish Medical Center found in a preliminary study of 15 women who had had a minimum of five yeast infections in the previous year. The doctor monitored the women for six months and found they averaged three yeast infections each. Then she asked them to eat a cup of acidophilus yogurt every day for six months. During this period, the number of infections dropped to less than one per woman.

Acidophilus also looks promising in the laboratory. The most intriguing studies by far hint that acidophilus may have cancer-fighting properties. Studies with lab animals suggest that it can repair the DNA damage done by cancer-causing nitrosamines and reduce both the size and number of colon tumors. (Nitrosamines form in the gastrointestinal tract when nitrites—a type of preservative used in prepared foods like bacon—interact with other naturally occurring chemicals called amines.) Tufts researchers found that oral supplementation with acidophilus suppresses the activity of fecal bacteria enzymes that convert chemicals into carcinogens. The effect was noted in humans, as well as in rats. The relevance of these findings to human health has yet to be established. *See also* **yogurt**

acne remedies   As skin conditions go, acne is a lot like fingerprints: No two cases are exactly alike. You may have to try different products, in different strengths, to find a remedy—or combination of remedies—that works for you. Here's an overview of what's available.

Benzoyl peroxide. The most frequently used antiacne compound, benzoyl peroxide seems to dry up blemishes and kill off the bacteria that cause them. More than two dozen creams, cleansing bars, gels, lotions, and masks containing benzoyl peroxide are sold. Some are available over the counter; some require a prescription. Even if you try a nonprescription product, a dermatologist can help you use it effectively.

Exfoliating lotions. These over-the-counter products contain salicylic acid, resorcinol, or sulfur, ingredients that dry the skin, strip off surface cells, and peel away accumulated debris from skin pores. They're useful for people who don't tolerate benzoyl peroxide.

POWERFUL PRESCRIPTIONS

If acne persists, your doctor may prescribe stronger medicine.

Antibiotics. Tetracycline and erythromycin are standard therapy for inflammatory acne—that is, for blemishes that have erupted, leaking their irritating contents into the surrounding skin and forming pustules and cysts. Antibiotics applied directly to the skin are best for mild or moderate inflammatory acne. Oral antibiotics are reserved for more severe cases or for people who don't respond to topical (on-the-spot) medicine.

Metronidazole. Sold under the trade name MetroGel, Metronidazole is a powerful antibacterial drug developed specifically for people with acne rosacea (often called adult acne) who don't respond to standard oral antibiotics. In clinical tests, rosacea inflammation faded rapidly within three weeks after the invisible water-based gel was applied to the skin.

Tretinoin. Sold under the brand name Retin-A, tretinoin is a topically applied compound of retinoic acid, a derivative of vitamin A. Tretinoin is available as a cream, gel, or liquid, in various strengths. (Retin-A is also used to treat wrinkles and sun-damaged skin.)

Use of tretinoin requires a healthy dose of patience: You may experience slight irritation and inflammation for a month or two, and you may not see any improvement for 6 to 12 weeks. (The liquid form is slightly more irritating than the cream or gel, so it's reserved for more stubborn acne.) Tretinoin may be combined with benzoyl peroxide, antibiotic therapy, or both, to treat acne at different stages of development.

Isotretinoin. Marketed under the brand name Accutane, isotretinoin is a synthetic form of vitamin A that's related to tretinoin. And it's revolutionized the treatment of severe inflammatory acne: Taken orally, isotretinoin often reduces acne lesions by 90 percent. Pregnant women should not take isotretinoin, however, because it poses an extremely high risk of birth defects.

acupressure   Press *here* for pain relief and muscle relaxation. That's the allure of this oriental system of massage. Acupressure, like acupuncture, is used to stimulate certain precise points on the body. But instead of needles, it relies on finger and thumb pressure.

If you want a quick introduction to acupressure, try it on yourself or a friend the next time a headache strikes,

suggests Norman C. Shealy, M.D., Ph.D., director of the Shealy Institute for Comprehensive Health Care in Springfield, Missouri. Headache relief is where acupressure shines, he says.

"Several points are worth serious consideration," Dr. Shealy says. "The most important ones can be located by bringing both of your index fingers to the base of your skull, where your second and third vertebrae meet. Now bring your fingers out to either side until you feel a painful, tense little notch. When you find the sore spots, press hard.

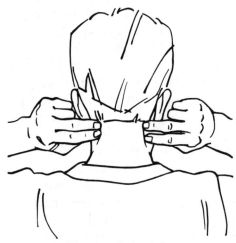

Acupressure self-treatment for headache

"If this doesn't relieve your headache, press hard on the web between your thumb and forefinger. Either of these methods should turn off acute headaches."

Stimulating the right pressure points can also relieve shoulder, back, and neck tension, as well as the pain of arthritis, claims Michael Reed Gach, author of *Acupressure's Potent Points: A Guide to Self-Care for Common Ailments* and head of the Acupressure Institute in Berkeley, California.

SHIATSU FOR RELAXATION

If you'd like a more complete experience of acupressure, consider shiatsu, a Japanese variation that works on points all over the body while gently stretching, rocking, and rotating the limbs. Dr. Shealy regards shiatsu as the ultimate technique of acupressure. "It's an excellent treatment for general relaxation," he says. "It will make you feel good all over."

Practitioners of shiatsu say that if it is done well, at session's end the body feels calm and revitalized and the mind clear. Flexibility is noticeably improved. It's not unusual to feel subtle, very pleasurable currents of energy coursing through the body for several hours—or even several days—afterward.

And while shiatsu is somewhat similar to acupuncture, the human touch factor gives shiatsu a whole different quality, says Saul Goodman, founder and director of the International School of Shiatsu in Doylestown, Pennsylvania, and author of *The Book of Shiatsu: The Healing Art of Finger Pressure.* "The body responds totally differently to human touch than to steel needles," he says. "It's very fundamental. When we were in the womb, we felt the pressure of the amniotic fluid on our developing bodies. That pressure helped stimulate the development of our respiratory, circulatory, and nervous systems. So pressure is a native experience for us. I don't think we ever stop needing it."

How does shiatsu work? According to classical oriental theory (the basis for acupuncture and acupressure), life energy called *ki* flows through the body along a series of pathways called meridians. Each meridian is said to be associated with a particular vital organ. It's also theorized that just under the skin, along the routes of these meridians, sit tiny cup-shaped energy conductors called *tsubos.* Their job is to keep energy circulating throughout the body, so that all the tissues are "fed." Poor diet, bad posture, and stress are said to cause the tsubos to malfunction. Acupressurists believe that if one or more tsubos stop doing their job, energy stagnates, initiating the process of disease.

Shiatsu practitioners say active tsubos give off a slight electrical charge, which skilled hands can sense. They apply sustained pressure to the inactive tsubos, "listening" with their hands for the energy shift they say accompanies reactivation of the point.

Western medicine does not accept this theory. But an explanation that can bridge both cultures may not be far off. A 1989 study by Yoshiaki Omura, M.D., Sc.D., medical director of the Heart Disease Research Foundation of New York, claims to have found, via a special imaging technique, a direct relationship among the meridians, the organs they serve, and the areas of the brain's cerebral cortex that govern those body systems. The study, published in *Acupuncture and Electrotherapeutics Research, The International Journal,* also found high concentrations of endorphins, enkephalins, and other pain-reducing natural substances within the boundaries of most areas traditionally regarded as acupuncture points and meridian lines.

That makes sense, given what science knows today about the ability of touch to stimulate the release of these pain-suppressing, mood-enhancing brain chemicals.

For more information on acupressure, contact the Acupressure Institute, 1533 Shattuck Avenue, Berkeley, CA 94709; the International School of Shiatsu at 22–28 South Main Street, Doylestown, PA 18901, or the American Oriental Bodywork Therapy Association, 50 Maple Place, Manhassett, NY 11030. *See also* **acupuncture; massage**

acupuncture Patients undergoing acupuncture may feel that they have something in common with a porcupine. That's because of the slender needles inserted at specific points in the skin and left in place during the treatment session. Although the procedure looks as if it would be very painful, it really isn't. In fact, pain *relief* is acupuncture's primary mission.

As it's practiced in America today, there are two camps in acupuncture, which was originally imported from Asia.

In the larger camp are traditionalists like Grace Wong, a Hong Kong native who practices acupuncture in Bethesda, Maryland. Hers is the classical oriental approach, which she learned at the Kowloon Chinese Traditional Medical College and the Hong Kong Chinese Acupuncture Research Center.

In the second camp are acupuncturists like George Ulett, M.D., Ph.D., a clinical professor of psychiatry at the University of Missouri School of Medicine who dismisses classical theory as so much "oriental hocus-pocus." They offer a system consonant with their understanding of neurophysiology, one based on stimulation—often electrical—of 80 "motor points," places where nerve enters muscle. (Classical acupuncture theory recognizes 365 points.)

Which method is best? There are no studies that answer the question definitively. Loyalties are divided even in medical circles. Dr. Wong, a doctor of oriental medicine (O.M.D.), shares her practice with a doctor of internal medicine who was won over to acupuncture after keeping meticulous records of how Dr. Wong's patients fared. After finding that 70 percent of the first 1,000 improved, he stopped counting.

Dr. Wong subscribes to the classical theory that life energy flows through the body along a series of pathways known as meridians. Along the merid-

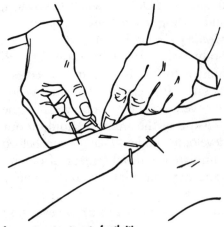

Acupuncture treatment of arthritis

ians are highly specific points, which sit just under the skin and conduct the energy. When one or more meridians become blocked, the energy stagnates and disease results. Acupuncture seeks to remove the blocks and help to restore the internal energy balance the body requires to heal itself.

A typical acupuncture session with Dr. Wong lasts half an hour. She takes six pulses, in the traditional Chinese way, and reviews CAT scans or x-rays to complete her diagnosis. Typically, she inserts 10 to 20 needles at a time, ¼ to 3 inches deep, depending on which part of the body she's treating.

"People come in very nervous," she says. "I tell them they will feel a pressure or numbness. Some people become so relaxed, they fall asleep on the table."

PAIN ERASED

Dr. Wong says acupuncture brings 50 to 70 percent improvement in many cases of chronic pain, and is particularly helpful for back and neck pain, tennis elbow, arthritis, sciatica, insomnia, migraines, stomach disorders, anxiety, and tendon and muscle injuries. Improvement is often seen within six to ten sessions, although additional treatments may be needed for maximum benefit, she says.

Dr. Ulett also uses acupuncture to combat pain, and he gets similar clinical results. Trained as a medical doctor, neurophysiologist, and acupuncturist, he views acupuncture as a neurophysiological phenomenon. To him, it's a "technique for getting a stimulus, preferably a pulsing DC current, into the central nervous system." This releases endorphins and enkephalins, natural substances that strengthen the body's own pain control mechanisms.

Dr. Ulett begins by feeling for trigger points, body hot spots that are tender to the touch. He says these are the ideal spots for needle insertion. If he can't find any, he places a few needles in a strategic relationship to the nerves that are delivering the pain impulse. He always connects the needles to a stimulator that delivers low-voltage electrical current, a technique that he says he's found makes acupuncture 100 percent more effective.

Again, six to eight treatments may be required before the patient sees improvement. If there's no change after ten treatments, Dr. Ulett says the condition isn't likely to respond to acupuncture. *See also* **acupressure**

acyclovir (ah-SI-klo-vir) At last, a treatment for herpes! This prescription drug has shown good results against herpes simplex viruses (which primarily affect the mouth and genitals) as well as herpes zoster infections (which cause shingles and chickenpox). Sold under the trade name Zovirax, acyclovir is the first of what have come to be known as specific antiviral drugs—that is, they are activated only when they come in contact with a specific enzyme released by a virus-infected cell. They don't affect uninfected cells.

Acyclovir doesn't cure herpes—the viruses can remain dormant for years—but it relieves pain and discomfort, speeds healing of sores (if present), and often prevents repeat attacks.

Acyclovir is available as either a topical ointment, oral medication (capsules, tablet, or syrup), or intravenous solution. In one study, taking acyclovir orally, beginning the day before a ski trip, helped skiers prone to sun-induced herpes attacks avoid lip sores. In the case of genital herpes, a doctor may ask patients to continue taking acyclovir orally for a year or more after an attack subsides. According to a study published in the *Journal of the American Medical Association,* long-term use of acyclovir seems to prevent repeat outbreaks of genital herpes more effectively than use during flare-ups only.

Remarkably Safe

Acyclovir is also being used to prevent cytomegalovirus (CMV), an opportunistic type of human herpes virus that can infect patients who have undergone either a kidney transplant or bone marrow transplant, people with Hodgkin's disease, or others whose immune system isn't working up to par. (But the drug isn't effective for established CMV.) "AIDS patients with hairy cell leukoplakia [white patches inside the mouth] also seem to respond to acyclovir," says Clyde Crumpacker, M.D., associate professor of medicine at Harvard Medical School and Beth Israel Hospital, Boston.

Because acyclovir's war against viruses is waged within cells and involves DNA—the genetic stuff of life—doctors use caution when prescribing the drug for pregnant women or newborns. But in general, acyclovir has an impressive safety record.

"Acyclovir is the yardstick by which new antiviral drugs are judged," says Dr. Crumpacker. "It really works, and it's almost unique in that it's so free of toxic effects." *See also* **lysine**

adrenaline. *See* **epinephrine**

Advil. *See* **ibuprofen**

aerobic exercise. *See* **exercise therapy**

affirmations Are you in the habit of talking to yourself? You should be. Self-talk can be healthy, provided your words build you up rather than tear you down. Affirmations, which are short, positive statements you repeat to yourself, can boost your confidence and encourage you to reach goals, and they may even help your body function at optimum level.

"Affirmations, also called 'positive self-talk,' are not wishful thinking or Pollyana-ish statements," says Richard Sackett, Ph.D., a psychologist in private practice in New York City. They can serve as an effective way to counterbalance negative thoughts.

Psychologists say we all have internal tapes that get switched on automatically. In some people, these tapes play self-defeating messages. For example: "I can't stop eating," "I'm terrible at public speaking," or "I'm a lousy mother." The purpose of affirmation is to gradually erase these destructive choruses and replace them with positive ones, such as, "I can eat just one serving at each meal and feel completely satisfied."

Whenever you catch yourself slipping into a negative mind trap, blaming yourself, or putting yourself down, counter it with a positive affirmation. "This statement will help you fight through the fog of negative thoughts and help you quickly regain perspective," says Dr. Sackett.

SHAPING YOUR FUTURE

You can also think of affirmations as expectations put down in words. By repeating them, your expectations will begin to guide your behavior. "Affirmations help you reprogram your subconscious mind to believe that you can succeed," says Douglas Bloch, a psychologist in Portland, Oregon, and author of *Words That Heal: Affirmations and Meditations for Daily Living.* "Your new belief will lead to corresponding behaviors which create the outcome you desire."

Some studies suggest that positive self-talk could help you reprogram your body for better health. After all, words illustrate your thoughts, and there is evidence that positive thoughts can encourage good health.

A study conducted by Michael Scheier, Ph.D., professor of psychology at Carnegie-Mellon University and Charles S. Carver, Ph.D., of the University of Miami, looked at 141 students under the stress of deadlines. They found that the students who were more optimistic reported being less bothered by headaches, stomach problems, depression, and other symptoms than students who were not optimistic.

"We assume that one of the reasons optimists remain healthy is their tendency to use positive self-talk during coping,"says Dr. Scheier.

Other researchers are attempting to show that thoughts and emotions are linked to biochemicals that influence your body's ability to resist illness. "This research has prompted many health specialists to incorporate affirmations in techniques that help people use their mind to fight infections, high blood pressure, allergies, and even cancer," according to Errol Korn, M.D., a gastroenterologist in San Diego who uses affirmations for physical healing.

GETTING STARTED

The beauty of affirmations is that you can use them to heal or improve any part of your life. To compose your own affirmation, choose an area of your life that needs improvement, such as health, work relationships, peace of mind, and so on, suggests Bloch. Decide what goal you would like to achieve. Write a statement in the present tense as if you have already reached your goal, such as "I am enjoying a new job in a pleasant work environment," "I have now found the perfect mate," or "My body is slim and trim."

Keep your statements short, clear, and crisp, and phrase your affirmations positively. Avoid negative affirmations such as "I'll never get angry again." Use words such as "I am" or "I can."

Be specific and realistic. "I am enjoying wealth" is too vague. "I am making seven sales calls a day" is better.

Being specific takes affirmations out of the realm of magic and into reality, says Dennis Jaffe, Ph.D., professor at Saybrook Institute in San Francisco.

"If the affirmation doesn't click with you, fine-tune it by altering a word or two," says Bloch.

Repeat the phrase several times a day, especially just before sleep or upon waking, when access to the unconscious is greatest, suggests Joan Borysenko, Ph.D., president of Mind/Body Health Sciences in Scituate, Massachusetts, and author of *Minding the Body, Mending the Mind.* Affirmations work best when you are relaxed, quiet, and not distracted.

When you repeat your affirmation, actually picture yourself changing. If your affirmation relates to being healthy, visualize yourself running. "Affirmations work the same way as goal-setting," says Dr. Korn. "By stating your goal clearly, and then picturing it happening, it will become reality more quickly."

Place copies of your affirmations on your bathroom mirror, your dashboard, your desk. Carry your written affirmation with you to glance at whenever you find yourself slipping into negative self-talk.

Give your affirmation several days or even weeks to take hold. You may be trying to replace negative thoughts or challenge beliefs that you've been holding onto for years. Meanwhile, work with it. If you are telling yourself that people respect you, act as though you respect yourself, too. Smile. Take pride in your appearance. Affirmation combined with af-firmative action is the best path to improvement.

An example that affirmations work? Think of Muhammad Ali, suggests Bloch. "By repeating the phrase, 'I am the greatest' countless times, a relatively unknown boxer became one of the greatest fighters of all time. Ali tapped into the power of affirmation."

You can, too. Pick up a book of sample affirmations to get you started. Just make sure that the affirmation you use is expansive, empowering, and supportive.

air cleaners   Many people with hay fever or bronchial asthma find they can breathe easy after installing a room air cleaner. But it seems that some breathe easier than others.

It's not that air cleaners don't work. They do. But they have limits.

Air filters are intended to remove bothersome particles from the air faster than they can fall to the floor or settle on other surfaces. (Larger particles, like pollen and house dust mites, fall to the floor far more quickly than animal dander or mold spores.)

Air filters come in two major types: high-efficiency particulate air (HEPA) filters and electronic precipitators.

Developed during World War II to remove radioactive dust from atomic energy plant exhaust, HEPA filters are made of fine, tightly woven glass fibers. They remove 99.97 percent or more of the particles in a room—and they become *more* efficient with use. Also, HEPA filters require no maintenance, although they do need to be replaced at regular intervals.

Electronic precipitators zap particles like dust, pet dander, and cigarette smoke with an electrical charge, then draw them to a collecting plate with an opposite charge. Allergy specialists say two-stage devices work considerably better than one-stage units. Electronic precipitators have a major disadvantage — they need to be cleaned frequently to remain efficient. Even then, they're less efficient than HEPA filters.

LIMITED BENEFITS

So electronic precipitators work pretty well, and HEPA filters work better. But can they help you breathe easier? It depends, say specialists.

So far, only one study, which compared an air cleaner with a dummy device in homes of allergic people, has shown measurable health benefits. But the results are positive and encouraging. "This is the first valid study to suggest that air cleaners have some potential health benefits," says Harold S. Nelson, M.D., a respiratory disease specialist at the National Jewish Center for Immunology and Respiratory Medicine in Denver, who reviewed data on air cleaners for the Food and Drug Administration a few years ago.

But whether or not an air cleaner can help *you* breathe easier depends on several factors — including what you're allergic to. "Just because you have asthma, for example, doesn't mean dust will bother you, so filtering the air may or may not help," says Dr. Nelson.

Even if an air cleaner gets rid of an airborne substance you're allergic to, symptoms may persist, for the simple reason that particles on surfaces — bedding, furniture, and floors — greatly outnumber particles in the air.

"An air cleaner can scrub dust or pet dander out of the air, and do it very thoroughly," says Dr. Nelson. "But it won't pick up what's embedded in bedding, carpeting, and so forth. So the minute you settle into an upholstered chair or walk across the carpet, you stir up particles."

REDUCE THE SOURCE

In other words, an air cleaner can scrub your air, but it can't scrub your floors. Regular, thorough cleaning of mattress covers, blankets, and pillowcases may also be necessary. For some people, eliminating the source of the allergens (be it a cat or a mite-infested carpet) may be the only way to decrease exposure — and symptoms.

"Reduce the source *first,* then try a filter," says Thomas A. E. Platts-Mills, M.D., Ph.D., professor of medicine at the University of Virginia in Charlottesville, who adds, "In fact, if someone has asthma, which is more serious than hay fever, we insist they get rid of the source of their misery, even if they want to try an air cleaner."

alcohol, drinking   Folk medicine is full of alcohol remedies: Wine aids digestion . . . whiskey at bedtime helps you sleep . . . you can ease a hangover by taking "the hair of the dog that bit you."

Most alcohol "cures" don't work, says James Roerig, Pharm.D., a clinical pharmacist at Ramsey Clinic in St. Paul, Minnesota. Alcohol (ethanol) may help you relax at bedtime, but it's more likely to disturb your sleep than improve it, he says. Nor is alcohol recommended for hangovers.

Small amounts of alcohol probably do stimulate saliva and gastric juices, he says, which may improve your digestion. On the other hand, too much alcohol probably will spoil your appetite—and your insides. But between "too much" and teetotaling there may be a "just right"—at least as far as your heart is concerned.

"There is fairly good evidence that one or two drinks a day may have some degree of a protective effect against coronary heart disease," says Harold Kalant, M.D., Ph.D., professor emeritus in the University of Toronto's pharmacology department.

Researchers at the University of North Carolina at Chapel Hill analyzed the drinking habits of 152 people who had suffered heart attacks. They discovered light to moderate drinkers (people who have more than a drink a month and fewer than four drinks a day) actually had fewer heart attacks than abstainers.

Alcohol may protect your heart by making your "good" HDL cholesterol feel *really* good—studies show that 1½ ounces of alcohol a day boosts HDL. These findings are still being debated, however—and no one is recommending that people at risk for heart disease get more exercise by raising a glass.

Alcohol's protective abilities clearly are offset by its dangers, Dr. Roerig warns. "It's very, very difficult for people to use alcohol on a daily basis in small quantities and to stay at that level."

alcohol, rubbing   The key ingredient in many cosmetics, rubbing alcohol (or isopropanol) quickly strips your skin of bacteria, as well as oily residues, leaving it feeling cool and fresh. A powerful cleanser, it's often used to disinfect metal surfaces and instruments.

Some doctors suggest dipping a cloth in rubbing alcohol when your face feels hot and grimy, or when acne raises its ugly head. People also apply rubbing alcohol to take the sting from insect bites and to cool hot skin.

Rubbing alcohol will dry your skin, so don't overdo it. It's also highly toxic, so don't drink it. But when you have a fever, or summer's heat is making you boil, cool off with a rubbing alcohol rubdown.

Alexander Technique   Neurosurgeon Jack Stern, M.D., Ph.D., found out about the technique by accident, when a physical therapist opened an office near his. He began referring back pain patients to her—and watched them get better fast. Her secret? The Alexander Technique, which she taught in addition to providing more routine physical therapy.

The technique teaches people how to sit, stand, and walk with greater ease. Students learn to change the thoughts that initiate movement and to eliminate unnecessary bodily tension, so they can overcome bad postural habits acquired over the years.

"I think it's an excellent system," says Dr. Stern, who is a professor of neurosurgery at New York Medical College. He credits his own Alexander lessons with helping him stay pain free while performing 20-hour operations. He also cites the case of a corporate executive who used the technique to help eliminate chronic low back pain after years of suffering. "There are many such cases," he says.

Dr. Stern thinks the technique can especially benefit people with muscle-related back and neck pain or small spinal disk bulges, as well as sports enthusiasts interested in improving their game. His one caution to people in pain is that they undergo a thorough medical examination first to rule out more serious causes of the pain, such as tumors.

Physical therapist and Alexander teacher Deborah Caplan, who wrote *Back Trouble: A New Approach to Prevention and Recovery*, says Alexander lessons can also bring relief to some people who suffer from pinched nerves or arthritis, and can strengthen the frame-supporting muscles of those with scoliosis—curvature of the spine—who are being "weaned from the brace."

LOST VOICE FOUND

The technique was devised 100 years ago by F. M. Alexander, an Australian actor who sought a way to end a series of mysterious episodes in which he lost his voice after performing. He found that his problems were a result of "a total pattern of misuse that involved his entire body," says Caplan.

When doctors couldn't help him, Alexander rigged up a series of mirrors so he could observe himself from several angles as he stood and spoke. He discovered that whenever he began a dramatic recitation he'd automatically pull his head backward and down, initiating a series of movements that ultimately compressed his larynx and lungs.

Even though he knew what he was doing wrong, it wasn't easy to stop. He'd gotten used to pulling his head down. Trying to keep his neck erect and relaxed felt wrong. He found he had to catch himself—at the moment he was about to pull his head down—and cut off the impulse. Then he could consciously correct himself. Eventually, the improved, erect posture replaced the old one.

As a result of Alexander's discoveries, teachers of the technique work with the whole body to solve specific postural problems. They also teach stu-

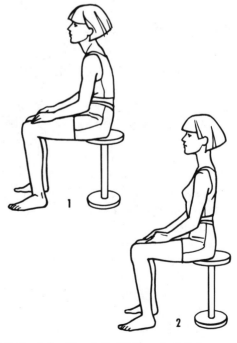

Posture before (1) and after (2) Alexander Technique

dents "to move more intelligently by thinking differently," says Bill Connington, president and chairman of the board of the American Center for the Alexander Technique. "Through this technique, you grow in understanding in the use of the body and how it interacts with your mind."

Apparently, physical changes can follow. Preliminary findings of a pilot study by John Austin, M.D., professor of radiology at Columbia Presbyterian Medical Center, indicate that healthy adults who took 20 Alexander lessons showed a slight but definite increase in lung volume and other measures of vital capacity. Twenty to 30 lessons, in fact, are considered optimal.

For more information or to find a certified teacher, contact the North American Society of Teachers of the Alexander Technique, P.O. Box 3992, Champaign, IL 61826–3992.

allergy shots   People with allergies are advised to steer clear of the plants, animals, or foods causing their symptoms. And that's good advice. It's the first and sometimes the only thing people need to do to minimize their sniffling, sneezing, and scratching.

People who get allergy shots, though, are *deliberately* exposed to the substances causing their symptoms. Purified versions of the substances are injected directly into their body, in controlled amounts and sometimes in a form slightly different from that found in nature.

Unlike occasional, uncontrolled exposure to allergy-producing sub-

stances, allergy shots (or immunotherapy, as doctors call it) are proven in scientific studies to reduce certain allergic symptoms.

The shots apparently have a dampening effect on the body's immune system, says Lawrence Lichtenstein, M.D., director of the Johns Hopkins Asthma and Allergy Center in Baltimore.

In an allergic person, the body's immune system is overprotective. It may mistake particles of pollen for infectious invaders and fight them off by releasing biochemicals that cause a runny nose, watery eyes, and itchy skin.

Allergy shots make the body's immune system less reactive. "The theory is that, over time, immunotherapy decreases the number of reactive antibodies and increases the number of protective antibodies that combine with the allergen and block the release of reaction-producing biochemicals such as histamine," Dr. Lichtenstein says. In other words, the shots make you less likely to have an allergic reaction to the substance that's being injected.

Good candidates for allergy shots include people who haven't been helped enough by symptom-reducing drugs such as antihistamines or those who have unpleasant side effects when they take those drugs; people who've had a life-threatening reaction to an insect sting; and sometimes people with bad, multiple, year-round allergies.

HAY FEVER CONTROLLED

Allergy shots work better for some conditions than for others, Dr. Lichtenstein says. "They definitely relieve hay fever, or allergic rhinitis, which is caused by inhaled grass, tree, or rag-weed pollens."

And over the past few years, shots have been developed that block severe reactions to bee or hornet stings. (Early versions of these shots used ground-up bodies of whole insects; now a much more effective version uses just the venom.) "We've been able to stop reactions in over 98 percent of the people we've treated, and the remaining 2 percent have very mild reactions," Dr. Lichtenstein says.

Shots that quell household dust reactions are also new and improved. These shots used to be formulated from the contents of vacuum cleaner bags, which included pet hair, molds, pollens, and anything else lying around the house. Now, though, they are made from ground-up dust mites, microscopic creatures that live everywhere, including *your bed,* and are now known to cause most dust allergies.

Shots for cat and dog allergies are still not particularly effective, Dr. Lichtenstein says. These injections used to be formulated from fur, skin, and dried saliva vacuumed from the hides of animals. Those now being tested are made from animal proteins known to be causing allergic reactions. (The allergy shot for cats, for instance, is a synthesized protein developed from a component of cat saliva.)

No allergy shots have been proven to be useful for food allergies, including severe allergic reactions to shrimp and peanuts, Dr. Lichtenstein says. Even so, "Some doctors give shots for food allergies that they believe are causing symptoms such as fatigue or head-aches," he says. "There is no proof that they work."

WHAT TO EXPECT

Allergy shots can be time-consuming. Most doctors start their patients on weekly shots for two or three months, then switch to monthly maintenance shots which may continue for years, depending on your symptoms. Most people stop their allergy shots, at least temporarily, after no more than four or five years of treatment, Dr. Lichtenstein says.

You should see improvements within two to three months, or if your symptoms are seasonal, the next time your season rolls around, Dr. Lichtenstein says. If your symptoms haven't improved, it's possible you aren't being given the proper injection or that you're being given a dose that is too weak to work.

Some people get shots that include only one or a few allergens. But shots can include up to 20 or 30 allergens, which cover most of the bases with most people. Pollen shots are formulated according to geographic region and season.

In some cases, allergy shots can cause allergic reactions. At Johns Hopkins, people stay at the clinic for half an hour after receiving their shot. That way, if they have a reaction, they can get prompt medical care.

If you're considering allergy shots, talk with an allergist. Be sure you've given allergy drugs a fair try first. And be sure you're allergic to things the shots work against. (Doctors say your allergy history and skin prick tests, *not* blood tests, are still the best way to pinpoint allergies.)

You can also be tested to see if you are allergic to insect stings. And that might be a wise thing to do if you've ever reacted to a sting with dizziness, faintness, or breathing difficulty, Dr. Lichtenstein recommends. *See also* **antihistamines**

aloe (AL-o) "Relief in a leaf" is one way of describing the healing powers of the remarkable aloe vera plant. Gel from its thick and fleshy leaves can soothe and help heal minor burns, scrapes, cuts, skin ulcers, cold sores, pressure sores, and sunburn. Purdue University medicinal herb authority Varro Tyler, Ph.D., credits aloe as "a handy, homegrown remedy for minor burns, abrasions, and other skin irritations."

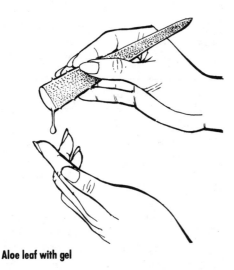

Aloe leaf with gel

In one study, aloe not only reduced pain and swelling in 18 patients recovering from dermabrasion (a technique used by cosmetic surgeons to sand away facial scars), it speeded up the healing process by three days. Patients treated with aloe on one side of the face and a usual wound dressing on the other experienced a 40 to 50 percent greater regrowth of skin after six days on the aloe-treated sides. Extracts of aloe are even showing promise in fighting viruses responsible for such conditions as herpes, measles, and possibly even AIDS. "Aloe is not a panacea, but it does have some very useful therapeutic properties," says Sheldon Saul Hendler, M.D., Ph.D., of the University of California, San Diego.

The biology behind aloe's palliative punch appears to be multifaceted: The plant contains salicylates, the same painkilling and anti-inflammatory compounds found in aspirin, and it also contains magnesium lactate, a substance that inhibits histamine reactions capable of causing skin irritation and itching. There's even evidence that an extract of aloe known as Carrisyn may stimulate the body to produce more immune-protective substances, including T-lymphocyte helper cells capable of combating infection. Aloe extracts currently can be found in products ranging from cosmetics, skin lotions, and soaps to suntan preparations and shampoos—yet gel squeezed directly from an aloe leaf appears to boast the greatest medicinal muscle.

HOW TO USE IT

Simply cut a thick, fleshy leaf lengthwise, squeeze out its clear gel (stopping short of squeezing out a yellowish substance that should *not* be used) and apply the gel directly to the wound in need. Aloe works best when exposed to open air, so leave the wound uncovered if possible.

Notes of caution: Aloe should not be used on burns that are more than skin-deep, nor should it be used on skin ulcers larger than a dime. Some people also are hypersensitive to aloe and will develop rashes in response to its use, so discontinue if this turns out to be true. Also consider it ill-advised to drink aloe, as research has yet to prove this to be effective or safe.

If you'd like to keep an aloe plant handy for possible first-aid duty, just remember this: Plants should be protected against temperatures below approximately 40°F, but otherwise are not fussy and will do well on any sunny, southern-facing windowsill. You can even give your aloe plant a vacation outdoors during the summer months. Plants can be obtained at most well-stocked garden centers or plant shops.

alum   Years ago, folks treated hemorrhoids with a homemade ointment of alum and lard. Today, alum—specifically, aluminum sulfate—is probably best known as the primary ingredient in styptic pencils, which are used to stop bleeding if you cut yourself shaving.

Alum is a catch-all term for a variety of aluminum compounds mainly used as astringents to tighten the skin, reduce swelling and inflammation, or stanch minor bleeding. Combined with boric acid and calcium acetate, aluminum sulfate, for example, is an active ingredient in soaking solutions (such as Bluboro Powder) used to relieve skin inflammation due to athlete's foot, allergies, insect bites, poison ivy, and minor bruises.

Another form of alum, aluminum acetate (also known as Burow's solution) is a main ingredient in drops used to prevent swimmer's ear. Yet another, ammonium alum, acts as a freshening agent in powdered douches.

Aluminum compounds are also used in many antiperspirants. Pharmacists report that people who are allergic to fragrances or other ingredients in commercial antiperspirants sometimes make their own by mixing alum with distilled water. They dab it on with cotton balls. Alum is sold at pharmacies, but you may have to special-order it.

amphetamines   Once known on the street as "speed," these powerful central nervous system stimulants are available by prescription only—if you can get them at all. Because of their potentially volatile side effects, physicians rarely prescribe them today, except for a select few medical conditions. The list of potential adverse effects is long and frightening, including excessive nervousness, insomnia, blurred vision, pounding heartbeat, and loss of appetite. They can possibly even lead to stroke or heart attack.

If amphetamines are used in appropriate clinical doses, however, many of these side effects are unlikely to occur. Amphetamines are also addictive—people who take them may experience distressing withdrawal symptoms when they stop.

Because amphetamines mask, delay, or alter perceptions of fatigue, some athletes have been known to use them to try to enhance performance or endurance. And once upon a time, diet doctors freely prescribed amphetamines to people who wanted to lose excess pounds.

Today, the U.S. Olympic Committee has banned the use of amphetamines by competitors. And reputable weight-loss doctors rely on diet, exercise, and behavior modification—not pills—to help overweight people reduce.

LEGITIMATE USES

Yet amphetamines still have a couple of legitimate medical uses. They're sometimes prescribed for narcoleptics, people who tend to fall asleep at the drop of a hat, anytime, anywhere. And pediatricians may prescribe dexedrine or other forms of dextroamphetamine for children with attention deficit hyperactivity disorder (ADHD).

"The current hypothesis is that children with ADHD have a deficiency of norepinephrine, a brain chemical that prevents stimuli from racing from nerve cell to nerve cell, unchecked," explains Julian Haber, M.D., member of the American Academy of Pediatrics and the National Committee for Children with Learning Disabilities. "Like Ritalin and Cylert [other, more commonly prescribed drugs for ADHD], dextroamphetamine increases levels of norepinephrine in children with a deficit, increasing their attention span." Once they can pay attention, they may be better able to learn.

ampicillin. *See* **penicillin**

analgesics. *See* **painkillers**

angioplasty (AN-jee-o-plas-tee) Should your arteries someday get jammed with fatty sludge, making your heart gasp for oxygen, a doctor with a little balloon may be your best ally.

Whether it's called angioplasty, balloon angioplasty, or percutaneous transluminal coronary angioplasty (whew!), the procedure is the same: A doctor very delicately snakes a thin, hollow tube up through your arteries until it reaches the criminal clog. A second, smaller, balloon-tipped tube is then passed through the first. Then the doctor oh-so-gently wedges this tube deep into the area of the fatty deposit and puffs up the balloon. If all goes well—presto—no more clogged artery.

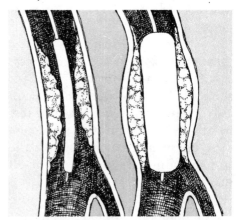

Balloon before and after inflation in plaque-blocked artery

How does it work? "We're not 100 percent certain why the procedure works, but there are a few probable explanations," says Howard S. Bush, M.D., a cardiologist at Fort Lauderdale's Cleveland Clinic in Florida. Inflating the balloon seems to compress plaque (that nasty sludge) against the artery wall. "It's like stepping on 10 inches of snow and scrunching it into an inch," says Dr. Bush. In addition, the balloon may also enlarge the artery by exerting force against its pliable walls.

Together, the scrunching and the stretching and possibly the breaking up of some of the plaque allow more room for blood to pass by—and that's all that *really* matters.

A STAR IS BORN

Balloon angioplasties were first performed in 1977. In 1990, about 200,000 heart patients underwent the procedure. Of these, the great majority, about 95 percent, came through with flying colors—a good reason for angioplasty's increasing popularity. Of the few who didn't fare well, the problem was either that the wire couldn't find its way to the problem, or worse, the abrupt intrusion caused a collapse of the artery.

As rare as such collapses are, angioplasties are typically done with a surgical SWAT team on standby, ready to rush in should the need arise. Even so, 1 percent of all patients expire on the table.

Still, angioplasty is safer than its most common alternative, bypass surgery. The procedure is also much cheaper (roughly one-third the cost of a bypass), simpler, and faster. Angioplasties are done under local anesthesia,

and you can be out of the hospital after a good night's rest (although some physicians may prefer to keep you in for an extra day). The procedure itself takes from 30 minutes to a couple of hours. There is usually not much pain.

GOOD WITHIN LIMITS

Despite their growing popularity, angioplasties are not the be-all and end-all of coronary care. One limitation, says Dr. Bush, is that the wire often can't penetrate an artery too jammed with plaque. The second limitation is "restenosis." That's what doctors call the process when a declogged artery starts to fill back up with sludge.

"From 30 to 35 percent of patients experience restenosis within three to six months [after an angioplasty]," says Dr. Bush. "It's the Achilles' heel of angioplasty. It's what turns a *great* procedure into a *good* procedure," he says. No one is clear why so many arteries fill back up, but doctors have been searching hard for ways to improve on the basic balloon angioplasty so that restenosis doesn't occur.

They've come up with, well, plaque "crackers, breakers, stretchers, drillers, scrapers, shavers, burners, welders, and melters," according to the title of one article in the *Journal of the American College of Cardiology.* Unfortunately, none of these new devices or new-fangled methods has proven much better than the usually reliable balloon, although some show definite promise.

Should you suffer from clogged arteries, how do you know whether it's best to have *your* arterial sludge cracked, drilled, scraped, burned, melted, or ballooned? Obviously you'll need to discuss it with your doctor.

The best answer for you may be one of the above—or it may be to grit your way through bypass surgery, or leave the situation as is, perhaps suffering an occasional angina attack and taking medications to reduce the clotting of your blood. Some researchers believe that this last option should be considered more often than it generally is.

Every clogged artery case is different, and you'll need the help of your cardiologist to make the best decision for you. *See also* **atherectomy; coronary bypass; laser surgery**

anise   (AN-iss) Any child will tell you that medicine often is too bitter to swallow. Anise, a sweet, licorice-like herb, is sometimes mixed with medicines to improve their unpleasant flavor. As Mary Poppins might have sung, "A spoonful of *anise* helps the medicine go down!"

This pleasant, aromatic herb isn't merely a nice taste, however. Medicine in its own right, anise traditionally has been used against flatulence, phlegm, and indigestion.

Like fennel, anise's healing powers generally are attributed to its primary constituent, the volatile oil anethole. "Some of the volatile oils are called antiflatulents," says pharmacist David Spoerke, director of POISINDEX Information System, a toxicology computer network in Denver, Colorado.

Spoerke adds, however, that *he* wouldn't raid the spice cabinet if he suffered a gas attack. "I wouldn't bother. If I really had flatulence, I'd take simethicone [an over-the-counter digestive aid]," he says.

A FOLK FAVORITE

Of course, anise was used in traditional medicine long before the advent of simethicone and related drugs. As with most folk remedies, anise's reputation runs well ahead of scientific validation. Herbalists have used anise as a diuretic, expectorant, stimulant, and galactogogue—a substance that increases a mother's store of breast milk.

There may be some biochemical factors that explain anise's traditional uses in folk medicine. It has been suggested, for example, that anise may flavor the taste of a mother's milk in a way that promotes enthusiastic suckling, which naturally boosts milk production.

The next time you have gas, you might want to give anise tea a try. Just steep a few tablespoons of seeds in hot water, to make a pleasant-tasting, and possibly therapeutic, beverage.

It's important not to substitute anise *oil* for anise seeds. The concentrated oil may cause skin irritations, nausea, or worse. Stick with the seeds. Of course, some people may have allergic reactions from the seeds, too. If you have any medical problems, leave anise alone, and tell your doctor. *See also* **fennel**

antacids   Heartburn? Sour stomach? Acid indigestion? Step into any drugstore, and you'll find a dozen or more different antacid products to soothe digestive distress. Most contain compounds of one or more minerals—such as calcium, magnesium, sodium, and aluminum—that neutralize excess stomach acid.

Doctors often prescribe antacids to help promote healing of peptic ulcers. But most people take them for occasional gastrointestinal upsets.

"No one knows exactly how much acid has to be neutralized to reduce minor ailments like heartburn," says Roy C. Parish, Pharm.D., an assistant professor at the University of Georgia College of Pharmacy, Athens. And not all antacids are equally potent. But generally, antacids neutralize about 90 percent of stomach acid—enough to get rid of that sour, queasy feeling you get after eating something that doesn't agree with you—or too much of something that does!

INGREDIENTS VARY

Antacids differ depending on the particular active ingredients they contain.

Sodium bicarbonate (as found in Alka-Seltzer) is basically plain old baking soda—a potent, fast-acting antacid for short-term relief of occasional indigestion or overeating. One caution: "The sodium content of products containing sodium bicarbonate is a concern for people with congestive heart failure, high blood pressure, or others on a low-sodium diet," says Dr. Parish. "Most other types of antacids have been reformulated, so they contain very little sodium. And those would proba-

bly be a better choice in such cases. Still, people who need to take antacids over the long term should check with their doctor."

Calcium carbonate compounds (such as Tums) also act quickly but the effects last longer than sodium bicarbonate. Constipation is a common side effect.

Some doctors suggest calcium-based antacids as a dietary supplement to help prevent bone-weakening osteoporosis. "Chewing three Tums a day, for example, will help supply the daily requirement for calcium," says Dr. Parish.

Aluminum compounds (such as Mylanta) neutralize less acid than calcium carbonate or sodium bicarbonate. Because aluminum compounds tend to be constipating, they are often combined with magnesium to counter the effect (Maalox is an example).

Magnesium compounds (such as Phillips' Milk of Magnesia) are more potent than aluminum compounds but less potent than sodium bicarbonate or calcium carbonate. Diarrhea may be a problem, but magnesium/aluminum combinations minimize this side effect. On the other hand, people with chronic constipation may benefit from a magnesium antacid.

Some antacids (such as Di-Gel, Gelusil, and Mylanta) also contain simethicone, to relieve excess gas. Other antacids (such as Alka-Seltzer) contain a pain reliever.

LIQUIDS WORK FAST

Antacids are available without a prescription, as liquids, powders, capsules, gum, wafers, lozenges, and chewable tablets.

"Liquid antacids are definitely more effective than tablets—the antacid is ground up, suspended, and ready to go to work," says Dr. Parish. Chewable tablets work best if they're chewed well before swallowing, and chased by a full glass of water. (Refrigerating an antacid may improve its slightly chalky flavor.)

As a rule, taking an antacid an hour after eating may counteract acidity for up to 3 hours, compared to only 30 minutes when taken on an empty stomach. Nevertheless, people with digestive problems may want to consult their doctor for special instructions.

"Lots of people who've been told they have a hiatal hernia, for example, are instructed to take antacids 'as needed,'" says Dr. Parish. "But they may get more relief if they take an antacid regularly—every 6 hours or so." *See also* **baking soda; bismuth; ulcer drugs**

antianxiety drugs For someone in the grip of an anxiety disorder, the world can seem like a scary place. Fortunately, the right prescription drug may be just the ticket back to normal day-to-day functioning. But while antianxiety drugs can bring panic attacks, irrational fears, and other symptoms under control, experts recognize that they seldom produce a cure. For that reason, some psychiatrists view antianxiety drugs as just one component of a larger comprehensive treatment. Other components include psychother-

apy, relaxation techniques, and a check for any medical factors that might be aggravating the anxiety.

Clinical evidence suggests that talking about the problem with a trained psychotherapist may shorten the length of time a person with chronic anxiety needs medication. Also, psychotherapy and relaxation techniques may extend the anxiety-free periods between attacks. Obsessive-compulsive disorder is the one condition that may require taking antianxiety drugs for life.

Several classes of medications are used to treat anxiety disorders. Here's a brief overview.

Benzodiazepines. These medications are so commonly prescribed for anxiety that they account for one in every 20 prescriptions written in the United States. The most familiar brand names include Valium, Librium, and Xanax. They're usually prescribed for chronic anxiety, otherwise known as generalized anxiety disorder. Xanax is also considered especially effective for panic disorders, which are often accompanied by rapid heartbeat, lightheadedness, and an extreme fear of losing control.

Benzodiazepines work by depressing activity in the part of the brain that controls emotions, effectively reducing the communication between brain cells. The drug reduces feelings of agitation and restlessness and may even induce drowsiness.

Benzodiazepines are available in two categories: Long-acting benzodiazepines, like Valium and Librium, remain in the body for days after the last pill is swallowed. The strength of the drug diminishes gradually, making withdrawal symptoms less severe. Short-acting benzodiazepines, like Xanax and Activan, are completely eliminated from the body a few hours after you take them. That makes withdrawal more abrupt. On the plus side, however, short-acting benzodiazepines taken before bedtime won't affect alertness the following day.

Both types of benzodiazepines are considered relatively safe. They are not known to be fatal in overdoses, unless mixed with alcohol—a combination that can be very dangerous. At least 50 percent of people on these drugs experience some degree of withdrawal when they stop taking them. Withdrawal symptoms, which can last for two weeks, include nervousness, insomnia, loss of appetite, a metallic taste in the mouth, and tingling sensations in the arms and legs.

Buspirone. Marketed under the name BuSpar, this drug is as effective as the benzodiazepines in treating generalized anxiety disorder, even though it works by a different mechanism. BuSpar has far fewer side effects: It doesn't make people sleepy, interact dangerously with alcohol, or produce withdrawal symptoms. It may, however, induce nausea, dizziness, headaches, nervousness, or excitement.

Beta blockers. Propeanolot (Inderal) and atenolol (Tenormin), two drugs in this category, can offer great relief to people who suffer from social phobia, who become severely anxious whenever they're the center of attention. Beta blockers reduce the amount of nervous system stimulation to the body,

helping to stop the flushing, sweating, or shaking that often accompanies such attacks.

Because they lower blood pressure and slow heart rate, beta blockers are not advisable for people with abnormally low blood pressure or certain heart conditions. Otherwise, side effects aren't much of a problem. On occasion, these drugs produce nightmares, depression, and tingling of the fingers and toes.

Monoamine oxidase inhibitors. Studies have shown that two drugs in this category, Nardil and Parnate, are 70 percent effective in relieving social phobia within four weeks. They are also prescribed for panic disorders. Their worst drawback is their dangerous interaction with certain foods and other drugs.

Anafranil. This new drug (known generically as chlorimipramine or clomipramine) has been shown to help at least half of those who suffer from obsessive-compulsive disorders—such as the need for constant hand washing. It may also be useful for panic disorders.

Anafranil may take four weeks or longer before its full effects are felt. Side effects include dry mouth, constipation, weight gain, dizziness after standing quickly, and drowsiness. Studies show the relapse rate is high when people stop taking this drug.

Prozac. Like Anafranil, this new antidepressant shows promise for obsessive-compulsive disorder and panic attacks. And like Anafril, it can take four weeks to work. But Prozac, which may also be useful in the treatment of social phobias, has relatively few side effects. These include jitteriness, nausea, stomach cramps, and diarrhea. Experts say much more research is needed to determine just how effective Prozac is for anxiety disorders. *See also* **antidepressants; sedatives; tranquilizers**

antibiotics Antibiotics haven't exactly turned us into a nation of long-lived George Burnses, but it has been estimated that, on average, these drugs have given each American another ten years of life.

Ironically—but significantly—the term "antibiotic" literally means "against life." That's because within the human immune system, these drugs are involved in a shootout for better health at the OK Corral. If the antibiotic drug works, it helps your own body's natural defenses (such as the white cells) kill or at least inhibit the growth of the bad-guy bacteria.

These germbusters generally do their work in one of four ways.

Some attack and weaken bacterial cell walls, causing the cells to rupture and spill their contents. That puts those particular germs out of commission fast. These include such drugs as the penicillins, cephalosporins, and bacitracin.

Another group sets up a roadblock inside bacteria so that genetic information cannot be exchanged. This makes it impossible for the germs to reproduce. These agents include griseofulvin and tetracycline.

A third group goes after the bacteria's cell membranes, putting a hole in the proverbial dike that makes the stuff of life leak out with fatal results.

Amphotericin B and polymyxin B do just that.

Finally, the fourth group wreaks havoc with a bacterial cell's metabolism. These include sulfonamides, aminosalicylic acid, and isoniazid.

The antibiotic that's extended our lease on life the longest is penicillin, but other antibiotics also deserve the thanks and hallelujahs of a grateful mankind. Some conditions that are zapped by antibiotics include pneumonia and other respiratory infections and urinary tract infections.

Most of the powerful antibiotics are administered by injection or taken orally. Some less powerful topical drugs are placed directly on the skin to treat problems such as the eczema-like minor skin infections that children often get.

MEDICINAL BOUNTY HUNTERS

The origins of these antibiotics make them sound more like antiquated folk remedies than high-tech medications. These sources include bread mold, catfish slime, and frog skin—just about everything but eye of newt.

For years, scientists have been running a rather unusual talent contest—they've been auditioning soil and water samples from all over the world in hopes of finding another wonder drug like penicillin. Through a simple chemical process known as semisynthesis, researchers take a basic molecule from these samples and manipulate it, perhaps by adding an extra carbon chain to it, thus modifying it in some chemical way.

What happens, in effect, is that

what started as an innocuous, weak antibiotic in nature is turned into a chemical strongman by simple chemical manipulation. Squibb researchers, for example, derived a new antibiotic called Azactam from the tea-colored water of the Pine Barrens forest in New Jersey. Before locating what they needed, these researchers spent a decade inspecting 200,000 soil and water samples. Researchers aren't beyond looking anywhere they think there's the faintest reason to suspect that something capable of killing germs may exist.

In fact, because antibiotics are synthetically derived from some pretty exotic soil and plant samples, it's feared that environmental destruction—including the burning and clearing of rain forests—may prevent researchers from locating the source of the next miracle drug.

"In a general way, future antibiotic discoveries may be affected if sources are destroyed before they can be identified and studied to determine if they have medicinal effects," says Enrique Forero, Ph.D., director of research at the Missouri Botanical Garden in St. Louis. In other words, he says, mankind may never know what medicinal breakthrough it will have missed should the rain forests and other habitats disappear.

BACTERIA ARE RESISTING

There are two good reasons why it is important that new antibiotics be discovered on a frequent and regular basis. For one thing, one person's cure may be another's poison—someone sen-

sitive to penicillin, for example, might very well tolerate some other agent perfectly well.

The other reason is that some bacteria learn to build up their biceps to the point where they can resist the antibiotics that routinely rub out weaker bacteria, says George A. Jacoby, M.D., associate professor of medicine at Harvard Medical School and physician with the Infectious Disease Unit, Massachusetts General Hospital in Boston. In other words, in today's war against germs, it's the germs themselves that are shooting back.

While not a public health disaster, bacteria resistant to antibiotics have "become a great problem," says Dr. Jacoby. For example, he cites gonorrhea as one disease that has defied standard therapy in recent years "because the frequency of resistance has gotten pretty high."

To fight the problem, medical experts since the mid-1970s "have been modifying existing antibiotics to improve their properties," says Dr. Jacoby. For example, researchers have modified penicillin to produce an "improved generation of antibiotics," he says.

It has been estimated that the problem of bacterial resistance costs the American economy anywhere from $100 million to $30 billion a year, says Dr. Jacoby. "One reason is because doctors must use more toxic and expensive antibiotics to treat infections that are resistant," he says.

In addition, resistance results in longer hospital stays, an increasing number of people whose diseases linger unnecessarily, and even deaths, says Dr. Jacoby.

The situation varies from antibiotic to antibiotic. "Some bugs have stayed sensitive [vulnerable] to antibiotics that they were sensitive to 50 years ago—they haven't changed at all," says Dr. Jacoby. "In other cases the resistance has accumulated to the point that there are drugs we can no longer use." *See also* **penicillin; tetracycline**

anticholinergics (an-tee-ko-lihn-ER-jiks) Your body's autonomic nervous system, like any efficient machine, tries to keep the parts it governs—the bowels, airways, and muscles of the glands—working together. It does this by balancing two different systems. The sympathetic nervous system, for example, relaxes the intestines and dilates the pupils. At the same time, the parasympathetic nervous system is *tensing* the bowels and *constricting* the pupils. Ideally it all evens out.

Problems can arise, though, when there's too much tension and not enough relaxation. This can cause muscle tremors, intestinal cramping, or poor bladder control. For all of these conditions—and many others—the anticholinergic drugs, sometimes called antispasmodics, can help. Here's how they work.

A neurotransmitter called acetylcholine is responsible for giving orders—"Contract! Constrict!"—to muscles in the bladder, airways, and intestines. Anticholinergic drugs, as the name suggests, block acetylcholine, preventing its orders from getting through. The muscles relax.

Perhaps the best known of the anticholinergic drugs is atropine, once widely used for asthma, ulcers, and the tremors of Parkinson's disease. Atropine has many side effects, however, and for the most part it's been replaced by a newer, safer generation of anticholinergic drugs, says James Roerig, Pharm.D., clinical pharmacist in the Department of Psychiatry at the Ramsey Clinic in St. Paul.

CRAMPS RELIEVED

One such drug is dicyclomine (Bentyl), sometimes used to relieve severe intestinal cramping. "Your bowel is constricting too much, and that hurts," Dr. Roerig says. "But if you block acetylcholine, you get a decrease in the activity of the bowel so it doesn't clamp down so much."

Similar contractions in the bladder can cause incontinence, or at least the need—sometimes urgent—to urinate frequently. Anticholinergic drugs can help by easing the contractions that force urine from the bladder.

The anticholinergics also are used to stop muscle contractions in the airways, which can block airflow. Loaded into inhalers, they quickly open tiny passageways called bronchioles, and they are used to relieve asthma attacks, Dr. Roerig says. They may be used during eye examinations to dilate the pupil, a process called mydriasis. Anticholinergics are also found in some over-the-counter allergy medications and sleep aids.

Today, anticholinergics are used primarily to counteract the side effects of some antipsychotic medications, Dr.

Roerig says, which tend to tip the all-important push/pull balance. "People taking these drugs might have muscle spasms, their eyes might roll up, and they may look like they have Parkinson's disease," he says.

In the past, the anticholinergic drugs often were used to relieve the symptoms—stiffness, shaking, and excessive salivation—that marked the early stages of Parkinson's disease. For the most part, a drug called levodopa has supplanted the anticholinergics for treating Parkinson's, Dr. Roerig says.

While the anticholinergics are a relatively safe class of drugs, they aren't without side effects. "People's pupils will dilate, and they may get some blurring of vision," Dr. Roerig says. "They get a dry mouth, and perhaps a rapid heart rate. Constipation is one of the more common side effects, especially in the elderly, and urinary retention also can occur." The elderly are also more likely to experience side effects such as confusion, visual hallucinations, and agitation when taking over-the-counter products containing anticholinergics.

Except in psychiatry, the use of the anticholinergics is slowly declining, he says. Newer drugs simply are more efficient and, for the most part, have fewer side effects.

anticoagulants　As every commuter knows, the best highway in the world doesn't always get you where you want to go. All it takes is a stalled car during rush hour, or a spilled crate of oranges, and traffic simply stops. *Cold.*

Of course, a traffic jam can be aggravating, but it isn't life-threatening—unless it occurs in your bloodstream. People can die when blood clots lodge in their arterial and venous highways, preventing traffic—blood—from getting through. Anticoagulant drugs prevent blood clots from forming, so the roads stay open.

Heparin is one of the most widely used anticoagulants. Given by injection, it's typically administered during or immediately after many types of surgery, times when blood clots are likely to form. If you've just had an artificial heart valve installed, you certainly don't want a wandering blood clot to gum up the works. In fact, doctors often use heparin when kidney disease patients undergo dialysis, so blood clots won't clog the machines!

If you're healthy, of course, blood clots are a crucial part of healing. "In most cases involving wounds, you *want* a barrier to blood flow, because it stops you from bleeding to death," says one scientist. "In other instances—such as in your coronary arteries—you do not want such a barrier."

HEART HELPERS

Unfortunately, the coronary arteries are precisely the places where blood clots often do form—and do the most damage by triggering a heart attack. Every year, Americans undergo more than 300,000 coronary-artery bypass operations. But a large percentage of those arterial detours—up to 30 percent—will close off within a year of surgery. Anticoagulant drugs improve the chances of those grafts staying clear.

Slower-acting than heparin, warfarin is an anticlotting agent that's taken orally. It's often used by people with long-term heart problems who are prone to developing dangerous blood clots.

Aspirin may be used in much the same way as heparin and warfarin. It helps keep the tiny, disk-shaped blood platelets from clumping together. Doctors often suggest that people take aspirin after heart surgery because it helps keep the blood flowing smoothly. In fact, researchers at Harvard Medical School found that people who regularly take aspirin (one pill every other day) may significantly reduce their risks for fatal heart attacks.

While anticoagulants prevent blood clots from forming, they don't eliminate clots that already have formed. Another class of drugs, the thrombolytics, actually dissolve blood clots already in place.

Because anticoagulant drugs inhibit or stop the clotting process, even minor cuts may bleed profusely. Nosebleeds commonly occur, as do bleeding in the urinary and gastrointestinal tracts. Doctors may advise people taking anticoagulants to avoid anything that might cause bleeding: razors, contact sports, power tools, and so on.

Today's anticoagulants are especially efficient, powerful drugs, but the basic concept isn't new. Warfarin, for example, is based on a chemical compound found in sweet clover. There are many other natural substances—leeches, ticks, and garlic to name just a few—that also hinder the clotting process. *See also* **aspirin**

anticonvulsants   Also known as antiepileptic drugs, anticonvulsants prevent seizures triggered by epilepsy, a chronic brain disorder with various causes. The seizures are brought on by sudden, excessive discharges of neurons (nerve cells) in different parts of the brain. The type of anticonvulsant prescribed depends on the type of seizure being treated.

Here's a brief rundown on the most commonly prescribed antiepileptic medicines.

Phenytoin (Dilantin) and carbamazepine (Tegretol). These drugs control most generalized tonic-clonic seizures (grand mal seizures), in which the arms and legs become rigid, followed by jerking of the entire body. They also control partial seizures (a less severe disorder). Carbamazepine is less apt to cloud thinking than phenytoin, and it's the most frequently prescribed anticonvulsant in the world.

Ethosuximide (Zarontin). This is useful for treating absence seizures (petit mal seizures), characterized by brief periods of altered consciousness.

Valproic acid (Depakene). This drug is effective against both absence seizures and generalized tonic-clonic seizures (including myoclonic seizures, or sudden muscle contractions). It's particularly hard on the liver, so doses should be monitored carefully.

STICK TO THE REGIMEN

If you have epilepsy, it's important to take your medicine every day. Many patients continue to have seizures because they forget to take their pills, prompting their doctors to prescribe higher and higher doses, increasing the risk of side effects. Also, anticonvulsants can interact with other drugs, so be sure to tell your doctor if you're taking any other medication. Carbamazepine, for example, may speed up breakdown of oral contraceptives, in which case extra estrogen may be needed to prevent unwanted pregnancy.

Growing evidence suggests that after two or three seizure-free years, some epileptics may be able to discontinue their medication with relative safety. And some patients with epilepsy would rather chance an occasional seizure than risk toxicity or endure side effects (like nausea or dizziness) from drug therapy. This is a controversial issue, however, so don't stop taking your medication without the advice of your physician. *See also* **barbiturates; phenobarbital**

antidepressants   This class of drugs is used to treat chemical abnormalities in the brain, which underlie many depressive illnesses. There are three main categories in use today: the tricyclics, monoamine oxidase (MAO) inhibitors, and the relatively new arrivals like fluoxetine (Prozac) or bupropion (Wellbutrin). Antidepressants are only available by prescription.

"Any single drug for depression on the market right now is likely to be effective for 70 to 75 percent of patients," says Sidney Zisook, M.D., professor of psychiatry and director of outpatient research and training at the University of California at San Diego. "But it is not always the same 75 percent. In other words, people who don't do well with Prozac may do well with Wellbutrin—or something else."

The key seems to be pairing the right drug with the specific depressive disorder, he says. For instance, clinicians find that Wellbutrin does a better job than other antidepressants with bipolar depression, an illness in which people occasionally experience manic highs as well as lows.

DELAYED EFFECT

Despite individual quirks, antidepressants do have some characteristics in common. One of the most troubling is that they can take up to four weeks to deliver full benefits. The reason for this still puzzles experts. Some speculate that the drugs may need that much time to help key groups of nerve cells reset the chemical balance.

Are antidepressants necessary for all varieties of depression? Apparently not. Studies have found that "talk" therapies such as cognitive, interpersonal, and behavioral psychotherapy may be just as good—or better—for mild to moderate depression. These newer therapies are shorter term and more problem focused than the therapies of the past. But experts still consider the drugs essential for more serious cases. For one thing, they're much faster than psychotherapy. Improvement can often be seen in weeks, rather than in the months it may take psychotherapy to bring relief. Even so, there's still a role for talk-oriented approaches.

"Often psychotherapy plus medication is better than drugs alone," Dr. Zisook says. "I think some form of supportive therapy is always useful."

Here's a rundown on the most widely-used antidepressants.

Tricyclics. So named because their molecules are composed of three rings, one of these drugs, imipramine (Tofranil, Jasimine), is still the standard against which the new drugs are judged, says Jack M. Gorman, M.D., author of *The Essential Guide to Psychiatric Drugs.* Other oft-prescribed drugs in this class include Tofranil, Norpramin, Elavil, Endep, Dapin, and Pamelor.

On the plus side, the tricyclics are "tried and true" and very effective against major depression, according to Dr. Gorman. But the side effects are considerable. They include dry mouth, constipation, drowsiness, blurry vision, difficulty urinating, dizziness after standing up quickly, and a tendency for weight gain.

Monoamine oxidase inhibitors. Nardil and Parnate are the two best-known examples of this class of drug, which accomplishes its mood-elevating effect by inhibiting the work of an important brain chemical. An unfortunate consequence of this blocking mechanism is that the liver can no longer metabolize a substance called tyramine. So that means that tyramine-rich foods like cheese and herring must be avoided by people taking MAO inhibitors. Otherwise, the potential is there for tyramine to enter the bloodstream, dangerously elevate blood pressure, and initiate a stroke.

It was for this reason that this class of drugs fell out of favor for a time. MAO inhibitors are now regaining their popularity because of clinical evidence that shows them to be more effective than other antidepressants in the battle against atypical depression, a condition characterized by mood swings and a tendency to overeat and oversleep. Possible adverse effects of these drugs include sleep disturbances, fluid retention, difficulty achieving orgasm, and a tendency for weight gain.

The new antidepressants. This is a catch-all term for new arrivals on the market that have a different chemical structure from the tricyclics and a different biological effect on the brain. In this group, Prozac, the top seller, is fast becoming the first-choice treatment. It is considered highly effective for major depression and has far fewer side effects than the cyclic antidepressants. Side effects include insomnia, nausea, diarrhea, stomach cramps, headache, and nervousness. One of its biggest drawbacks is its price. A single capsule can retail for more than $3.50.

Wellbutrin has shown satisfactory antidepressant action in clinical trials, as well as fewer side effects than the tricyclics. Its adverse effects include insomnia, agitation, and a tendency to cause seizures. Long-term effects are not yet established. *See also* **behavior therapy; cognitive therapy; interpersonal psychotherapy**

antiemetics People vomit when they're sick, eat the wrong foods, or simply take too many rides on the merry-go-round. Because throwing up expels potentially harmful substances from the body, it's often a necessary, even life-saving, reflex.

Sometimes, however, vomiting only makes people miserable. On those occasions, antiemetics may help. When people with cancer receive chemotherapy, for example, they often take antiemetics to keep vomiting at bay. Antiemetics help people prone to motion sickness get through long car trips. They also offer pregnant women welcome relief from morning sickness.

BLOCKING THE REFLEX

The nausea and vomiting that accompany cancer chemotherapy are sometimes so severe that people actually stop the treatments—treatments they need, in some cases, to save their life. To counter those side effects, antiemetic drugs—metoclopramide and haloperidol are two examples—commonly are used during chemotherapy. They work, in essence, by preventing the brain from pulling the trigger that fires the vomiting reflex.

Dronabinol, another antiemetic drug sometimes prescribed for chemotherapy patients, contains one of the active substances found in marijuana. Since dronabinol affects the brain in some of the same ways marijuana does, doctors generally prescribe it only when other antiemetics don't do the trick.

Motion sickness, as queasy travelers know, can make even the shortest trip, well, a little messy. For many people, dimenhydrinate, better known

as Dramamine, is the drug of choice for all types of motion sickness—from driving coast to coast to sailing on the QEII. An antihistamine, dimenhydrinate works by making the vomiting center inside the brain less sensitive.

PLANNING AHEAD

Even though antiemetics will *prevent* vomiting, they aren't so good at *stopping* it. When it's time for your annual vacation, start the Dramamine an hour before you start the car, advises Robert M. Stern, Ph.D., a professor of psychology at Pennsylvania State University who has performed numerous studies on motion sickness. "If a slightly older sibling throws up in the car, then it's very, very hard to keep the younger kid from getting sick, too," he says.

Dr. Stern says you can combat motion-induced vomiting by staying active, watching the scenery (in a car, look out the window; on a boat, go on deck), and nibbling bread or crackers.

In recent years, researchers have begun to investigate the antiemetic properties of acupressure. In one study, pregnant women who pressed a precise spot above their wrists—in acupuncture terminology, the P6 position—several times a day reported feeling less nausea and morning sickness. In another study, postsurgical patients experienced less nausea and vomiting when they wore wristbands designed to exert constant pressure on the P6 spot.

Antiemetics aren't foolproof, however. So if all else fails, just remem-

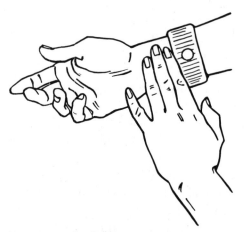

Antinausea wristband at P6 acupressure point

ber the one good thing about vomiting: it doesn't last forever. People get sick, throw up, and, most of the time, start feeling better. If vomiting persists, see your doctor. *See also* **ginger; motion sickness remedies; soda crackers**

antihistamines The next time you find yourself eyeing antihistamines in the drugstore, wondering which of these allergy-relief medications will *really* keep your nose from running and your skin from erupting into hives, remember this little secret that doctors know: There is no one best choice for everyone. The brand that works for you might make life downright miserable for your Aunt Maude. Experts say it's all a matter of personal chemistry.

Fortunately, your chances of finding the one that works without troubling side effects—like making you dangerous behind the wheel—are better than ever, thanks to new antihistamines, such as Seldane and Hismanal, that don't cause drowsiness or loss of coordination in most people. "These are available only by prescription right now," says antihistamine expert Eli O. Meltzer, M.D., clinical professor of pediatrics in the Division of Allergy and Immunology at the University of California at San Diego.

So you've got a decision to make. Should you opt for the convenience of buying a product from your druggist's shelf or see your doctor about getting a prescription?

"Just because the over-the-counter products are found next to the toothpaste doesn't mean they're any safer [than prescription antihistamines]," Dr. Meltzer cautions. In addition to drowsiness, these products may cause blurred vision and dry mouth. Of course, the new drugs aren't perfect either. Hismanal, for example, may cause weight gain. Seldane, a more popular drug in this category, has been reported to cause headaches, nausea, and dry mouth in some people.

Here's what else you need to know to make an informed choice.

GOODBYE, RUNNY NOSE

Studies show that antihistamines—which are made to relieve allergy and hay fever symptoms—do best at stopping you from developing a runny or itchy nose, sneezing, and skin disorders like hives and itching. They do less well at clearing stuffy noses. Of course, if you can avoid the substance that triggers the allergic attack, so much the better. But if that's impractical—as it is when a little house dust or some ragweed pollen is all it takes to set you off—antihistamines may offer you a measure of protection.

Antihistamines work by competing with a substance in the body called histamine for special histamine H1 receptors. Not surprisingly, you'll find these receptors on the small blood vessels in the skin, nose, and eyes—the very places where allergy misery strikes. All histamine needs to do to start trouble, once an allergen triggers its release, is dock in these receptors.

Once absorbed into the bloodstream, antihistamines attach themselves to the histamine receptors, blocking histamine from attaching. They don't harm or change the histamine; they simply prevent it from causing trouble. That's why antihistamines are best used *before* you have symptoms. Once the histamine settles into the receptors, you may have to wait a while for relief.

The biggest difference between the old and new antihistamines is that while the old are capable of crossing into the brain via the cerebral capillaries, the new ones cannot. Once in, these first-generation antihistamines may somehow depress the central nervous system, which is what accounts for that sleepy feeling they bring on. Studies show that up to one-fourth of the people who take them complain of drowsiness. The newer drugs aren't able to make their way into the brain, so they're considered safer in this regard.

These new drugs have other advantages, too, Dr. Meltzer says. "They're quicker acting. It may only take you 1 hour or 2 to get relief, as opposed to 2 to 4 hours for the others. The effects tend to last longer, too."

TRIAL AND ERROR

Whether you opt for the newer prescription antihistamines or the older over-the-counter ones, you may have to test your reactions to a few to find the one you like. "If you pick one that seems to really zonk you, or bothers you in some other way, try another," advises Roger Maickel, Ph.D., professor of pharmacology and toxicology at Purdue University School of Pharmacy and Pharmacal Sciences. Just be careful to compare the ingredients list of the one that didn't work to that of the one you're considering.

Some allergists even send their patients home with a sample pack of antihistamines and instructions to log their reactions to the various products over the next few weeks. If you're going to buy yours at the store, you might want to choose trial sizes and log your reactions, too.

Until you find an antihistamine that doesn't make you sleepy, don't use it when you have to drive or use heavy machinery. Don't mix antihistamines with alcohol, either, because alcohol tends to make them even more sedating, Dr. Maickel says. And always check with your pharmacist to make sure you can safely combine an antihistamine drug with other medication you may be taking. *See also* **allergy shots; antiemetics**

antihypertensives   Doctors can choose from almost 50 different drugs to treat high blood pressure (hypertension). Yet physicians prescribe antihypertensives less readily than they did years ago.

"We used to tell patients, 'Your blood pressure's high. Take these pills, goodbye,'" says Charles P. Tifft, M.D., associate professor of medicine at Boston University School of Medicine. "Now we think it over. To begin with, does the patient really have high blood pressure? If so, is drug therapy appropriate, or should nondrug measures, such as losing weight and giving up cigarettes, be tried first?"

One elevated reading—systolic (upper) value of 140 or above and/or diastolic (lower) value of 90 or above—doesn't necessarily mean you have high blood pressure. To be certain of the diagnosis, your doctor may take a couple of readings on several different occasions—each time after you've been sitting quietly for 5 minutes.

If diastolic blood pressure is persistently high (95 or higher), or between 90 and 95 with other risk factors (such as high cholesterol), medication is probably in order, especially if nondrug therapy has failed. Generally, the goal is to control blood pressure with as few drugs as possible, at the lowest possible doses, in order to minimize side effects. Sometimes, smaller doses of two or three drugs work better and cause fewer side effects than a single medication. And of course, some people simply respond better to one drug than to another.

But an effective drug regimen *should* be found, because left uncontrolled, high blood pressure can damage the blood vessels of the brain, heart, and kidneys, resulting in a stroke, heart failure, or kidney failure.

A RANGE OF CHOICES

Here's a rundown of the most commonly used antihypertensives and how they work.

Diuretics (such as chlorothiazide). By forcing the kidneys to excrete more sodium, diuretics lower the volume of blood and thereby decrease blood pressure.

Thiazide-type diuretics, in particular, pay major lifesaving dividends. "They are probably the most effective antihypertensive agents studied so far for reducing the risk of stroke," says Dr. Tifft. "I prescribe thiazide diuretics for hypertensives with a previous stroke or a strong family history of stroke." Side effects include the possibility of impaired sexual response.

Angiotensin converting enzyme (ACE) inhibitors. These types of drugs (such as captopril) are among the newest antihypertensives. They block production of angiotensin, a hormone that raises pressure by constricting blood vessels and promoting salt and water retention. Side effects may include rashes and a dry, hacking cough.

Centrally acting alpha agents. By telling the brain to send fewer impulses to the blood vessels, these drugs, such as clonidine, cause the vessels to widen and blood pressure to go down. Clonidine may also help reduce the craving for nicotine, making it a good choice for smokers who are trying to quit.

Peripheral-acting adrenergic antagonists. These drugs, which include reserpine, block the effects of adrenaline (a hormone) at nerve endings, widening blood vessels. They may be combined with diuretics. Lethargy or depression may occur.

Beta blockers. Beta blockers, including propanolol, reduce blood pressure by interfering with responses to certain nerve impulses, thus prompting the heart to pump less blood. They are the second most widely prescribed antihypertensives, following diuretics. But they're not for everyone. They may interfere with sexual functioning. "Beta blockers also tend to reduce exercise tolerance," says Dr. Tifft. "So if a patient jogs regularly, an ACE inhibitor, calcium blocker, alpha blocker, or centrally acting drug may be a better choice."

Calcium channel blockers. These drugs, such as verapamil, block the entry of calcium into small blood vessels, which then relax, lowering blood pressure. Major side effects may include headache, flushing, local swelling, and constipation.

Vasodilators. Acting directly on blood vessel walls to widen them—or at least keep them from narrowing— vasodilators such as minoxidil aren't usually prescribed unless other drugs have failed. Side effects include fluid retention and excess hair growth.

For some people, nondrug measures, such as sodium restriction or relaxation therapy, may improve the effectiveness of antihypertensive drugs.

USE THEM WISELY

Many people with high blood pressure have to take antihypertensives for the rest of their life, even if they feel well. To help patients stick with their medication, Dr. Tifft offers the following advice.

Take your pills at the same time every day. Keep a few pills at work, clearly labeled. Make sure you have enough medicine on hand to last you through the weekend, a vacation, or business trip. And if side effects bother you, speak up.

"If you experience side effects, don't adjust the dosage on your own, and don't be afraid to discuss the problem with your doctor," says Dr. Tifft. "The problem may or may not be drug related. In some people, for example, just being labeled 'hypertensive' is enough to cause sexual problems. And even if the drug is to blame, lowering the dosage or switching to another type of drug may solve the problem." *See also* **beta blockers; calcium channel blockers; diuretics; low-sodium diet; minoxidil**

anti-inflammatories You expected *some* discomfort when the dentist pulled your tooth, but nothing like this. What's worse, your entire face has puffed up. It feels like you have an eggplant in your cheek. It hurts!

There are many anti-inflammatory drugs that can help knock that eggplant down to peanut size. Aspirin is one of the most effective anti-inflammatory drugs you can buy. Ibuprofen also works well, as do indomethacin and the other nonsteroidal anti-inflammatory drugs (NSAIDs). Fast-acting and hard-working steroids, of course, may be the toughest inflammation fighters of all.

Anti-inflammatory drugs are selective. Aspirin may work for you, but not for your husband. *He* may need to try ibuprofen, indomethacin, and a dozen others before finding the right drug for him. When it comes to beating inflammation, doctors advise patience.

Where to begin? First, let's take a closer look at inflammation. Then we'll see how *anti*-inflammatory drugs beat it down.

CURBING PROSTAGLANDINS

Inflammation begins when you're hurt. When the dentist yanks that tooth, or arthritis flares, or you bop your head on the freezer door, compounds called prostaglandins sound the alarm in your body. Pain signals speed to your brain; white blood cells rush to the injury. Swelling starts.

Anti-inflammatory drugs inhibit your body's production of prostaglandins. That means fewer white blood cells arrive, so swelling goes down. Fewer pain signals make it to your brain, so you hurt less, too.

If, for example, you twist your knee and there is serious swelling, steroids may be injected straight into the injured joint. Not only do steroids inhibit prostaglandins, they also permeate the joint lining, preventing inflammation-causing cells from getting inside.

Doctors agree that steroid drugs such as cortisone and prednisone are indefatigable inflammation busters. However, they may cause serious side effects—bone damage, for example, or suppressed adrenal functions.

For many types of inflammation, NSAIDs are recommended. (See "Nonsteroidal Anti-Inflammatory Drugs" on the opposite page.) Indeed, NSAIDs are among the most widely prescribed medications in the world.

Aspirin, the prototypical NSAID, reduces pain and swelling so well that Americans take billions of tablets every year.

Doctors recommend aspirin as a first-line defense for many types of swelling. People with rheumatoid arthritis, for example, often take aspirin to control the swelling.

But some people can't take aspirin because of side effects. Even regular users sometimes complain of stomach pain, and peptic ulcers aren't uncommon.

ASPIRIN ALTERNATIVES

Fortunately, the new generations of NSAIDs seem to work as well as aspirin, sometimes producing fewer unpleasant side effects. In one study, people with rheumatoid arthritis took either aspirin, ibuprofen, fenoprofen, naproxen, or tolmetin. All the drugs worked, but people had the most problems with aspirin.

Some aspirin formulas are designed for sensitive stomachs. When people with that problem take enteric-coated aspirin (aspirin that dissolves in the small intestine, not in the stomach), they seem to tolerate it better than noncoated aspirin.

Selected with care, most over-the-

Nonsteroidal Anti-Inflammatory Drugs (NSAIDs)

aspirin (Anacin, Ascriptin, Bayer, Bufferin, Easprin, Ecotrin, Zorprin)
diflunisal (Dolobid)
fenoprofen (Nalfon)
ibuprofen (Advil, Midol, Motrin, Nuprin)
indomethacin (Indocin)
ketoprofen
meclofenamate (Meclomen)
mefenamic acid (Ponstel)
naproxen (Naprosyn)
phenylbutazone (Azolid, Butozolidin)
piroxicam (Feldene)
sulindac (Clinoril)
tolmetin (Tolectin)

---

counter anti-inflammatory drugs are safe and effective ways to treat temporary inflammation. A flare-up of arthritis can make life miserable. Why suffer when aspirin, ibuprofen, or one of the many NSAIDs may help take the kinks out? *See also* **aspirin; ibuprofen; steroids**

antispasmodics. *See* **anticonvulsants**

antitussive agents. *See* **cough medicines**

apple   It's 3:00 P.M. Although you can't believe it, you hear the office snack machines calling your name—and it's not a faint cry. But instead of turning to what some consider the sinful chocolate bar, you reach for what's not an evil fruit.

Crrrunnnch.

Whether at home or at work, for a meal or for a snack, you'll have trouble finding anything better for nutrition and taste than the apple's sweet/tart mix. And this fruit can do more for you than just satisfy your appetite.

Apples have been cultivated for at least 3,000 years and are grown in temperate zones throughout the world. While you're familiar with Red and Golden Delicious, McIntosh, and Granny Smith apples, thousands of varieties exist.

An average apple registers about 72 calories, with 17 grams of carbohydrate, 175 milligrams of potassium, just 0.3 gram of fat, and virtually no sodium. About 5 grams of dietary fiber are also present, with about 81 percent in the form of soluble fiber, explains Jack Hegenauer, Ph.D., a research professor in biology at the University of California at San Diego. Most of this soluble fiber is pectin, says Dr. Hegenauer, who has studied the nutritional makeup of apples and other fruits.

CHOLESTEROL DROP

Pectin is important because it has been shown in several studies to help lower blood cholesterol levels. Researchers at Central Washington University found that people who ate three cookies with added apple fiber daily had a 7 percent drop in cholesterol levels in six weeks, with no other dietary changes.

While almost everyone can benefit from the cholesterol-lowering effects of apples, dieters get an extra boost from the apple's bulk.

"It's a very real effect, and I would certainly recommend to people that, if they are considering fiber supplements, they can get exactly the same effect— filling themselves up without giving themselves too many calories—by eating readily available fruits and vegetables," Dr. Hegenauer explains.

Apples also can be used to fight bruxism or nighttime tooth grinding, reports Harold Perry, D.D.S., Ph.D., of Northwestern University Dental School. Eating one apple before bed tires jaw muscles, helping to alleviate the nocturnal grinding.

APPLE PICKING

What's the best way for you to utilize the apple's healthy qualities?

"We always recommend the whole fruit over the juice," explains Heidi Dufner, a registered dietician with the University of Vermont extension system in Burlington. "Apples are a good source of fiber, especially when eaten with the skin. When you remove the skin, you reduce the fiber content."

Most researchers believe that applesauce and apple butter have some fiber, but less than raw apples. "The further you process anything, the more you lose. For example, applesauce is hardly ever done with the peel, unless you do it at home," Dufner says. As the fiber content of the final product lessens, so does its cholesterol-lowering ability, Dr. Hegenauer says.

But you can add powdered apple pectin (available at health food stores) to foods that don't necessarily contain apples or fiber. About 2 teaspoons of pectin—which has the texture of powdered sugar and a citruslike taste—is all you need for a dozen muffins, for example.

As for the idea of eating an apple a day to keep the doctor away, Dr. Hegenauer says, "I take that advice pretty seriously, not only for health reasons but for sensory reasons. I like the taste, sweetness, and crunch." *See also* **pectin**

apple cider vinegar This longtime folk remedy got lots of press a few years back as nature's answer to any number of ailments. Some people still swear that a daily swig of apple cider vinegar and honey can cure rheumatism and arthritis. A weight-loss diet combining lecithin, cider vinegar, B_6, and kelp has also had its heyday, thanks to a *New York Times* beauty writer.

Of course, there's not a shred of evidence that either of these "cures" works.

People have used apple cider vinegar in some creative ways. It has been pressed into service as an astringent to help tone the skin, as a salve for sunburned skin, as a home treatment for dandruff, as a soap substitute to relieve anal itching, as an ingredient in a gargle for sore throats, and as a rinse for swimmer's ear.

"I use it so much I keep gallons of it in my pantry," says herbalist Nan Koehler of Sebastopol, California. "It's especially good for infections. When I treat a puncture wound, I'll wash it with soap and water first and then put the apple cider vinegar on straight. It's an acid, and bacteria can't grow in an acid environment." Her husband, Donald Solomon, M.D., agrees that apple cider vinegar is useful as a disinfectant for cuts and scrapes.

That's not to say he is overly enthusiastic about its therapeutic value—nor were the other doctors who were queried. There's no scientific basis for any of these uses, they agreed. Still, they doubted that apple cider vinegar could be harmful even if you added some to your diet every day. (At least one dentist, however, has expressed concern that the acid in apple cider vinegar could wear away tooth enamel.)

"The normal pH of the stomach is extremely acid. But the acid in the vinegar is relatively weak," says Andrew Diehl, M.D., professor and chief of the Division of General Medicine at the University of Texas Health Science Center in San Antonio.

"It shouldn't cause problems for most people," agrees Lynn Goodrich, R.N., a certified poison control expert with the Maryland Regional Poison Center. But people who are taking the medication antabuse to help them curb their drinking problems should avoid it, she says. The chemical interaction between the two could make you very sick.

aromatherapy Few would argue that a fragrant bath or spritz of scent can help you feel better. But aromatherapy goes a step further, using essential oils extracted from plants for medicinal, psychological, and aesthetic purposes. Practitioners incorporate aromatic—such as cedarwood, jasmine, and lavender—in baths, inhalations, compresses, teas, lotions, skin creams, and massage.

Some aromatherapists claim that essential oils diffuse through the skin

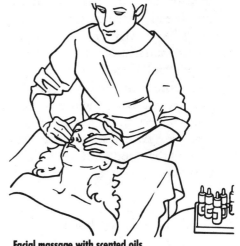

Facial massage with scented oils

and membranes and penetrate deeply into the tissues and circulatory system. By applying an oil topically to certain zones of the body, they claim you can activate your lymphatic system and treat diseases related to the lungs, the heart, the brain, and the blood. Arthritis, menstrual pain, respiratory problems, depression, jet lag, hair loss, herpes, varicose veins, cystitis, gallbladder problems, and memory loss are just a few of the countless ailments aromatherapists say can be treated.

"WISHFUL THINKING"

Nevertheless, you won't find aromatherapy in any medical dictionary. The aromatherapy methods used today evolved in France during the 1920s, and most therapeutic claims made for it are based on folklore passed down through the years by European herbalists. From a scientific standpoint, aromatherapy is just "wishful thinking," says Varro E. Tyler, Ph.D., an expert at Purdue University on the biological effects of natural drugs.

"We do know that odors can affect people, directly and indirectly, in various ways," says Alan Hirsch, M.D., a psychiatrist and neurologist who heads the Smell and Taste Treatment and Research Foundation in Chicago. "Researchers are studying the use of odor to reduce anxiety and relieve insomnia, for example." Also, researchers at Yale have found that food odors, especially a spicy apple scent, can calm your nerves.

But it's still quite a stretch from intriguing but isolated laboratory findings like these and the kinds of healing claims aromatherapists make. "By the year 2000, aromatherapy may be a legitimate therapy," says Dr. Hirsch. "But at the present, it has no scientific basis."

The prudent course is to use aromatherapy for aesthetic purposes only. If you get a lift from a lavender-laced bath, fine. If a massage with aromatic oil relaxes you, enjoy yourself. But if you have a health problem, seek medical help.

The American Aromatherapy Association certifies massage therapists, aestheticians, chiropractors, and other licensed health professionals who have been properly trained in the use of essential oils and is trying to standardize training for aromatherapists. Many practice in spas and salons.

If you want to sample aromatherapy at home, be sure to use pure, high-quality oils that haven't been diluted with synthetic compounds and that have been stored in airtight brown bottles, away from sunlight, advises Mark Blumenthal, executive director of the American Botanical Council in Austin, Texas. And be prepared to spend some cash: Most pure, undiluted essential oils are expensive. *See also* **lavender**

arthroscopy (ahr-THROS-kah-pee) All you really wanted was a leisurely game of touch football with your friends. You had a great time, too, until you tripped on a sprinkler. "Pop!" said your knee. "Surgery," said your doctor.

Make that arthroscopy, a procedure that allows doctors to evaluate and repair injured joints without cutting you wide open. Arthroscopic surgery generally requires only a few holes—holes sometimes as small as 2 millimeters in diameter.

Here's how it works: The surgeon opens two or three holes in the flesh covering the injured joint. In one hole goes the arthroscope, a hollow, flexible tube fitted with lenses and lights that "sees" inside the injured joint. The surgeon manipulates his scalpels, forceps, and other instruments in the other holes.

The joint is filled with a solution (often saline), which spreads things out and gives the surgeon room to work. The circulating solution also irrigates the wound, clearing blood and debris from the arthroscopic lens. Some arthroscopes project images of the injured joint to a television screen in the operating room. Others, similar to telescopes, are fitted with an eyepiece, allowing the surgeon to peer inside.

Most arthroscopic knee operations are finished in an hour or two, says Ward Casscells, M.D., editor-in-chief of *Arthroscopy: The Journal of Arthroscopic and Related Surgery.* "Sometimes the person stays awake and watches the operation on the monitor," he says.

Arthroscopy generally works as well or better than open-joint surgery, Dr. Casscells says. But it's less traumatic because the entry wounds are so much smaller. Most people go home the same day.

In the United States, knee arthroscopy is one of the most frequently performed elective surgeries. How-

ever, surgeons are increasingly guiding arthroscopes into hips, shoulders, and jaws—tight joints that were inaccessible just a few years ago.

PAIN TODAY, GONE TOMORROW

Arthroscopic success stories are legion. People who have had open-joint surgery often spend weeks or months recovering. After arthroscopy, patients sometimes return to work the next day.

"I remember a man who had a badly torn meniscus [the protective cartilage in the knee]," Dr. Casscells says. "Forty-eight hours after the surgery, he went on a business trip to the West Coast."

Arthroscopy gets more versatile all the time. "You can remove parts of a torn cartilage or suture it," Dr. Casscells explains. "Arthroscopy can be used to assist in the repair of ligaments and the removal of loose pieces in the joint."

One drawback to arthroscopy is training: Doctors need a lot of it. Manipulating tiny surgical instruments in tiny holes takes practice. "If you've done or watched 25 open-joint meniscus operations, that's fairly good experience," Dr. Casscells says. "Arthroscopically, that's almost nothing. You need far more experience to be good at it."

Using arthroscopy, doctors these days are finding ever-smaller niches to work in. Take the jaw hinge, for instance. The protective cartilage pad in this joint sometimes gets loose, causing painful clicking and popping, says James H. Quinn, D.D.S., professor of oral and maxillofacial surgery at the School of Dentistry at Louisiana State University.

"Before arthroscopy, we had to open the joint when the patient had painful clicking and popping," he says. "The potential for problems with arthroscopic surgery is much less than with open-joint surgery." What's more, arthroscopic images may be magnified 10 to 20 times, he says, giving the surgeon a good view even of tiny joints.

For all its benefits, arthroscopy isn't the answer to all joint problems, Dr. Casscells warns. Nor is arthroscopy risk free.

"There's always the danger of damage to the major blood vessels. If you use an anesthetic, in both types of surgery the risk is about the same," he says.

However, in the future, arthroscopy probably will be the surgery of choice for many orthopedic conditions, Dr. Casscells says: "It's very sophisticated." *See also* **endoscopy**

art therapy   At the Graham Headache Centre in Jamaica Plain, Massachusetts, people with migraine headaches paint self-portraits depicting flashing lights, zigzags, blackouts, and other bizarre effects that migraines often trigger. The resulting "migraine masterpieces" graphically express the pain of migraine in a way that words can't.

But they do more than that. Since headaches, like other kinds of pain, don't show up on a CAT scan, a painting can actually help doctors diagnose the problem. People who suffer migraines might draw self-portraits show-

ing a spike boring into their skull or a vise squeezing their head—images that tell doctors, "This is no ordinary headache." And the act of painting is cathartic, helping migraine sufferers confront their pain and vent their anger.

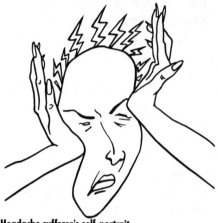

Headache sufferer's self-portrait

In art therapy, people doodle, draw, paint, or sculpt not merely for pleasure but for a purpose. Under the guidance of trained therapists, art becomes a versatile tool that can help diagnose or treat many complex health problems, from headaches to emotional disturbances.

WINDOW TO THE SOUL

You might say that art therapy for emotional problems dates back to the development of the Rorschach inkblot tests in the early 1920s, which psychiatrists use to diagnose thought disorders or other psychological problems. "The way people interpret varying designs and colors reveals a lot about their mental state," says Linda Gantt, Ph.D., registered art therapist and president of the American Art

Therapy Association. "And the way they use design and color to create art can be equally revealing.

"A lot of subconscious material surfaces in people's drawings," says Dr. Gantt. "Art is an alternative for the person who can't—or won't—talk. It bypasses the intellectual defenses."

When words don't come easily, art can break through psychological barriers. Counselors at Veterans Administration hospitals, for example, use art therapy as a gateway to psychotherapy, to help Vietnam War veterans deal with the nightmares and flashbacks of posttraumatic stress disorder. Art therapy is also a vital part of some recovery programs for drug and alcohol abusers, as well as for children who have been traumatized by mistreatment. For children who've been sexually molested and warned not to "tell," for example, drawing what happened to them is a safe way to communicate. Adult victims of incest who have trouble talking about their experience say they're relieved to be able to express their anger, shame, and other feelings through art.

But art is more than a window to the soul. It's a tonic and a tool.

"Making art is a soothing process," says Dr. Gantt. "Art diverts attention away from pain and provides emotional release. For people with terminal cancer or AIDS, art is a way to leave behind something tangible of themselves."

RETRAINING THE BRAIN

Because the physical act of creating artwork activates brain/nerve/ muscle connections, art therapy is a useful aid for teaching learning-disabled children. Also, drawing can help adult stroke victims who've lost the use of their dominant hand. With practice, their other hand becomes more dexterous and useful. Similarly, people with spinal cord injuries may be able to overcome some of their physical disabilities by drawing or sculpting.

Most art therapists are educated in both psychology and studio art and have practical training. And most work for community or mental health agencies.

If you'd like to try art therapy, it's important to check out the therapist's qualifications. Look for someone who is a registered art therapist (A.T.R.). Such individuals have had a minimum of two years postgraduate training in art therapy. Or contact the American Art Therapy Association, 1202 Allanson Road, Mundelein, IL 60060, for the location of a chapter in your state or region.

aspirin   You probably don't have to think too far back to remember the last time you popped an aspirin. Most of us rely on it frequently to relieve our everyday aches and pains. Take a look in your purse, or in the medicine cabinet, or in your old suitcase. You found some aspirin, didn't you?

Aspirin, short for acetylsalicylic acid, is used for just about everything. Aspirin cools fevers, heads off headaches, and eases painful, swollen joints. Aspirin takes the edge off colds and flu. It eases the pain of twisted ankles, sore shoulders, and wracked-up lower backs. In fact, some doctors now think aspirin helps ward off strokes and heart attacks.

Aspirin, to put it simply, is good stuff. That's why we take billions of the humble little tablets every year. That's not bad for a simple painkiller approaching its 100th birthday—a drug so common it's one of the cheapest over-the-counter remedies you can buy.

Let's take a closer look at aspirin's abilities—and at its shortcomings.

STOPS HEADACHES

Headache is a word that tells tales—tales of late nights and hearty parties, office stress and domestic strife. Tales of 50 million people who every year suffer their painful way through tension headaches and migraine skull-busters.

You know the signs. You're stuck in traffic, perhaps, and pain starts in your shoulders. It moves to your neck. You can just feel that tension, fuel for headache fire, swimming upstream.

"Hold everything!" you cry, fumbling in your purse. "I've got some *somewhere.*"

And you do—thank goodness! Aspirin can beat tension headaches by inhibiting your body's production of prostaglandins, chemical messengers that help carry pain signals from your body to your brain. Kill the messenger and you kill some of the pain, too.

Aspirin also can ease vascular headaches, the stuff of migraines. In fact, one study of doctors with migraines showed that those who took low doses of aspirin every other day had 20 percent fewer migraines than those who took placebos (nontherapeutic lookalikes). Here's how aspirin is thought to help.

Your body at rush hour is a crowded maze of arterial highways, avenues, and interstates just packed with traffic. Blood flows right along—until, somewhere, a blood clot forms. Traffic g-r-i-n-d-s to a halt. Serotonin, a nerve messenger, is released, redirecting traffic and causing vessels to expand. If conditions in the brain are right, and you're migraine prone . . . ouch!

Aspirin, an antiplatelet drug, inhibits clot-producing cells in your blood from clumping together. In a sense, aspirin "thins" your blood and thus helps keep serotonin levels down. So migraines are held in check.

REDUCES SWELLING – AND MORE

Aspirin is one of the best anti-inflammatory drugs you can buy. (Better yet, it's one of the *cheapest* drugs you can buy.) Thats why, when the bee stings, the ankle twists, or the arthritis flares, we pop the top on the aspirin container.

Aspirin reduces swelling the same way it eases pain: by inhibiting production of prostaglandins. These versatile chemicals not only send pain messages, they also "invite" white blood cells to mob the places where you're hurt. Get rid of the white blood cells, and the swelling goes down.

There's not much you can do to stop a fever, but aspirin can lower your temperature by a few degrees. In effect, aspirin turns down the dial on your internal thermostat, the hypothalmus. As you get cooler, of course, you feel a little bit better.

What else? Well, aspirin has been found to inhibit some influenza viruses. Taken in low doses (75 milligrams a day), aspirin lowers pregnancy-induced hypertension, according to a British study reported in *Lancet*. Some researchers have even suggested aspirin may reduce the risk of cataracts.

BLOCKS HEART ATTACKS?

Get ready for aspirin's curtain call. Doctors now suggest it helps prevent heart attacks.

In a five-year, double-blind study led by researchers at Harvard Medical School, 22,071 participating physicians took either placebos or 325 milligrams of aspirin (one tablet) every other day. The conclusion: Doctors in the aspirin group reduced their risk of cardiovascular mortality by 44 percent.

The results looked so promising, in fact, that 74 percent of doctors in the placebo group asked to be switched to aspirin!

It may seem unlikely that aspirin, the stuff of everyday use, now belongs on the cardiology cart. But aspirin, remember, is a powerful antiplatelet drug. That is, it helps to keep your clot-producing blood cells, called platelets, from clumping together. The less your platelets clump, the lower your chance of having a heart attack.

Of course, doctors don't all agree that an aspirin every other day keeps heart attacks away. British researchers, for instance, following a six-year study,

concluded aspirin has little effect on the risks for myocardial infarction. In addition, aspirin's antiplatelet activities appear more effective for men than for women. All the participants in the Harvard study were men—and relatively healthy men, besides.

What to believe? The U.S. Preventive Services Task Force in Washington, D.C., offers this advice: "Low-dose aspirin therapy (325 milligrams every other day) should be considered for primary prevention in men aged 40 and over who have risk factors for myocardial infarction," and who *aren't* at risk for hypertension, liver or kidney disease, gastric disturbances, or cerebral hemorrhage, among other things.

Aspirin, alas, isn't without problems. It has been associated with gastrointestinal discomfort, ulcers, and Reye syndrome, a children's disease that sometimes is fatal. Aspirin may compromise liver and kidney functions in adults as well.

Ironically, many of aspirin's complications stem from the very mechanisms that make it work—its ability to inhibit platelet aggregation and prostaglandin production. For example, blood with less clotting power may not block cerebral arteries; it may, however, contribute to the type of stroke caused by blood leaks in the brain.

In fact, doctors often ask people *not* to take aspirin starting five days before some surgeries or dental procedures because they might bleed more.

Remember the pain-causing prostaglandins? Well, they also help your stomach maintain its protective lining. Get rid of prostaglandins, as aspirin does, and you endanger your stomach lining. That's partly what makes aspirin so hard on your insides.

For most people, low doses of aspirin—say, one or two tablets every other day—aren't likely to cause serious side effects. If you are sensitive to aspirin, you might try buffered aspirin or timed-release formulas.

If you plan on taking aspirin regularly, even if you aren't especially sensitive, you should seek your doctor's supervision. Aspirin is about as safe as any high-powered drug can be. But it isn't without dangers. *See also* **anti-inflammatories; painkillers**

assertiveness training   Have you ever had difficulty saying "no" to an unreasonable request from your boss, your spouse, your kids, or your parents? If the answer is "yes," what you may need is a strong dose of assertiveness training.

According to behavioral psychologists, assertiveness training is based on the premise that your self-assertion determines your self-esteem. When you consistently fail to assert your own needs and rights, you may end up feeling not very good about yourself—dishonest, manipulated, even victimized by others.

"A lack of assertiveness can show up in a person in all kinds of large and small ways," says Dennis Nagel, a marriage, family, and child counselor from San Rafael, California, who has used assertiveness techniques in his therapy for more than two decades. "Some

people simply cannot speak their mind openly, especially when they feel they have negative communications to make. Others are reluctant to make eye contact or small talk because they are socially shy and awkward."

Non-assertive behavior—whether it be reluctance to seek a refund you are entitled to or inability to say no to requests from friends—is often based on a fear of rejection, anger, or even intimacy. That nice-guy strategy, however, can backfire by trapping you in unwanted situations and leading you into depression.

Fortunately, help is available. Proponents of assertiveness training claim that through self-observation, simple behavioral "homework assignments," and role-playing (in therapeutic situations or with friends), anyone can learn to be more assertive in intimate relationships, on the job, at the car dealership, and in other everyday social situations. "It's a way to break through limits on self-expression and get out of the rut of repeating behaviors that lower your own self-esteem," says Nagel.

Assertiveness training can begin on your own or with a therapist. The first step is to ask yourself some simple questions that can help identify your own potential problem areas. Counselors recommend that you start with key issues like these:

• Do you procrastinate on difficult projects at work?
• When you are going to be late for an appointment, are you afraid to call and tell the other person?
• Are you holding on to a prob-

lem that you want to discuss with your boss or your colleagues?

● Are you afraid to return defective merchandise or bargain with a salesperson?

● Are you satisfied with your sex life?

● Are you willing to ask to be paid what you deserve?

● When your schedule is overloaded, do you still have trouble refusing work or social engagements?

Supplement your answers to these questions with a list of all the situations that make you feel insecure, worried, or upset.

Once you've identified all the situations where you are consistently failing to assert yourself, therapists recommend that you get in touch with your rationalizations for why you "can't" be more assertive. "Check out the fears you have—whether it is fear of being angry, getting put down, or being vulnerable," says Nagel. "Then consider ways of changing your behavior that will empower you to be more direct and get what you want."

Finally, when you are clear on where you are now and where you want to go, you are ready to do the actual "homework" of assertiveness training. This homework involves learning to express your full range of feelings— from indignation to love—and acting in ways that are consistent with a positive self-image. The exercises are also designed to teach you to strike the right balance between assertiveness and passivity.

TIME TO SPEAK UP

Whether you work by yourself, with a friend or support group, or with a therapist, you will need to follow through on specific assignments that require you to stretch to fulfill personal goals. Homework assignments usually involve cutting through resistance to difficult interpersonal communications. A woman who is dissatisfied with her husband's aggressive, confrontational style might be asked to make her feelings known to him in a non-threatening way. A man who feels overworked and underpaid might take on the assignment of scheduling a real conversation with his boss to resolve the issues.

Another typical assignment might involve changing a humble pattern of non-assertiveness—such as always lending out your car to a friend even though you feel uncomfortable about it. In this example, once you inspect the pattern of non-assertive behavior (the first step in the training process), you may discover your own belief that you must have solid, logical reasons before you can say "no" to someone. Since nothing bad has ever happened when you have lent your car out in the past, you don't feel you can justify denying future requests.

This is an ideal time to reclaim your rights and stand firm on the basis of your *feelings*—not just your logic, therapists say. Of course, they are quick to point out the difference between assertiveness and aggressiveness. Being assertive is about being vulnerable in the most positive and strong sense—

expressing your own feelings and commanding other's respect through your own honesty and courage. Unlike aggressiveness, assertiveness need not be abrasive, dominating, or vindictive. If you are denying your friend's request to borrow your car, for instance, you don't want to alienate him in the process. Rather than getting angry with him or turning a cold shoulder, or meekly offering false excuses, you use the assertiveness skill of self-disclosure. You reveal your own feelings by saying, "No, I get too worried when I lend my car to anyone." Because this is a personal feeling, it is hard to argue with.

Assertiveness training teaches that by respecting such feelings as worry and uncertainty, and sharing those feelings, others will tend to respect you.

If your friend does choose to argue, it may be time to employ the assertiveness skill called the "broken record." Be persistent. Stand firm with your feelings. And do not be afraid to admit your own weaknesses. In this case, you might simply keep repeating, "Maybe you're right that I should lend out the car. I realize this isn't very logical, but it's just the way I feel."

Nagel says that "by letting other people know how *you* feel, you actually become stronger, not weaker. It's very hard for people to argue with *your* feelings. And by opening up yourself, you invite the same kind of vulnerability in the other person."

Assertiveness training is taught by many psychologists and other private therapists and is offered in university training programs and classes, weekend seminars, and professional workshops. Impressive results have also been achieved with children in school training programs. *See also* **behavior therapy**

atherectomy (ATH-er-EK-tum-ee) This is the Stealth bomber of cardiology: sleek, super high-tech, and designed for surgical strikes.

The target is plaque, a kind of fatty sludge. It is blockading your coronary arteries, and your heart isn't getting the blood it needs. Enter the atherectomy. This relatively new medical procedure is similar to the more common angioplasty, a procedure where a small balloon is inserted into the artery and expanded to crunch up plaque and widen the opening. The atherectomy goes one step further. Using a tiny swirling blade attached to a balloon, doctors can actually *remove* the offending plaque.

The most common device for the procedure, the only one approved for general use, is known as the Simpson Coronary AtheroCath. By the end of 1990, this device and others had been used to treat roughly 3,000 patients nationwide, says Matthew R. Selmon, M.D., attending cardiologist at Sequoia Hospital in Redwood City, California, clinical instructor of medicine at Stanford University Hospital, and one of the co-developers of the procedure.

Cutting Edge Techology

Because of the obvious parallels, atherectomies are often referred to as "coronary Roto-Rooter jobs." But what do the doctors who perform the procedure think of that nickname? "We dislike it," says Dr. Selmon. "It conjures images of this big device spinning and knocking off debris in a very random way." In contrast, the Athero-Cath gently slices off shavings of plaque and spits them back into a tiny receptacle. (Its cutting action is more similar to that of an electric shaver than that of a plumber's snake.) After the plaque has been removed, the device is pulled back through the artery and out a small incision in the groin area where it originally entered the body. The entire procedure takes about 90 minutes, and the patient is usually discharged from the hospital the next day.

But is the procedure really reliable? Studies show that atherectomies are roughly as effective as angioplasties at clearing the arteries—there is cause to celebrate in about 95 percent of all cases. And, although angioplasties are not considered very dangerous (about one percent of patients suffer lethal complications), atherectomies are even safer, says Dr. Selmon.

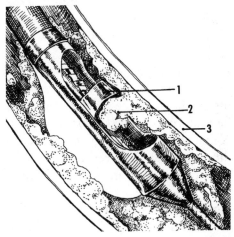

Atherectomy: (1) blade, (2) plaque, (3) artery wall

Atherectomies also seem to have a slight advantage over angioplasties at reducing restenosis rates. That's when the arteries fill back up with sludge after the procedure. It happens in roughly one-third of all angioplasties, while the rate for atherectomies seems to be under one-quarter, says Dr. Selmon.

Despite those advantages, atherectomies are not for everyone. The size of the device limits its usefulness to only those arteries that are fairly large and straight. And "for patients with severe buildup of plaque in the arteries, a bypass operation is still often the best option," says Dr. Selmon. *See also* **angioplasty; coronary bypass**

athlete's foot remedies   The fungus that causes athlete's foot infection doesn't care if you run the Boston Marathon or are confined to marathon work sessions at your desk. What this irritating microbe craves is a warm, moist, dark environment—just the climate found in many shoes, from sneakers to wingtips. But you can foil this fungus with topical antifungal medications.

The key to stamping out athlete's foot is to catch the infection in its early, mild stages. "Look between the fourth and fifth toes. If you notice white, peeling, moist skin, it's a sure sign that a fungus is underfoot," says Michael Ramsey, M.D., clinical instructor of dermatology at Baylor College of Medicine in Houston. It's also your cue to dash to the drugstore for an over-the-counter athlete's foot medication.

Any antifungal product can help as long as its label lists an ingredient ending in -*zole*, says Dr. Ramsey. Those letters indicate the product contains some form of imidazole, the most effective antifungal agent on the market. Tolnaftate and undecylenic acid are also effective antifungals, says Dr. Ramsey, who suggests that you buy an antifungal cream to apply directly on your infection and a powder to sprinkle in your socks and shoes.

Antifungals do their work by weakening fungus cell walls, forcing the cell contents to leak out. The fungus dies and your infection clears. But this fungicidal action doesn't happen overnight or without some help from you.

KEEP SKIN DRY

Before applying the medication, it's important to clean your toes and remove flaking skin with a terry washcloth. Then dry between the toes thoroughly. A hair dryer can help remove every drop of moisture. Finally, apply the antifungal cream. Repeat this routine twice a day.

If you are prone to sweaty feet, or if your athlete's foot has advanced to the oozy, itchy, inflamed stage, you may also need to add a drying solution to your antifungal attack plan. Simply dissolve a packet of Burow's solution powder (available in drugstores) in a pint of water, soak a clean cloth in the solution, and drape it on your feet and between your toes, says Dr. Ramsey. When you remove the compress, allow the skin to dry, and then apply a thin film of antifungal cream.

For advanced cases, soaking your feet in vinegar is another good way to dry your skin, increase acidity, and stamp out fungal and bacterial growth. Soak in a basin containing 1 cup of vinegar and 4 cups of water for 10 minutes twice daily.

If your feet continue to perspire profusely, your doctor may prescribe Drysol, a superpotent antiperspirant that works both as a treatment and preventive for athlete's foot.

In addition to applying antifungals, choose footwear that will keep your feet as cool and dry as possible. Wear only white cotton socks that wick away moisture, rather than wool or synthetics that trap moisture. Change your socks often and wash them in hot water to kill the fungi. Wear breathable shoes made of leather or canvas, and avoid rubber-soled shoes. Go barefoot whenever you can or wear open-toed sandals.

Typically, it may take about two weeks of applying antifungals before your skin returns to its pink, smooth self. But when that happens, don't stash the cream in the medicine chest, Dr. Ramsey warns. Continue applying the medication for at least two more weeks after your athlete's foot appears to be healed.

If your feet don't show any improvement at all after a week of applying medication, see a doctor. It could be that your flaky skin or red rash is contact dermatitis or some other condition or that you need a more powerful prescription antifungal product.

atropine   (AT-ro-peen) One of the oldest treatments for asthma and bronchitis, atropine is sometimes still used when people need a powerful, fast-acting bronchodilator. This drug goes to work inside the brain, where it stops chemicals called neurotransmitters from triggering muscle contractions—contractions that, in an asthma attack, obstruct the flow of air through the tiny passages, called bronchioles, in the lungs.

While atropine sometimes is injected, it is often administered with an inhaler, puffer, or nebulizer. It goes to work in minutes, relieving airway spasms and reducing the sputum that often accumulates with bronchitis.

MULTIPLE USES

Ophthalmologists sometimes give atropine as an eyedrop during eye examinations, because it dilates (widens) the pupil, permitting inspection of the interior of the eye. Because atropine may temporarily impair the eye's ability to focus, patients may need a friend to drive them home after the examination.

Atropine also boosts electrical conduction in the heart, so cardiologists sometimes use it to treat sinus bradycardia (slow heartbeat) or complete heart block.

Atropine may be dangerous for people with high blood pressure or heart disease. Its potential side effects—including dry skin and mucous membranes, tachycardia (rapid heartbeat), and restlessness—have led some doctors to seek newer, better-tolerated drugs. "Atropine has been replaced, to a certain extent, by a drug called Atrovent (ipratropium bromide), which does not pass through biological membranes as readily as atropine does, so it has less of a systemic [whole body] effect," says Henry Milgrom, M.D., staff physician at the National Jewish Center for Immunology and Respiratory Medicine in Denver and an associate professor of pediatrics at the University of Colorado.

"I wouldn't say atropine is completely out of use, but it's used much less than it used to be," Dr. Milgrom says. "In asthma therapy, at least, it's fairly low on the list." *See also* **bronchodilators**

autogenic training   If you think only crazy people talk to themselves, perhaps autogenic training isn't for you. But if you're willing to keep an open mind, some therapists say that you won't find a more powerful technique for calming both body and soul.

Autogenic training (autogenic means "self-generating") was developed by a German physician early in this century. It is somewhat akin to meditation, self-hypnosis, and deep relaxation exercises. The crux of the technique is to rest in a comfortable position and give your body a series of instructions, such as "My body is calm . . . My body is relaxed . . ."

As you say these phrases silently to yourself over and over (a typical session takes about 20 minutes), amazing things may start to happen. Ideally, "your mind and body enter the same state of repair that normally you only enter for a short time during deep sleep," says Mohammad R. Sadigh, Ph.D., director of psychology and psychophysiological services at the Gateway Institute, a center for pain and stress management in Bethlehem, Pennsylvania.

As the body's natural healing mechanisms are activated, participants often find themselves functioning better "physically, emotionally, and psychologically," says Dr. Sadigh. "They think better, feel better, and rest better."

TURN YOURSELF INWARD

To get an idea of what autogenic training feels like, lie down, gently close your eyes, and repeat to yourself, "My body is calm . . . My body is calm . . ." Pause for several seconds between statements. After four or five repetitions, say to yourself, "My body is quiet . . . My body is quiet . . . My body is beginning to relax . . . My body is beginning to relax . . ." (Again, repeat each phrase four or five times.)

As your autogenic training progresses, you'll soon move on to statements such as, "My hands and arms are getting warm and heavy . . . My feet and legs are heavy and warm . . . My breathing is deep and even . . . My heartbeat is calm and regular . . ." You'll find that your hands and arms actually *will* get heavy and warm (as your thoughts direct more blood into the area), and your heartbeat *will* get more regular, says Dr. Sadigh.

Part of the trick of making your body and brain respond is to take a *passive* attitude. Don't *try* to make your arms heavy and warm—just repeat the phrases and allow it to happen. Be forewarned that autogenic training is not a quick fix for stress or anything else. Therapists who use it say six

months or more may be needed before mastery can be achieved. Afterward, however, you should be able to summon the technique's effect by repeating only a phrase or two.

"I know a physician, an internist, who practices autogenic training. When things get too hectic he sits down and practices for 3 to 5 minutes, then walks away feeling completely relaxed and energized," says Dr. Sadigh.

Autogenic training is most effective if taught by a professional. But the technique has always been more popular in Europe than in North America, so finding an instructor on this side of the Atlantic may not be simple. Dr. Sadigh suggests starting your search by checking with your family physician. In addition, many biofeedback practitioners are familiar with autogenic training. *See also* **biofeedback; hypnosis; meditation; progressive relaxation; Relaxation Response; stress management**

aversion therapy   Pretend for a moment you're a cat. And there's nothing you would like better than to sink your claws into the living room furniture for a good, long scratcheroo. But every time you try—whoosh!—a spray of cold water lands on your whiskers! You learn quickly to confine your scratching to official scratching posts. That's because you have been an unconsenting participant in one of the most controversial types of behavior modification around: aversion therapy.

Aversion therapy is designed to eliminate unwanted behaviors, and it's effective for people as well as animals.

It works by helping you build a psychological aversion to something you do by linking it in your mind with something unpleasant.

Aversion therapy has been used to treat thumb sucking, sexual deviance, criminal behavior, severe overweight, cigarette smoking, alcoholism, drug abuse, and other bad habits. It also has been used to treat self-destructive behavior in autistic people.

THE REVULSION FACTOR

Here's an example of how it works in practice. If you're a kid who sucks your thumb, a therapist may apply a terrible-tasting but otherwise harmless solution to your thumb. Eventually, just thinking about sucking your thumb leaves you with a bad taste in your mouth—literally.

When it comes to cigarette smoking, drug addiction, and alcoholism, "the idea is to make the sight, smell, and taste of the particular substance unpalatable," explains James Smith, M.D., chief of staff at Schick Shadel Hospital in Seattle, the oldest chemical dependence treatment hospital in the United States.

Several kinds of aversion therapy can be used. With chemical aversion, for example, a person with alcohol dependency is given a medication that causes nausea, then given alcohol. By the end of the five-session program, the sight, smell, and thought of alcohol should no longer be appealing.

There's also faradic aversion. Here the person is hooked up to an electric stimulator. "We turn it down to zero," says Dr. Smith, "then slowly turn it up to the intensity that the person determines is unpleasant for him. Not painful, just uncomfortable." As the person engages in the undesirable act—lighting up a cigarette, for example—a therapist administers the electrical stimulation in the form of a mild to moderate electric shock to the person's forearm.

Using both chemical and electrical aversion techniques, the Schick Shadel program boasts a total success rate of more than 50 percent. Although results from other chemical dependence treatment centers are mixed, some report similar success.

SMOKING MADE HER SICK

"Aversion therapy worked for me!" attests June Nickerson, a Long Islander who tried "quick puff" aversion therapy to beat her 40-year cigarette habit. On five consecutive days Nickerson and three others rapidly smoked three cigarettes at a time in a small, windowless room. By the fourth session, the four puffers were literally sick of smoking. "Graduation day, we all threw up, got our diplomas, and that was it!" remembers Nickerson, who hasn't smoked since she completed the program.

Can a modified, self-administered form of aversion therapy help you overcome a bad habit on your own? Maybe—*if* you have a vivid imagination. If you want to stop overeating, for example, try imagining gobs of extra fat on your thighs every time you're about to binge. "There is a problem of compliance with self-administered aversion therapy," explains John Donahoe, Ph.D., a professor in the psychology department at the University of Massachusetts. And according to research, this type of self-inflicted mental punishment used on problems like weight control may work best as just one part of a larger program.

In the case of serious addictions, however, therapist-directed aversion techniques are certainly worth a try. "Aversion therapy helps give people back their free will," Dr. Smith says. "When patients first come to us, alcohol, cigarettes, or drugs are forcing them to jump through a hoop. And they find themselves jumping even though they absolutely hate it." After the treatment, harsh as it may seem, "they are calling the shots again."

In fact, going for help is the first step toward regaining personal control and self-reliance, because nobody can force you into aversion therapy. These programs require what doctors call "informed consent." "This is all strictly voluntary," says Dr. Smith. "Patients know exactly what the treatment is and can stop at any time."

Ayurvedic medicine (ah-yoor-VAY-dik) Loosely translated from Sanskrit, *ayu* means "life" and *veda* means "knowledge." An ancient system of healing, Ayurveda is based on the collective folk wisdom of more than 5,000 years in India.

But Ayurveda has an interesting twist that sets it apart from other cultural medicine chests. It defines the physical world—including the human body—as a moving stream of submolecular particles that can be arranged and rearranged at will, explains endocrinologist Deepak Chopra, M.D., president of the American Association of Ayurvedic Medicine. And it defines disease as a state in which your particles are out of the order in which they normally flow.

How do you get these scrambled particles back into their natural order? How do you achieve, as an Ayurvedic physician might say, "harmony" or "balance"?

Any one of your five senses can be used by the mind to reorder your physical state at the submolecular level, asserts Dr. Chopra. Now that may sound a bit odd to Western ears. But scientists certainly have plenty of evidence that the mind can influence the health of the body. Today they know that, stimulated by thoughts and emotions, naturally occurring chemical transmitters called neuropeptides can carry orders from the brain to disease-fighting immune system warriors throughout the body—warriors that will then attack bacteria, obliterate viruses, even destroy cancers.

But can the mind simply tell the body to get well? Yes, says Dr. Chopra. In a particularly Ayurvedic way, it can.

THE POWER OF SOUND

Certain "primordial" sounds, for example, may stimulate chemicals that are transmitted to particular organs throughout your body, suggests Dr. Chopra. There they could cause the submolecular structure of the organ to resonate in a way that either maintains the health of that organ or, if there's a problem, heals it. It's almost as though the sound acts as a molecular template to show the organ how it should be operating, Dr. Chopra says.

The sound "Ma," for example, resonates in your sinuses. Give it a try and see how it feels, Dr. Chopra suggests. Take a deep breath through your nose and, as you exhale through your mouth, let the syllable "Ma-a-a-a-a-a" just roll out of your mouth along with the expelled air. Repeat the syllable three times.

If you have digestive problems, says Dr. Chopra, use the syllable "Huh." Take a deep breath and, as you exhale, forcefully expel the syllable as a series— "Huh! Huh! Huh!"—out of your mouth. Feel how the sound bounces off your stomach and seems to resonate throughout your gut. Repeat the exercise three times.

If you have a migraine headache, use the syllables "Ya-Yoo-Yay" as you exhale, says Dr. Chopra. And repeat the exercise three times. Sense the sound stretching out your lower jaw and releasing tension.

If you suffer from tinnitus (ringing or other sound in the ear), Dr. Chopra suggests putting your tongue against your bottom teeth and, on the exhale, letting the syllable "Na-a-a-a-a" roll out of your mouth along with your breath. Repeat three times.

THE THREE DOSHAS

Just as a Western doctor types and matches blood before he uses it, an Ayurvedic doctor will type and match the way in which he believes your mind and body speak to one another

before attempting to heal. That's why knowing your mind/body type—or *dosha*—is as important in Ayurvedic medicine as knowing your blood type is in Western medicine. An Ayurvedic doctor can literally not write a prescription without knowing it.

Generally, says Dr. Chopra, most people fall into one of three categories: *pitta, vata,* or *kapha.* And although there are all sorts of complicated tests that Ayurvedic doctors use to determine a person's type, the following story may give you a basic understanding.

One day Dr. Chopra was in an airport waiting for a plane. The plane's departure had been delayed by a snowstorm, and eventually, a ticket agent announced that the flight had been canceled.

When that happened, says Dr. Chopra, one group of people immediately surrounded the ticket agent and forcefully insisted that the plane could and should take off. Another group ran to the ticket counter of another airline and tried to catch a different flight. A third group simply walked over to a snack counter and ordered ice cream cones.

The group that surrounded the ticket agent was typically *pitta,* says Dr. Chopra. *Pitta* are intense people who are characteristically very bright, very critical, and very quick to anger. The group that ran to another airline was typically *vata,* he adds, changeable people who are generally enthusiastic, excitable, and quick to grasp new information. The third group, the ice cream lovers, was typically *kapha*, relaxed people who are usually tranquil, affectionate, and forgiving.

Once an Ayurvedic physician has diagnosed your illness, he may write a prescription for specific foods, herbs, massage techniques, exercises, or even aromas that are thought to "balance" the disease-scrambled particles of your particular mind/body type, says Dr. Chopra.

When using aromas as a treatment, for example, Ayurvedic physicians say that *vata* people become balanced and relaxed when exposed to warm, sweet aromas like basil, orange, rose, geranium, and clove. *Pitta* people are balanced by cool, sweet aromas like sandalwood, rose, cinnamon, and jasmine. *Kapha* people are balanced by warm and spicy aromas such as juniper, eucalyptus, camphor, clove, and marjoram.

AZT Also called zidovudine, this promising new drug can delay the onset of symptoms of AIDS (acquired immune deficiency syndrome) for people in the early stages of this viral infection and prolong survival in more advanced cases. But the million-dollar question—can early initiation of AZT treatment help people beat AIDS?—remains to be answered.

The drug works by interfering with the ability of the AIDS virus to synthesize its own DNA, or cellular genetic material. With viral DNA production disrupted, the virus cannot replicate itself. This slows the spread of the virus to other susceptible cells.

How useful is AZT? Physicians involved in a 1990 state-of-the-art review of the drug found "unequivocal benefit from early initiation of zidovudine therapy in delaying progression to advanced disease."

Experts say AZT may hold the greatest benefits, and the least risk, for people who've tested positive for the AIDS virus but have no symptoms, or only mild ones. Numerous clinical trials show that the drug can delay the onset of both AIDS-related complex (the stage when the first physical symptoms appear) and full-blown AIDS. The results suggest that early detection of the disease may be the key to survival.

Patients with mild symptoms suffered minimal side effects from AZT. Nausea was the most common. The more serious side effects, anemia and a blood disorder called neutropenia, occurred in 5 and 4 percent respectively.

Studies of people in advanced stages of the disease suggest that AZT can minimize the frequency and severity of infections, temporarily boost the number of protective lymphocyte cells, and improve brain and nervous system function. Side effects for this group were more frequent, however.

AZT, marketed under the name Retrovir, received Food and Drug Administration approval in 1987.

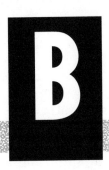

baking soda That powdery white stuff you add to biscuit and bread batters to make them rise has some intriguing therapeutic properties—inside the body and out. The "soda" in baking soda is actually pure sodium bicarbonate, a substance that dissolves in water and, because of its slightly alkaline nature, has the ability to neutralize acid.

You'll find sodium bicarbonate in over-the-counter antacid preparations like Alka-Seltzer and Citrocarbonate that are designed to help relieve occasional episodes of indigestion and heartburn. Doctors sometimes recommend sodium bicarbonate for cystitis, too, because it minimizes the acidity of urine, helping to prevent infection. Gout sufferers have used it to reduce the risk of kidney stones.

In hospitals, doctors sometimes administer sodium bicarbonate by injection to treat acidosis, a potentially fatal condition of the blood and tissues that may result from cardiac arrest or other life-threatening illnesses. Some doctors mix baking soda with certain local anesthetics, which are generally quite acidic, to reduce the pain that follows injection.

TONIC FOR QUITTERS

The Mayo Clinic recommends sodium bicarbonate tonics for short-term relief of nicotine withdrawal symptoms. To make the tonic, dissolve 2 tablespoons in a glass of water. Try taking the tonic in the morning, afternoon, and evening, the Mayo Clinic suggests. But don't do it if you're on a low-sodium diet or suffer from peptic ulcers.

Before you take sodium bicarbonate products internally, there are a few things you should know. Because it is a salt, sodium bicarbonate is taboo for people on salt-restricted diets. For the rest of us, even a single dose can cause belching and stomach pain, a result of the carbon dioxide produced as sodium bicarbonate neutralizes stomach acid. For this reason, never take sodium bicarbonate in any form when you're flying. The gas produced may expand, bloat your stomach, and give you a bad case of belching.

Sodium bicarbonate can also interfere with the absorption or excretion of a wide range of drugs. Consult your doctor if you're taking tetracycline, steroid drugs, oral anticoagulants, antipsychotic medication, or iron preparations, for example.

Baking soda is also useful in external applications. Use it to reduce the pain and swelling of sunburn or to relieve sore muscles by sprinkling a liberal amount in a tub of warm water and then taking a good soak. Soothe itching from insect bites or poison ivy by dissolving a teaspoon in a glass of water, dipping a cloth in the solution, and applying it to the affected area for 15 to 20 minutes. A mouthwash made of ½ teaspoon baking soda dissolved in 6 ounces of water may help relieve canker sore pain.

balm of Gilead   This resinous, sweet-smelling herbal remedy was well known for its healing powers in the Middle East thousands of years ago. It was so common, in fact, that one biblical prophet suggests a *shortage* of balm is as unlikely as a bride forgetting her wedding dress.

Balm of Gilead—also called *Populus gileadensis, Populus candicans,* and *Populus balsamifera*—contains resins, volatile oils, and salicin, a chemical relative of aspirin. Harvested in the spring from the closed buds of poplars and related trees, it's said to reduce pain, fever, congestion, and inflammation.

"Taken internally, balm of Gilead has been used for coughs and chest conditions," says Mark Blumenthal, executive director of the American Botanical Council in Austin, Texas. "Externally, it's been used for rheumatic arthritis and muscle soreness."

Balm of Gilead also appears to contain an antioxidant. That's why it's sometimes added to certain ointments to prevent rancidity.

As you might expect, folklore lends balm of Gilead some rather special powers. In this old spiritual, for example: "There is a balm in Gilead to make the wounded whole; There is a balm in Gilead to heal the sin-sick soul."

As with most balsams, balm of Gilead doesn't appear to have dangerous side effects, although skin rashes and allergic reactions aren't uncommon.

Balm of Gilead is commonly used in Europe, but it's a rarity in American medicine chests, Blumenthal says. That doesn't mean it doesn't work, says Leonard Grayson, M.D., a skin allergy specialist and clinical associate allergist and dermatologist at Southern Illinois University School of Medicine.

"As the circulation increases and the area gets warm following application, there's a feeling of improvement," Dr. Grayson says. "When you boost the flow of blood to the site of an injury, you're sending in a lot of blood cells, and that might do some good," he explains.

Dr. Grayson dug through his medical books to find references to balm of Gilead; none appeared. "I'm one of the old-timers, but that's one remedy that's before my time," he says.

banana   It's the bicycle rider's best friend, a potassium pipeline that instantly picks up a sagging pumper.

It's the diarrhea sufferer's ally, a soothing substance that may stop what you most want stopped and help replace what you've lost.

It's a helping hand against high blood pressure that may help keep your numbers low.

It's a tropical fruit, a large berry, that's handy and healthy, providing 451 milligrams of potassium, 33 milligrams of magnesium, and just over 2 grams of fiber.

The banana shares many benefits of its fruity brethren: It's low in calories, fat, and sodium, and much of its fiber is soluble—the kind that can help lower cholesterol. It stands out, however, because it has lots of potassium and a respectable amount of magnesium. That's why it's the favorite fruit of most athletes and often is recommended for people with diarrhea or high blood pressure.

ELECTROLYTE SOURCE

"Bananas have always been recommended as a way of replacing electrolytes," says Jack Hegenauer, Ph.D., a research professor in biology at the University of California at San Diego. Electrolytes are minerals that, when dissolved in fluids, provide the very tiny electrical charges needed to power the body and maintain fluid balance. "You have to be very aggressive about replacing electrolytes when you have diarrhea—especially severe diarrhea—or you run out of water completely," Dr. Hegenauer says.

Bananas are helpful because they restore lost potassium and add fiber to absorb water in the stool.

The soft yellow fruit also is help-ful for athletes, especially long-distance types who should be concerned with mineral replacement. Bananas are often the only extra weight bicyclists want to carry and are a postrace staple at most fun runs.

"There's not a lot of breakdown that needs to occur when you digest bananas," Dr. Hegenauer explains. "Many of the carbohydrates are in the form of fairly simple starches that are broken down without a lot of fuss in the intestine. The starch, which is converted directly to glucose, is a good, quick source of energy for athletes while they are working out, not just afterward to replace what they've burned."

Some doctors recommend including bananas in the diet to combat high blood pressure. Studies have shown that people with high levels of potassium in their diet have a lower incidence of hypertension, even if they don't watch their salt intake.

Bananas also are a very good source of vitamin B_6, providing one-third of the daily requirement in a single serving. Studies suggest this vitamin may help fight a form of kidney stone disease, as well as carpal tunnel syndrome—a painful condition that affects the wrist and hand.

If the idea of eating a banana straight leaves you cold, or if you can't get your spouse to partake of the fruit, be creative.

"Bananas incorporate themselves very well into things like breads and pancakes," says Heidi Dufner, a registered dietitian with the University of

Vermont extension system in Burlington. She adds that you shouldn't worry about bananas losing their health benefits after cooking.

How many bananas is it safe to eat?

"You really can't get too much potassium," Dr. Hegenauer says. "You couldn't eat enough bananas in a day to overdose on potassium." *See also* **electrolytes**

bandages   If Scarlett O'Hara had had today's wound dressings, she wouldn't have had to roll all those cotton bandages in the blazing Atlanta sun.

Today, cotton gauze bandages are practically gone with the wind. The best-dressed wounds are often covered with see-through plastic, elastic, or liquid gels. What's more, these new bandages do more than protect wounds from germs; they actually promote healing.

A good example is the artificial-skin bandages now being used to cover serious burns. The synthetic coverings reportedly work better than even natural skin grafting for healing deep wounds. The reason? "Skin grafting replaces only the outer layer of skin," explains Richard Knutson, M.D., an orthopedic surgeon at Delta Medical Center in Greenville, Mississippi. "But the artificial bandages stimulate the natural skin cells to grow in the deeper layers of the skin."

Here's how they work: A plastic outer layer seals out infection while a spongelike inner layer made of collagen substitutes for the skin's naturally thick, fibrous, inner layer. The colla-

gen acts as a scaffold for new skin to grow into. The new skin eventually replaces the fake stuff completely as the collagen dissolves. When the process is complete, the artificial outer layer is peeled off and covered with a standard skin graft.

"Essentially, the artificial-skin bandage melts into the skin and provides good coverage until the real skin can grow," says Dr. Knutson.

WRAP UP SWELLING

Not all modern bandage options are that sophisticated. A simple stretchy elastic bandage (or compression wrap), for example, can be a valuable healing aid for a pulled thigh muscle, tennis elbow, and other sprains and strains. Compressing an injury with an elastic bandage in the first 48 to 72 hours can minimize swelling and stimulate the flow of healing white blood cells to the area, according to Glen Halvorson, M.D., medical director of Sport Training and Rehabilitation of Tempe/Tucson (START) in Arizona. At the very least, compressing an injury restricts full movement. And that's good. "A wrap forces you to rest an injury, which is also very important in the early phases of healing," says Dr. Halvorson.

Elastic bandages come in a variety of widths for use on virtually any part of the body. Some wraps have pouches for inserting ice packs to further reduce swelling and aid healing.

When wrapping an elastic bandage, follow this rule: Overlap each layer of bandage by half its width to apply even pressure. The bandage

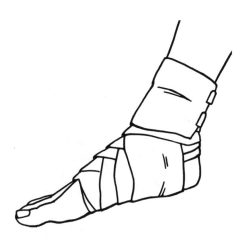

Compression bandage for ankle strain

should be snug, but not too tight, or you could cut off the blood supply and cause tissue damage. Remember, swelling of an area may cause a tight bandage to become tighter, notes Dr. Halvorson. "If you feel a tingling or your fingers, ankles, or toes turn blue, rewrap the area less tightly," he says. Take the wrap off for an hour or so at night to allow the blood to circulate. Gently move your injury. If there is still swelling or pain after two or three days, see your doctor.

Once your injury is healed, you can use a compression bandage as a way to prevent overextending muscles and joints, mimimizing the chance of getting a new sprain or strain. "A wrap is not a brace or support for an injury-prone ankle, for example. But it can help your body become more aware of joint movement," says Dr. Halvorson. Theoretically, this awareness causes your muscles to tense and relax at appropriate times, lessening reinjury risk. Put

simply, if you wrap your bum knee before skiing, it might prevent you from limping to the lodge with another sprain.

Keep the Air Out

Thanks to occlusive (airtight) bandages, kids who suffer skinned knees may never know the exquisite pain of peeling a bandage from a crusty scab.

Thirty years ago, doctors thought the best way to heal an open wound was to cover it with breathable gauze. Those porous bandages allowed air to dry the wound, creating a crusty cover. "The idea was that a dry environment helped prevent possible bacterial growth and infection," explains Vincent Falanga, M.D., associate professor of dermatology at the University of Miami School of Medicine.

Fortunately for everybody, the "let the air get at the wound" idea went out the window when studies showed that wounds heal faster—as much as 40 percent faster—when kept moist and scab free instead. Moreover, the minute amounts of bacteria in the moist wounds did not seem to cause infection.

Doctors can only speculate as to why occlusion speeds healing. "Possibly, when there is no scab, new skin cells can move freely on the wound surface and form a healthy layer of skin," says Dr. Falanga. "Sealing a wound may also seal in healing fluid instead of allowing it to evaporate or be absorbed into gauze." It's theorized that this fluid contains substances that help stimulate new skin cells.

What's more, the fluid may also

contain antiprostaglandins, natural pain-killing substances. Very possibly, the occlusive bandage keeps the natural painkiller in the wound, says Dr. Falanga. That could be why a covered wound throbs less than one that's exposed to the air. "When a kid says that bandaging his knee makes his boo-boo all better, it's probably true," says Dr. Falanga.

TAKE YOUR PICK

So you've slipped on the front step and scraped your knee. Fortunately, you have your pick of semiairtight dressings to tend to your wound.

"An ordinary-looking plastic-backed bandage or gauze impregnated with petroleum jelly can provide good occlusion,"says Patricia Mertz, a research associate professor of dermatology and cutaneous surgery at the University of Miami School of Medicine.

Or you could try one of the transparent, self-adhesive bandages. These nonabsorbent strips create an artificial, blisterlike covering. They let you actually watch the wound fluid building up. In time, the fluid evaporates through pores in the dressing and the wound heals.

Along these same lines, so-called liquid bandages also are available. They coat your wound to form a waterproof, flexible, transparent film.

Somewhat different are the hydrogels. These opaque membranes made of water and polyethylene oxide "look like strips of plastic wrap with gelatin in the center," says Mertz. "You cool them in the refrigerator until you're ready to apply them." Currently, only a nonsterile hydrogel is available over the counter, and it's intended for abrasions rather than open cuts.

KEEP IT CLEAN

Even the best bandage is going to have its work cut out for it if you don't take care to clean the wound site first. Like your mother's best china, wounds are fragile. So clean them gently. "Rinse your cut with plain water or a weak saltwater solution," says Mertz. "It may sting a bit, but it won't harm healthy tissues as some soap can."

And skip the harsh antiseptics. You're better off applying an antibiotic ointment, studies show. Researchers at the University of Pennsylvania tested antibotic ointments against traditional antiseptics such as iodine and merthiolate. They found that the antiseptics *slowed* healing time to an average of 16 days. Untreated wounds took 13 days to heal. But the various antibiotic ointments healed wounds on an average of just 9 days—that's more than 25 percent faster.

Why the difference? "Unlike antiseptics, the broad-spectrum antibiotic ointments such as Polysporin kill just the microbes and not healthy skin cells," says Mertz.

DRESS CORRECTLY

You don't have to be a Red Cross volunteer to know how to apply a bandage to cuts and scrapes. Just remember to make it snug, but not too snug. Never apply a tourniquet. "You could completely shut off the blood supply to a limb," says Dr. Knutson. And never try to bandage a deep cut that is more than ½ inch long, a puncture wound, or a very dirty scrape. You might be at risk for infection, and you should see your doctor.

Change a bandage every two or three days. If your wound is red, painful, odorous, or swollen, it may be infected: You should see your doctor.

Finally, the ouchless way to remove an adhesive bandage strip is to soak it in water. "Pulling adhesive could tear your skin," warns Dr. Knutson. Simply trim the loose parts. If it still sticks, soak it some more. Eventually it will work itself loose. *See also* **skin grafts**

barbiturates They're commonly thought of as sleeping pills, but any reputable doctor will tell you that barbiturates really are too powerful, and too dangerous, to be used merely to facilitate pillow time. Drugs such as phenobarbital, secobarbital, and amobarbital, which depress all parts of the central nervous system, most often are used to control seizures, induce anesthesia, and, in some cases, relieve short-term anxiety.

Phenobarbital often is prescribed to stop, or prevent, the dramatic, grand mal convulsions characteristic of some types of epilepsy. Effective for long-term use, phenobarbital may be used in such low doses that unwanted sedation, a side effect common to all the barbiturates, is minimized or absent.

In emergencies, however, when epileptic convulsions may be life-threatening, doctors administer faster-acting barbiturates such as secobarbital or sodium pentothal. Both drugs depress the central nervous system in as little as 10 seconds—the time it takes for them to reach the brain.

The fast-acting barbiturates are also used for anesthesia, says E. Don Nelson, Pharm.D., professor of clinical pharmacology at the University of Cincinnati. In oral surgery, for example, the doctor may inject thiopental sodium (truth serum) for fast sedation, and then finish the operation with a longer-lasting anesthetic.

LOSING FAVOR

As anxiety fighters, the barbiturates have been largely replaced by a safer class of sedatives called the benzodiazepines, which include drugs such as diazepam (Valium) and flurazepam (Dalmane).

"If you consider the whole sedative market, only about 10 percent of it is comprised of barbiturates," Dr. Nelson says. "It used to be all barbiturates." The change has occurred, he says, because barbiturates are difficult to control.

It's not uncommon for people taking barbiturates, even in small doses, to complain about feeling tired and lethargic. Many people say the drugs make them feel slow—as if their mind isn't working at full capacity. This sedation often diminishes over the course of treatment, but it rarely disappears entirely as long as you're taking the drug.

In larger doses, of course, the barbiturates may be extremely dangerous.

They commonly depress breathing, and if combined with other drugs or alcohol, they may be deadly.

"There aren't any safe barbiturates," Dr. Nelson says. "If people take too much, they'll stop breathing and die. In addition, these drugs are profoundly addicting."

In fact, when people addicted to barbiturates suddenly *stop* taking the drugs, the withdrawal symptoms may be fatal. That's why people who have been taking barbiturates for a long time often check into a hospital for a few days while they kick the habit.

Even the conservative use of barbiturates may cause problems, Dr. Nelson says. For example, barbiturates commonly interfere with rapid eye movement (REM) sleep, the sleep stage during which dreams occur. They also cause unusually fast brain wave activity during sleep. So even if people get the same *amount* of sleep as previously, the *quality* of their sleep goes down, and they wake up feeling fatigued.

"There are about 100 billion neurons [nerve cells] in the brain, and a lot of them are inhibitory neurons," Dr. Nelson says. "When you sedate them, they quit inhibiting the other nerves, which all go wild."

People on barbiturates often experience subtle alterations in mood and performance. In addition, the barbiturates are hyperalgesic—they actually can heighten the sensation of pain. Because of all these side effects, Dr. Nelson says, it's not surprising that many doctors prefer other types of drugs. *See also* **phenobarbital; sedatives**

bed rest Few doctors prescribe extended bed rest these days—and with good reason.

"Before World War II, anyone who was hospitalized was told to stay in bed until they healed," says Jerome B. Kornfeld, M.D., specialist in preventive medicine and chief of family practice at Northridge Hospital in Northridge, California. "During the war, however, beds were in short supply, so injured soldiers were released quickly. And doctors discovered that injured people did better when they got out of bed *sooner.*"

Since then, the emphasis on getting patients up and moving has grown stronger and stronger. Years ago, for example, anyone who suffered a heart attack (and survived) was hospitalized for at least three weeks. Now they're often discharged within seven days. Even postoperative patients are encouraged to get out of bed quickly—often as early as the evening of the day of surgery. It's little wonder that you won't find bed rest listed in the index of most modern home medical guides.

EXCEPTION: BACK PAIN

"Except under rare circumstances, I generally don't recommend absolute bed rest," says Dr. Kornfeld. "One exception is low back pain caused by muscle sprain or trauma. An injured area won't heal if you continue to use it. So you have to immobilize it. If you tear a hamstring muscle or sprain your wrist, you can immobilize the joint with a splint or cast. But with back injury, complete bed rest is the only way to immobilize the back. Otherwise, it won't heal as rapidly."

Anyone with severe back pain probably doesn't need much coaxing to stay put. Just don't feel guilty about taking to your bed. "Rest relieves pain and promotes healing," says Robert L. Swezey, M.D., in his book, *Good News for Bad Backs*. "Bed rest for severe pain means 90 percent or more of the day is spent in bed. . . . Your only outing is to see the doctor."

For moderate back pain, Dr. Swezey says, "Initially, you should be up only to go to the bathroom, for meals and other essentials, and for doctor visits. With improvement, increase 'up' time progressively from 10 to 90 percent of the day." (Check with your doctor about when to increase your activity level, and by how much.)

If you have arthritic pain, you may be tempted to stay in bed. But your doctor may advise otherwise.

"For arthritis, bed rest is self-defeating," says Dr. Kornfeld. "An inflamed joint becomes frozen—that is, *more* immobile—if you immobilize it. Instead, you want range of motion."

Even a cold or flu attack may not call for bed rest, according to Dr. Kornfeld. "Anytime you have a viral infection, you should rest," he says. "Because with a fever, your body temperature rises and your metabolism speeds up, so you want to decrease your activity. But rest doesn't necessarily mean *bed* rest. Often what doctors really mean when they say 'Take two aspirin and go to bed' is 'Take it

easy. Don't go to work or participate in physical activity.' "

beds. *See* **mattresses and beds**

bee pollen   First the good news: Bee pollen contains vitamins, minerals, carbohydrates, and protein.

But now the bad: "The very same nutrients contained in bee pollen can be obtained much more cheaply and safely from a balanced diet of conventional foods," says John Renner, M.D., president of the Consumer Health Information Research Institute in Kansas City, Missouri. Worse yet, bee pollen can be dangerous for people who suffer from allergies—one of the very conditions the stuff has been alleged to treat!

Bee pollen is a mixture of plant nectar, pollen, and bee saliva—unusual ingredients, indeed—but there is no sound scientific evidence that these ingredients can do anything unusual for the health of the human body. Advocates claim bee pollen can boost energy, improve athletic performance and physical endurance, rejuvenate the skin, regulate the bowels, aid weight loss, enhance the immune system, and protect against heart disease, cancer, arthritis, and even stress. "But most of these claims rest on personal testimonials rather than controlled scientific studies," Dr. Renner points out. "That's the same technique once used to sell snake oil."

The controlled studies that have been done with bee pollen, moreover, have produced some rather stinging results. One experiment found no measurable difference whatsoever in 46 people who received 400 milligrams of bee pollen daily for 75 days as compared to people who received a placebo (nontherapeutic substance). Other studies of college swimmers and high school cross-country runners have produced similar results.

FULL OF ALLERGENS

What has been discovered regarding bee pollen has been decidedly negative, in fact: The material is composed largely of pollens that bees have collected from plants, and it can be a veritable warehouse of allergens capable of raising Cain with allergy sufferers. One examination of bee pollen capsules found pollens of five different varieties—sunflower, clover, amaranth, ragweed, and sage. Allergy relief, nonetheless, remains one of bee pollen's chief boasts.

"People with allergies should avoid bee pollen," states allergy specialist Fang L. Lin, M.D., of the San Diego Naval Hospital in California.

People looking to avoid having their pocketbooks stung should refrain from the stuff as well, Dr. Renner says. "None of the identified constituents of bee pollen has been linked to any significant treatment benefits."

behavior therapy If you'd rather face a firing squad than that spider on your wall . . . if you'd rather crawl from Chicago to Chattanooga than board a plane . . . if you'd sooner enter a coliseum full of lions than climb a ladder to fix a light bulb—you probably have a phobia. Fear not. Phobias are among the most common of psychological problems, and experts have a therapy that can usually tame them in a matter of months. It's behavior therapy.

Although most notable for its effectiveness in squashing phobias, behavior therapy (sometimes called behavior modification) has also proven beneficial for a large number of other psychological, emotional, and even physical problems. These include addictive habits (like smoking or overeating), stress, insomnia, and headaches.

Behavior therapy is to traditional psychoanalysis what dusting is to spring cleaning. Behavioral therapists don't ask you about early life experiences. "We mostly look for what's happening in the present. We don't analyze your childhood, which can be distorted by memories anyway," says Philip C. Kendall, Ph.D., professor of psychology, head of the Division of Clinical Psychology, and director of the Child and Adolescent Anxiety Disorders Clinic at Temple University in Philadelphia.

Many therapists today combine the techniques of behavior therapy with those of cognitive therapy. In fact, 70 percent of the members of the Association for Advancement of Behavior Therapy now consider themselves "cognitive-behavioral" therapists, says Dr. Kendall, who is past president of the association.

FACING YOUR FEAR

Behavior therapists believe that behaviors are learned and can be *un-*

learned. To alter unwanted behaviors, they use a number of tools, among which—contrary to the common conception—electric shock is typically *not* one! Stories of rats in cages having their paws zapped for pulling the wrong levers date back to the early history of behavioral science. Things have come a *long* way since then.

One technique used by some of today's behavior therapists, particularly for phobia treatment, is called systematic desensitization. The patient is ever so gradually exposed to the object of fear, whether it's snakes or public speaking or elevators. It's like entering an icy pool: You do it a little at a time—feet, knees, waist—until you're used to the cold.

In one case, a woman was so afraid of lightning that she hid in her basement every time she heard a storm warning on the radio. Eventually she went to a therapist and underwent desensitization training. First she learned deep-muscle relaxation techniques. Then, over several sessions, she used the techniques while the therapist gradually introduced the idea of lightning in a controlled, safe environment. This helped her to gradually associate lightning with relaxation instead of terror. She began by just talking about lightning, then later imagining that a storm was coming, then listening to tapes of thunder. Her treatment culminated in a full-scale thunder-and-lightning show at a planetarium! Today, she's able to weather storms—real storms—by recalling the relaxing feelings she learned to associate with lightning.

How typical is this case? Very. Studies show that behavior therapy knocks out phobias fast in the great majority of cases. "In 20 to 30 sessions, most people, while they won't be 'cured,' will learn the skills to manage their problem," says Dr. Kendall.

As a treatment for problems other than phobias, the track record is also impressive. These problems are not always strictly psychological, either. One study, published in the *Journal of the American Medical Association,* showed good results against urinary incontinence, which is often associated with emotional distress. After 13 weeks of behavior therapy, 65 nursing home residents were able to reduce their involuntary urination by 26 percent. How? Residents who remained dry were given praise and special attention. This technique is called reinforcement.

PUSHING ASIDE PAIN

Similarly, reinforcement has been used to treat asthma, allergies, and chronic pain, says John N. Marr, Ph.D., a professor at the University of Arkansas and a psychologist in private practice in Fayetteville. He explains that families of those with chronic pain can unwittingly reinforce that pain by doting on the individual every time he groans. Dr. Marr favors a different kind of reinforcement. "When I work with a pain problem, I work with the entire family," he says. "I tell family members not to pay attention when a person starts to groan, except to give him help he directly asks for (such as a pillow). I then ask them to increase the amount of attention they pay the person when he is not complaining." This may sound like harsh treatment—but it does often reduce the patient's pain. And it's done *with* the patient's full cooperation and consent, says Dr. Marr.

When is behavior therapy *not* appropriate? "It's not good for treating symptoms like delusions or hallucinations, nor is it the best method for treating antisocial behavior," says Dr. Kendall. Likewise, "some clients have strong beliefs that human behavior is so complicated that nothing simple can change it; others are obsessed with things that happened to them at three years old. Behavior therapy may not be for these people," he says.

CHANGING *YOUR* BEHAVIOR

Like most therapies, this one works best with the help of a professional. But certainly people can change some behaviors on their own. If you have a behavior you'd like to change, such as backing off when you see a spider, Dr. Marr suggests a simple technique: Make a fist with both hands and squeeze real hard for several seconds. Then, as you release, try to realize seven progressive levels of relaxation. Feel the tension drain not only from your hands but also from your arms and shoulders. Do this exercise whenever you're faced with the fear. Soon you should start to associate the feeling of calm with the source of your fear, and the fear itself may fade.

To locate a behavior therapist, talk to your family physician, check with a local university, or contact the Association for Advancement of Behavior Therapy, 15 West 36th Street, New York, NY 10018. *See also* **aversion therapy; cognitive therapy**

beta blockers Whether you're stretching your legs or running from a bear, neurotransmitters in your body make sure everything gets done. Let's suppose you really do spot a bear. Billions of these chemical messengers dash for beta receptors—the cellular equivalents of telephone booths—where they make their calls: Your heart beats faster, your airways expand, and—thank goodness!—your legs get moving.

But what happens when your body can't take all that excitement? People with chest pains, for example, don't *want* a speeding heart; people with stage fright don't want tense muscles or sweaty hands. The beta blockers, among the most widely prescribed drugs in the world, simply slow things down. Here's how.

Beta blockers—short for beta-adrenergic receptor blocking agents—occupy your body's beta receptors *before* the neurotransmitters arrive. That means the calls—"More blood! More pressure!"—don't get through. Muscles relax, anxiety drops, and the heartbeat slows down.

While there are many different beta blockers—all of which do essentially the same jobs—they are divided into two main categories: cardioselective beta blockers, which act primarily on beta-1 receptors in the heart muscle, and noncardioselective beta blockers, which act on beta-2 receptors in the airways and blood vessels.

ANGINA PAIN RELIEVED

The cardioselective beta blockers most frequently are prescribed for high blood pressure and angina—chest pain produced when the heart muscle doesn't get enough oxygen.

"Beta blockers decrease the strength of the heartbeat and also the rate at which the heart beats," says Norman Kaplan, M.D., professor of medicine and head of the Hypertension Division at the University of Texas Southwestern Medical School at Dallas. "That diminishes the amount of work the heart has to do, so it doesn't require so much oxygen."

Easing the heart's workload does more than help relieve angina. Because the heart contracts with less force, high blood pressure is also reduced. In addition, the slower, weaker heartbeats are less prone to cardiac arrhythmias, heartbeat irregularities that in rare cases can be fatal.

Every cell in the body has hundreds of thousands of beta receptor sites, Dr. Kaplan says, and the "beta blockade" goes to work throughout the body. Even small doses of beta blockers, for example, are thought to stop blood vessels in the brain from dilating, which helps stop migraines from getting started.

Beta blockers sometimes are used to treat glaucoma, which occurs when pressure in the eye builds to abnor-

mally high levels. Beta blocker eye-drops—timolol commonly is used—reduce the fluid secreted by the eye and thus reduce the pressure. Beta blockers also are useful for treating the "thyroid storm" that sometimes accompanies an overactive thyroid gland (hyperthyroidism) and that sends the metabolism and cardiovascular system spinning out of control.

Although not approved by the Food and Drug Administration for this use, beta blockers increasingly are being taken by lawyers, musicians, and other public performers to curb the racing heart and elevated blood pressure that accompany stage fright. The drugs appear safe for this use, Dr. Kaplan says, but as in the situation mentioned earlier, dangerous side effects sometimes occur.

SOME PRECAUTIONS

Perhaps most dangerous is the tendency of beta blockers to constrict the airways, particularly in people with asthma or bronchitis. That's not so bad if you're ready for it, Dr. Kaplan says, but it may be hazardous for people who aren't accustomed to breathing problems.

Because beta blockers slow the rate and pressure at which blood moves through the body, athletes may notice more fatigue when they take the drugs, Dr. Kaplan says. Nonathletes also may experience fatigue. Depression and impotence also have been reported.

The beta blockers may be especially dangerous for people whose heart is already weak, Dr. Kaplan says. "If you've got a borderline state where the heart muscle is just barely working hard enough to keep you going, and then you knock down the activity a bit, you can produce heart failure," he says.

It is ironic that a class of drugs used to reduce many heart risks actually *contributes* to one: high cholesterol. In fact, people who take beta blockers for a long time increase their serum cholesterol levels, on average, by about 20 percent, Dr. Kaplan says.

"Almost all the beta blockers raise the serum triglycerides and lower the [protective] HDL cholesterol levels," Dr. Kaplan says. "So even though they have a lot of advantageous effects on the heart and lower the blood pressure, they may *increase* the risk of heart attacks at the same time."

Beta blockers should not suddenly be discontinued without medical supervision. Severe angina, heightened blood pressure, or even a heart attack may result. *See also* **antianxiety drugs; antihypertensives; nitroglycerin**

biofeedback Master biofeedback and you can protect yourself against a variety of stress-related illnesses. You can learn to increase or decrease your heart rate at will, direct blood to any area of your body, relax your muscles, and alter your brain rhythms. Through this process of learning to consciously control many normally automatic body functions, you can directly harness the mind's hidden power to influence the course of disease.

The term *biofeedback* is rather broad. It describes the process of self-regulation, the instruments you use to measure physiological processes, and the information these instruments feed back to you about your progress.

Biofeedback works like this: You sit hooked to a monitoring machine that measures one or more of your vital signs, translating them into audio or visual cues, or "feedback." (Often the monitor is an electrical device that reads the information obtained from electrodes placed on your body.) As you practice altering the cues that the machine gives you, you learn to influence the body function they reflect. Ideally, you reach a level where you no longer need the machine, and you're able to effect these body processes on your own.

Biofeedback is used primarily as an adjunct therapy for stress-related disorders such as tension, migraine headaches, high blood pressure, and panic attacks. It is not meant to be the only treatment for most problems.

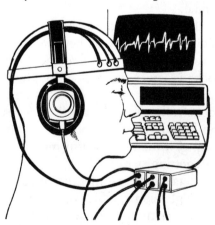

Biofeedback session

In a joint Russian and United States study of 59 men with mild high blood pressure, those who practiced a biofeedback relaxation technique twice a week for ten weeks showed a significant short-term decrease in diastolic pressure. Those who kept practicing the technique after the study ended maintained the decrease.

The men practiced a technique called "thermal biofeedback," which makes use of a machine that measures skin temperature. They were asked to concentrate on feelings of relaxation, heaviness, and warmth while learning to direct blood flow to either their feet or hands. This process of increasing blood flow and warmth in the extremities—known as peripheral vasodilation—is also helpful for sufferers of Raynaud's syndrome, the "cold hands and feet" disease. "By learning to increase blood flow to the fingers (and feet), you can warm them," says biofeedback expert Lynn Becker, Ed.D., clinical psychologist at the Veterans Administration Medical Center in Battle Creek, Michigan. And the machine, by feeding back temperature data, tells you when you're on the right track.

MIGRAINES FORESTALLED

Strangely enough, the same machine is used to help treat vascular headaches and migraines. The secret is that once you learn to influence blood flow to one extremity (the hands), the others, including the scalp and cranial vessels involved in headaches, will be influenced along with it.

In a study examining the effec-tiveness of biofeedback in forestalling classical migraines (the kind that come with warnings) and common migraines, Canadian researchers found that biofeedback helped reduce the intensity, duration, need for medication, and number of headache days. However, it worked most successfully for the classical migraine sufferers, who put it into practice at the first signs of an approaching headache.

Other studies have shown that biofeedback can help reduce the frequency of tension headaches, as well as anxiety and depression in headache sufferers.

Just how good is biofeedback's track record in helping solve health problems? Research suggests that it has indeed been moderately effective for stress-related conditions like tension and migraine headaches, insomnia, and hypertension.

Still, there seems to be a very individual response to biofeedback. Some people can master it, while others have trouble. "If you try too hard or are worried about failing," Dr. Becker says, "your stressful feelings will sabotage your attempt."

bismuth "For $100, the answer is: This chemical element, with an atomic number 83, atomic weight 208.980, symbol Bi, treats upset stomach, diarrhea, and ulcers, and prevents traveler's diarrhea."

"What is bismuth?"

"That's correct."

"For $200, the answer is: This liquid, developed in the early 1900s by a New York country doctor and produced in 20-gallon wooden tubs, contained oil of wintergreen, bismuth, and medicinal salts and was called 'Mixture Cholera Infantum,' then 'Bismosal.' After another name change, it is now found in nearly 60 percent of U.S. homes."

"What is Pepto-Bismol?"

"Right again."

Bismuth subsalicylate is the leading active ingredient in Pepto-Bismol. You know about the coating, soothing effect that pink liquid has on a grumbling gut. When you've eaten something you shouldn't have eaten, Pepto-Bismol may be able to help your upset stomach.

Bismuth subsalicylate can also play a role against diarrhea, provided the condition is mild, says Charles D. Ericsson, M.D., a professor of medicine at the University of Texas Health Sciences Center at Houston who has studied the medication. Dr. Ericsson defines mild diarrhea as two or three loose, controllable bowel movements in a day.

Taking Pepto-Bismol according to package directions should be helpful, he says. Possible side effects—darkened stools or tongue—may seem alarming but are not harmful, he adds. If your diarrhea is more severe, however, you should contact your doctor.

TURISTA CONTROLLED

Pepto-Bismol also can be used to treat traveler's diarrhea or turista, an uncomfortable condition caused by bacteria. When this ailment strikes, your vacation companions may include diarrhea, vomiting, abdominal cramps, and fever. Pepto-Bismol, in a dose of 1 ounce every half hour (no more than 8 ounces total per day) is effective against mild forms of the problem and may be taken for one or two days, Dr. Ericsson says.

"If you have moderate to severe diarrhea, though, I think there are better things to turn to," he says. Loperamide, available over the counter in Imodium A-D, has been shown to work better and faster than the bismuth subsalicylate in Pepto-Bismol, he adds.

The chief benefit of bismuth for the traveler is *preventing* the upsets caused by foreign food and drink. In a study involving almost 200 U.S. college students in Guadalajara, Mexico, Dr. Ericsson and other researchers found that two Pepto-Bismol tablets taken four times each day reduced the incidence of traveler's diarrhea for up to three weeks. Bismuth kills the germs that cause the problem. "We think it beats taking antibiotics because of their potential side effects," he says.

Travelers are advised to carefully follow directions, taking two Pepto-Bismol tablets four times daily, including two before bedtime. (Dr. Ericsson recommends Pepto-Bismol tablets over the liquid for convenience.) "If you take four tablets two times a day, it does not work as well. If you take one tablet four times a day, it doesn't work as well either," he explains. Keep taking the tablets for about two days after your return, because you may have something suspicious incubating in your stomach that the last-night-of-vacation dose didn't kill. In all, you should not exceed three weeks on the tablets, he says. Ask your doctor what to do if you'll be on vacation longer.

Be warned, however, that you still can get traveler's diarrhea even when taking Pepto-Bismol. "It doesn't give you carte blanche to eat anything you want. You're not off the hook," Dr. Ericsson says. "You can make the medication work even better by being cautious about what you eat."

When you're eating in a foreign country, Dr. Ericsson advises that you seek reputable restaurants where food is prepared "fresh and piping hot."

USED AGAINST ULCERS

Stomach upset and diarrhea aren't the only complaints for which bismuth is helpful. Ulcers are treated effectively in Europe with bismuth subcitrate, a form of bismuth not yet approved for use in the United States, says Howard Mertz, M.D., at the Center for Ulcer Research at the University of California in Los Angeles.

In 1982, two Australian researchers discovered a link between ulcers and a specific bacterium, now called *Helicobacter pylori*. These researchers believe this type of bacteria causes ulcers, although not everyone agrees that it is the sole cause. In any event, bismuth can kill the bacteria.

"Almost all studies show that bismuth compounds heal ulcers as well as other forms of therapy and that the relapse rate for duodenal ulcers is less in bismuth-treated patients," says Dr. Mertz.

Dr. Mertz believes that bismuth subcitrate formulas will be available in the United States within five years. Still, many U.S. doctors are already advocating Pepto-Bismol to kill the bacteria that may cause ulcers.

"Doctors won't prescribe Pepto-Bismol alone for an ulcer. But if they heal the ulcer with traditional therapy, they may then prescribe Pepto-Bismol along with antibiotics to eradicate that bacteria," Dr. Mertz explains. "We think now that if the bacteria are eradicated, the ulcers may not come back."

Dr. Mertz and other doctors caution it's too early for the general public to start chugging Pepto-Bismol as an ulcer cure. "The bottom line is that bismuth is effective for ulcers. But before widespread treatment in this country is begun with bismuth, we should do trials with Pepto-Bismol itself or wait for other bismuth compounds," he says. "I think it's important that patients and doctors don't start using Pepto-Bismol on a widespread basis unless we can really show that it's effective and safe." *See also* **Imodium; ulcer drugs**

bitters If you've ever sipped a Manhattan or an old-fashioned, then you've tasted Angostura aromatic bitters, a liquid flavoring extract made from a variety of herbs that's sometimes added to cocktails, fruit juices, desserts, and other dishes. But bitters weren't always taken for refreshment. Traditionally, bitter herbs were used to improve the appetite and aid digestion.

There are many bitter herbs. Gentian, chamomile, and dandelion are a few of the better-known bitters, while varieties such as scullcap and cinchona are fairly obscure. Angostura bitters, incidentally, actually contains gentian bitters and *not* angostura (a bitter South American tree bark).

"Originally, bitters were used as a stomach remedy for troops in Venezuela in the early 19th century," says Bob Hanson, president and CEO of Angostura International Ltd., the company that makes the bottled bitters. In the 1920s, he adds, bitters commonly were added to Prohibition's bathtub gin because they "tamed it down."

In Europe, people still consume large quantities of distilled bitters to improve their appetite. They also take bitters to settle their stomach after heavy meals. "All bitters reflexively stimulate the activity of the digestive glands," particularly the flow of bile and gastric juices, says Daniel B. Mowrey, Ph.D., director of the American Phytotherapy Research Laboratory in Salt Lake City and author of *The Scientific Validation of Herb Medicine.*

Various bitters have been credited as folk remedies for diarrhea, menstrual problems, hiccups, and dog bite. Herbalists have recommended chamomile both as a sleep inducer and an inflammation reducer. Dandelion commonly is taken both as a laxative and to settle the stomach.

"All that has been said about the bitter herbs, but I don't know how much proof there is," says James Duke, Ph.D., a botanist and toxicology specialist with the U.S. Department of Agriculture in Beltsville, Maryland. "Much of it is hearsay." *See also* **chamomile; dandelion**

black cohosh (KO-hosh) To say that natural childbirth is uncomfortable is like saying a tornado is breezy.

But the Algonquin Indian women relied on something more than huffing and puffing exercises to help them through the ordeal. Their secret weapon: black cohosh, otherwise known as squawroot, a medicinal herb that is said to gently stimulate uterine contractions and speed delivery.

Today, the practice of giving black cohosh to ease childbirth is still a part of some modern midwives' repertoire.

Black cohosh is also a favorite herb among natural health practitioners for stimulating the female system in other ways. It's claimed that this herb helps bring on a late menstrual period, eases heavy bleeding, relieves painful cramps, and cools menopausal hot flashes.

Black cohosh (Latin name, *Cimicifuga racemosa*) is also said to work as a sedative—an action that would no doubt add to its value as an aid during the throes of childbirth.

Until recently, black cohosh was

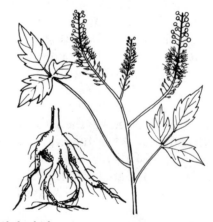

Black cohosh

a major ingredient in Lydia Pinkham's Vegetable Compound formula. This popular women's tonic was introduced decades ago to relieve uterine difficulties and other "female complaints."

Black cohosh is not regarded strictly as a gynecologic herb, however. "Besides relaxing the uterine muscle, the antispasmotic properties of the black cohosh root make it ideal for easing bronchial spasms," claims Cathy Rogers, a naturopathic doctor (one who treats without drugs or surgery) in Seattle. "And the powdered root mixed with massage oil makes a good liniment for overused muscles."

Some modern herbalists also recommend black cohosh tea to settle the stomach and ease sore throats.

CLAIMS ARE UNPROVEN

As with many herbal remedies, however, scientific studies to confirm black cohosh's supposed benefits are lacking. When researchers tested the plant on mice, they could not find any special estrogenic effects (which would indicate the herb acts like the female sex hormone estrogen). One extract of the plant did seem to reduce levels of the leutenizing hormone in rats, however. The leutenizing hormone plays a part in regulating the menstrual cycle.

There is also some evidence that black cohosh extract lowers blood pressure in animals. On the other hand, no such effects on humans with high blood pressure were noted.

Because black cohosh has yet to be proven safe or effective, experts do not recommend experimenting with the herb on your own. Large amounts could produce nausea, vomiting, and dizziness.

"You should definitely not use this herb for self-induced childbirth," says Ara Der Marderosian, Ph.D., professor of pharmacognosy and medicinal chemistry at the Philadelphia College of Pharmacy and Science. In addition, people with heart disease or those who take high blood pressure medicine should avoid ingesting black cohosh, he says.

If you want to use the herb externally as a liniment, just make sure you apply it when you are alone. *Cimicifuga* (which means bugbane) smells so awful it keeps bugs *and* people far away.

bleaching cream   Skin-bleaching products work by fading those oversized freckles known as "age" or "liver" spots, lightening brown patches, evening out splotchy skin tone, and depigmenting areas that are overly pigmented due to sun exposure, hormonal imbalance, or scarring.

Some over-the-counter skin lighteners have glamorous names such as Porcelana and Esoterica, which make them sound like cosmetics. In truth, these products are drugs containing the active ingredient hydroquinone in a 2 percent concentration, says Jerome Z. Litt, M.D., assistant clinical professor of dermatology at Case Western Reserve University School of Medicine in Cleveland. Hydroquinone does not actually bleach the skin. Instead it works by inhibiting the skin's pigment-producing cells, or melanocytes, which lie deep in the skin. Hydroquinone prevents the melanocytes en route to the surface from getting their full quota of pigment.

It may take weeks, and often months, for the new, lightened skin cells to finally arrive at the surface. That means you have to be diligent (and patient) in using your skin lightener, applying it twice a day, every day.

SUBDUED, NOT REMOVED

By following this regimen, 80 percent of users will show some lightening effect after three to six months, studies show. Just don't expect the spots to vanish entirely—the amount of hydroquinone in OTC products isn't great enough to work that kind of miracle, says Eugene Van Scott, M.D., clinical professor of dermatology at Hahnemann University Hospital in Philadelphia. "You can get spots to fade to some degree, depending on your skin type and the type of spots you want to lighten," he says. "But depigmented spots won't completely match your normal skin color."

Skin lighteners work best on people with lighter skin tone. They're also more effective against small, flat, frecklelike brown spots than raised spots or larger darkened areas.

Something else to keep in mind: While the Food and Drug Administration has determined that skin lighteners are safe and effective, that doesn't mean you should smear them on willynilly. Skin lighteners are not to be used on inflamed skin, bruises, birthmarks, moles, or blemishes that appear to be changing shape, color, or size. You could possibly disturb the skin's melanin production and trigger a cancerous condition called melanoma.

A final important rule: Always cover your dark spots with a sunblock (or use a skin lightener containing one). Otherwise the sun could undo the lightening action and spots may redarken.

If you have a brown or splotchy spot that doesn't fade at all after three months, Dr. Litt advises that you put a lid on your lightener and see your dermatologist. For stubborn spots, your doctor may prescribe a double-strength hydroquinone solution and also add a little tretinoin (Retin-A) cream or another acid. These additional substances help thin out the skin, allowing the hydroquinone to penetrate more deeply. Such a skin-lightening duo could make age spots disappear entirely after three to six months. As for those raised brown spots or resistant pigment patches, your doctor can freeze them off with liquid nitrogen, desiccate them with an electric needle, peel them off with trichloracidic acid, or zap them with a laser.

blood pressure monitors Despite the old saying, ignorance *isn't* bliss. In fact, it can be deadly if you suffer from high blood pressure.

Untreated, high blood pressure (or hypertension) can lead to heart attack, kidney damage, and stroke. Some people with hypertension have symptoms such as dizziness, nosebleeds, and headaches. Unfortunately, most people don't get such warnings. Because they are symptom free, they remain unaware of the problem. Often even a physician can't determine if you have hypertension until your blood pressure is measured by a device called a sphygmomanometer.

A sphygmomanometer is a rubber cuff with a gauge attached that is wrapped around your upper arm. The cuff is inflated to temporarily cut off blood flow through the large artery in your arm. As the air is slowly released from the cuff, a doctor or nurse listens with a stethoscope for the first sound of blood flowing. The reading on the gauge when that first sound is heard represents the systolic pressure, the maximum pressure of blood flow. Then more air is released from the cuff, until the pulse sound fades. The gauge reading at that point represents the minimum blood pressure, called the diastolic pressure. The harder it is for blood to flow, the higher both those numbers will be.

USEFUL AT HOME

Once a doctor diagnoses high blood pressure, he might recommend exercise, dietary changes, and if necessary, medication. He also might suggest that you use a sphygmomanometer to keep track of your blood pressure at home, says Richard Reeves, M.D., an assistant professor in the Department of Medicine at the University of Toronto.

Dr. Reeves is among a growing number of physicians who believe that patients who regularly monitor their own blood pressure are more likely to exercise and comply with other suggested treatments for hypertension.

"There's some reasonable evidence that people who do their own blood pressure monitoring may feel better because they're more involved in their treatment and have more control and understanding of the situation," Dr. Reeves says. "If they see an effect by taking their own readings at home, that's much more reinforcing than having to wait a month or two to have a reading taken at a doctor's office."

Home blood pressure monitoring also gives the doctor a better idea if the patient really has hypertension, he says.

"There are a number of people who get very nervous in a doctor's office, so naturally their blood pressure is elevated there. On the other hand, there are a number of people who have lower blood pressure readings in the office than in the real world. So if we just use office measurements, we may be treating some people we don't need to be and not treating others who really need it," Dr. Reeves says.

But there also is evidence that home monitoring could be a therapeutic tool.

In a small study of 15 people who had elevated systolic blood pressure, researchers found that home pressure monitoring helped the subjects significantly lower their readings.

During the seven-month trial conducted by the National Institute on Aging, the seven men and eight women were first instructed to measure their blood pressure nine times a day using a traditional arm cuff, gauge, and stethoscope. Later they were told to inflate the cuff up to the level of their previously measured systolic blood pressure reading. Then if they heard artery sounds through the stethoscope (indicating their systolic pressure was still high), they were told they should try to make those sounds disappear. They weren't told how to do that, but just to experiment until they could regularly make the sounds dissipate.

If the sounds disappeared, it meant that the patients had learned to lower their systolic blood pressure. Later, the patients were instructed to notice the sensations they felt when they successfully lowered their blood pressure. They were told to practice their blood pressure lowering by trying to duplicate those sensations—without monitoring—in stressful situations, such as in a traffic jam.

By the end of the trial, the patients had succeeded in lowering their systolic blood pressure an average of about 8 points.

GAUGE GUIDELINES

Even with its many potential advantages, doctors caution that home blood pressure monitoring should be done with a physician's approval.

"People shouldn't monitor their blood pressure in isolation. If it's done as part of a comprehensive care program, then it's useful. But if a person goes to a drugstore and buys a blood pressure monitor to diagnose and treat himself, then that's no good at all. The patient needs someone to help him interpret the data," says Bernard Engel, Ph.D., chief of the Laboratory of Behavioral Sciences at the National Institute on Aging in Bethesda, Maryland.

Dr. Reeves agrees. Taken out of context, a blood pressure reading can either unnecessarily worry a patient or give him a false sense of security.

"Some will measure their pressure and get nervous if it goes up 2 millimeters. They start taking their blood pressure constantly and think they're going to die," Dr. Reeves says. "On the other hand, there are people who will take their pressure a couple of times, see that it's gone down a bit, and then they'll stop taking their medication without consulting their doctor. That can be a very big mistake."

People who don't have high blood pressure really don't need a home monitoring unit, Dr. Reeves says. Instead, those folks should have their blood pressure taken when they visit the physician for routine checkups.

People with hypertension might find the devices useful, however. It takes practice to learn to use a traditional sphygmomanometer and stethoscope correctly, but they are more accurate than automatic digital monitors.

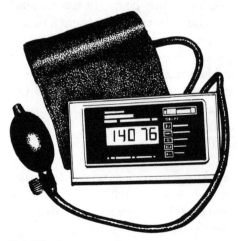

Digital blood pressure monitor

Avoid blood pressure monitors that rely on readings taken from your fingers. "Those finger monitors are dreadfully inaccurate," Dr. Reeves says.

No matter which type of monitor you buy, you should have it checked for accuracy by a physician or nurse before using it.

body wraps Picture this: You go to a spa to shed a few pounds, get a facial, and sweat off a year's accumulation of cigarette smoke and pollution. As part of the regimen, you are swathed from head to toe, mummylike, in towels impregnated with herbs, vitamins, seaweed, or cream. Then you are wrapped in plastic to seal in the magic ingredients while fat and toxins presumably melt away.

You've been body wrapped. Supposedly, body wraps can rejuvenate aged skin, flush toxins out of the body, get rid of cellulite, and whittle inches off your waist or thighs in as little as an hour.

"In reality, all you'll lose is money," says Peter D. Vash, M.D., assistant clinical professor of medicine at UCLA. Body wraps do nothing more than promote fluid loss, he says, which may account for a slight but temporary weight loss. But you won't lose fat. And there is no evidence that they get rid of toxins, rejuvenate your skin, or relieve any other conditions—except, perhaps, stress and tension.

"Body wraps appeal to people who aren't committed to losing fat but persist in trying to fool themselves by resorting to painless, passive attempts to lose weight—something they know

full well they can only achieve by exercising and reducing calories," says Dr. Vash, president of the American Society of Bariatric Physicians. He calls body wraps "fraudulent, misguided, and misrepresented."

But are they dangerous, too?

"If you wrap yourself excessively and sit in a steam room, they can be," says Dr. Vash. Also, if you're taking diuretics, a body wrap might cause a dangerous drop in blood pressure. And because body wraps can alter fluid balance, they're not advisable for pregnant women or anyone with circulatory problems.

bran We hear a lot about bran these days, but it's really nothing new.

Bran was a staple in everyone's diet until the 19th century, when whole grain cereals fell into disfavor. Peasants ate bran; aristocrats feasted on white flour. "White bread was the food of royalty," says Barbara Harland, Ph.D., a nutritionist at Howard University in Washington, D.C. Unfortunately, royalty (and those who mimicked the meal habits of royalty) also started having digestive problems from not eating enough dietary fiber.

Today, of course, many of us are trying to eat more bran. Not just wheat bran, but oat, rice, and corn bran as well. But what exactly *is* bran? Bran is actually the outer layers of the grain—layers packed with minerals, vitamins, and fiber. All whole grain cereals have it. Sprinkled on soup or baked in a muffin, bran can provide an efficient shortcut to meeting your daily fiber requirements. And bran doesn't have to be boring. With so many varieties to choose from, you can experiment with different tastes and different textures. Let's take a look.

WHEAT BRAN

Few foods smell—or taste—quite as good as a crusty loaf of bread fresh from the oven. If you used whole grain flour or added some additional wheat bran, that loaf would be especially good for your digestive system, too.

Researchers have noted that constipation is a frequent (and most unwelcome) guest in many American homes. Why? Because constipation thrives in people who don't eat enough fiber. Wheat bran, packed with insoluble fiber, soaks up water like a sponge in your lower intestine, which makes stools bulkier, softer, and easier to pass. (As with other kinds of fiber, it's important to increase your daily fluid intake when adding wheat bran to your diet.)

Hard stools cause more than constipation. Hemorrhoids flourish when people push and strain to pass hard, unwilling stools. What's more, hemorrhoids usually don't go away until the irritation stops. Wheat bran gives hemorrhoids a chance to heal.

A bout with irritable bowel syndrome can make the shortest journey—to the corner, say—seem fraught with danger. What if you get caught away from your bathroom? Then there's the cramping, the painful (and embarrassing) gas. What's more, you can't seem to stop it.

Wheat bran may offer relief in some cases. In a study at the University of Munich, volunteers with irritable bowel syndrome consumed 15 grams of wheat bran a day. About 12 percent reported their abdominal pains subsided. Ten percent reported less flatulence, and 22.5 percent said their bowel movements had become more regular. The researchers concluded, "The treatment of first choice should be bran."

People with non-insulin-dependent diabetes also may benefit from adding wheat bran to their diet. Wheat bran appears to smooth out blood sugar swings by slowing the absorption of glucose into the body. If your blood sugar supply is steadily replenished, you'll feel less jittery (or sleepy) before and after you eat—uncomfortable times for many diabetics.

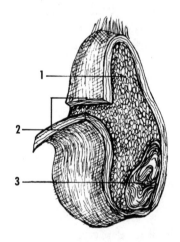

Wheat kernel: (1) endosperm, (2) bran, (3) germ

OAT BRAN

If we're paying homage to high-fiber foods, oat bran deserves a 21-gun salute. Once fodder for horses, now it's dished up in muffins, poured into cereals, and baked into meat loaf.

Oat bran grabbed the headlines several years ago when doctors at the the University of Kentucky College of Medicine and the Veterans Administration Medical Center gave volunteers 100 grams (about 3½ ounces) of oat bran a day in muffins and hot cereals. The volunteers lowered their cholesterol 18 percent. Studies since then have found similar results.

The oat bran equation seems simple. Eat oat bran and lower cholesterol; lower cholesterol and cut your risk for heart disease. How it works is not so simple.

Researchers suggested that oat bran's magic lies in its rich supply of soluble fiber. Some doctors believe the fiber ferments in the colon and inhibits cholesterol production. Others think the soluble fiber binds and helps eliminate bile acids, forcing your liver to collect extra cholesterol from your blood to make more bile acid. Voilà— your blood cholesterol goes down.

But these theories aren't without dissenters. For instance, when researchers from the Harvard Medical School gave 20 volunteers either oat bran supplements or low-fiber, refined wheat supplements, they found *both* regimens lowered cholesterol levels by about 7 percent.

The Boston researchers concluded that oat bran had little cholesterol-lowering effect of its own. Rather, both the high- and low-fiber supplements may have reduced the volunteers' cholesterol simply by replacing fatty foods in the diet.

These controversies shouldn't make you swear off fiber, says Dr. Harland.

Nor is oat bran the only good bran. All brans and whole grain cereals can be beneficial for the digestive system, she says. What's more, most appear to help people lower their cholesterol.

RICE BRAN

Watch out, oat bran, there's a new kid on the block. Rice bran is gaining ground as the grain to watch for lowering cholesterol. It's also vying with wheat bran to relieve constipation and calm irritable bowels.

Researchers still aren't sure how rice bran lowers cholesterol, but early studies look promising. When volunteers at Louisiana State University ate 3½ ounces (100 grams) of rice bran a day, they lowered their cholesterol by 7 percent.

In addition, researchers at Western Regional Research Center, U.S. Department of Agriculture, have been conducting studies feeding rice bran to hamsters on a high-cholesterol diet. In one study, the animals' cholesterol levels were lowered by 17 to 20 percent.

Antoinette A. Betschart, Ph.D., director of the hamster studies at Western Regional, suggests, however, that the fiber component of the bran can't take all the credit for lowering cholesterol. The oil in rice bran also appears to be important, she says.

At Louisiana State University, associate professor Maren Hegsted, Ph.D., also resists giving fiber the credit. Dr. Hegsted speculates there may be chemicals in rice bran that somehow fool your body into believing it's already produced all the cholesterol it needs. Production would therefore decrease, and total cholesterol levels would drop.

Because rice bran is "gummier" than wheat bran and oat bran, Dr. Hegsted says, it may be a bit difficult to get used to. She suggests baking it in muffins and cookies. But don't expect to get the same cholesterol-lowering results as the studies. "We used 100 grams a day, which is a lot of rice bran," she says. "It's one more thing that can be a contributor to good health, but it's not a magic food or anything like that—no more than oat bran is a magic food." She says a high-fiber diet incorporating all types of fiber is the best for overall good health.

If constipation is your problem, keep in mind that you don't have to load up on rice bran as heavily as you would on wheat bran to feel an effect. One study showed rice bran "increased stool mass and frequency by over twice the increase caused by wheat bran."

That's especially good news for people sensitive to the gluten found in wheat products. Rice bran seems to offer some of the advantages of wheat bran without the side effects.

CORN BRAN

How about some corn on the cob? Well, how about some bran on the cob?

Okay, it doesn't sound the same. But when you eat corn on the cob, you also eat the bran. And corn bran, however you eat it, is good for you. Overwhelmed by its more famous bran cousins, corn bran has gone nearly unnoticed as a cholesterol-lowering agent. That may change.

In a study at Georgetown University Hospital, seven volunteers ate first 18 and then 36 grams of corn bran a day. After 12 weeks, some lowered their cholesterol by as much as 20 percent. That compares favorably both with rice bran and with oat bran—until recently the undisputed cholesterol-lowering champ.

Of course, corn bran also offers a rich supply of insoluble, stool-bulking fiber. When constipation and hemorrhoids make the bathroom seem less a comfort station than a place of pain, a little corn bran may help.

Corn bran isn't yet widely available (except on the cob). Eventually it may be a welcome, high-fiber alternative for people who simply don't like (or who can't eat) wheat or rice bran. But the best approach of all might be to eat a wide variety of fiber-rich foods. "I would encourage people not to focus on one source of fiber," says Dr. Betschart of Western Regional. "I would have a wonderful smorgasbord, tapping into a number of them." *See also* **fiber**

breathing techniques Most of us breathe without giving it much thought. In comes the oxygen. Out goes the carbon dioxide. We breathe a little more deeply when we pass a hedge of honeysuckle, we breathe a little more shallowly when we pass someone who needs a bath.

Other than that, most of us don't pay much attention to our breathing. But maybe we should. Maybe we should, experts say, because how we breathe can reduce anxiety, boost our immune system, and help overcome debilitating respiratory diseases such as emphysema, asthma, and bronchitis.

DON'T GUZZLE GAS

Most people with breathing ailments can neither inhale deeply enough nor exhale fully enough, explains Diane Kreimer, R.N., a registered respiratory therapist who is director of respiratory care for United Health Care Services in Philadelphia. As a result, the least exertion—sometimes just walking up a flight of stairs—can cause them to run out of air.

Because their airways are often constricted or filled with gunk, "I tell people they've only got half a tank of gas," says Kreimer. And they'd better learn to use it wisely. They can be a gas guzzler that gets 16 miles to the gallon. Or they can be a compact car that gets 40 miles to the gallon.

As a gas guzzler, she adds, they'll race through activities and become short of breath. As a compact car, they'll learn how to force every bit of power possible out of the fuel they've got and avoid or diminish episodes of shortness of breath.

One technique that can help those with respiratory disease exhale more fully is pursed-lip breathing, says Janet Burda, manager of respiratory care at the University of Colorado Health Sciences Center. Just inhale through your nose, Burda says, then pucker your lips—pretend you're blowing out a candle, if you like—and exhale slowly. This type of exhalation builds up pressure in your airways, explains Burda, that helps to keep them open.

SAVE YOUR BREATH

Diaphragmatic breathing is a second technique that those with respiratory disease often find helpful, adds Kreimer. Most people don't breathe deeply enough because they normally breathe only from the chest. In the case of someone whose airway is already handicapped by respiratory disease, that may not be efficient enough.

Diaphragmatic breathing, which uses the band of muscle sandwiched between the lungs and abdomen, allows you to inhale and exhale more fully, increasing the amount of air available to your body. To try it, says Kreimer, inhale, letting the air slide past your chest toward your abdomen. Then slowly exhale.

How do you know you're doing it right? One way to tell is to place your fingertips just below the base of your rib cage, says Kreimer. When you breathe in, you'll feel your fingers lift as your abdomen rises.

If you want to make the technique even more effective, however, combine diaphragmatic breathing with pursed-lip breathing: Inhale with your diaphragm and exhale through pursed lips.

Another way to save your breath is to coordinate your activity with your breathing, says Kreimer. To climb a flight of stairs, for instance, take a deep breath, then exhale as you climb two steps. Pause, then try it again: Inhale, exhale as you climb two more steps.

Use diaphragmatic and pursed-lip breathing if possible as you do this.

"It takes some people only a couple of days to see how well this works," says Kreimer. "Some people, on the first day, go up the stairs and say 'I didn't get short of breath at all.'"

Where can you learn these techniques? Probably at your local community hospital, says Kreimer. Just call the hospital and ask for the director of respiratory care services or the department of pulmonary medicine.

BREATHE WITH THE YOGIS

The yoga masters of ancient India were so convinced of the power of breath that they developed a science of breathing. *Pranayama,* as they called it, emphasizes a number of breathing techniques—techniques that several studies say may help relieve asthma symptoms and stress.

How? Although there is little scientific work to support the effect of *pranayama* on respiratory problems, a British study of 18 patients with mild asthma does suggest that yoga may reduce symptoms and the need to use an inhaler. Researchers suspect that the deep relaxation produced by this type of breathing may calm parts of the nervous system that directly affect the lungs. Moreover, the increased amount of oxygen available during *pranayama* may cause the body to release natural tranquilizing hormones called endorphins.

Maybe that's why yogic breathing techniques can also be used to relieve stress, adds Jeffrey A. Migdow, M.D., an instructor at the Kripalu Center for Yoga and Health in Lenox, Massachusetts, and coauthor of the book *Take a Deep Breath.*

Want to give it a try? Inhale deeply and then, as you exhale, let the sound "Ah" just roll out of your mouth along with the air. Think of the sound vibrating all the way down your throat to your abdomen and on down to your toes. Repeat the "Ah" exercise three times.

Now inhale again, but when you exhale this time, roll the sound "O-o-o-o-o" out of your mouth along with the air. Feel the sound vibrating through your chest and down your arms all the way to your fingers.

When all the air is out of your lungs, inhale, and as you exhale this time through your nose, keep your lips together and make an "Mm" sound. You'll feel the vibration start in your throat, then continue on up into your nose and face.

End the exercise by saying "Om" three times and feeling the vibration throughout your body.

RELAX WITH QIGONG

Qigong is a traditional Chinese mental, physical, and spiritual exercise that combines breathing with a series of sitting and standing postures and movements that are designed to enhance the flow of air into and out of your body. According to its teachers, qigong has been used as an aid in the treatment of stress, immune disorders, asthma, paralysis following stroke, and neuromuscular conditions such as multiple sclerosis.

Although there are no studies to

support these claims in Western science, researchers have found that the type of deep relaxation promoted by qigong does seem to boost the immune system. In a series of studies at Ohio State University, for example, researchers found that students who learned a deep relaxation technique actually *de*creased their susceptibility to viral invaders by 18 percent and *in*creased their number of immune system fighters by 38 percent.

Want to give qigong a try? Here's an exercise from Effie Chow, Ph.D., a qigong master instuctor at the East West Academy of Healing Arts in San Francisco.

Stand up straight with your feet together and look straight ahead. As you inhale, lift your arms up above your head, stretching as high as you can, allowing your stretch to pull you up onto your toes. When you've reached the top of your stretch, turn your palms down and allow your arms to float back down to your side as you exhale.

Eight of these delightfully relaxing stretches a day can help make your body more resistant to stress, claims Dr. Chow. If you're interested in learning more about qigong, contact East West Academy of Healing Arts, Qigong Institute, 450 Sutter Street, Suite 916, San Francisco, CA 94108. *See also* **yoga**

bronchodilators Dashing to the bus. Cuddling the cat. Cutting the grass. If you have asthma, these everyday activities could take your breath away. During an asthma attack the muscles encircling your bronchioles (small passageways in the lungs) tighten. At the same time the mucous linings of the bronchioles swell. The result: Your air supply is squeezed off.

Fortunately, an episode of breathlessness need not always result in a panicky, wheezy race to the hospital for an adrenaline shot to dilate (expand) your airways. Today a number of bronchodilating drugs are available that can be either inhaled or taken orally to restore your breathing quickly and conveniently.

Familiar, over-the-counter inhaled bronchodilators such as Primatene and Bronkaid Mist contain a synthetic form of epinephrine (another name for adrenaline, the hormone that ignites your nervous system.) Sprayed from their portable inhaler canisters, they may relieve chest tightening and wheezing if you have an occasional, mild episode of breathlessness. But experts warn that because these products are so handy, they could be detrimental if your asthma is more severe. "Epinephrine is short-acting. To control your wheezing, you may need to take another hit from your inhaler sooner than the recommended interval of 3 hours," says Allan Weinstein, M.D., assistant professor of medicine at Georgetown University and author of *Asthma: A Complete Guide to Self-Management of Asthma and Allergies.* And use of these inhalers could be hazardous if abused. The reason? Epinephrine doesn't just act on the smooth muscles in the airways. It also acts on the heart and can cause tremor, irregular heartbeat, and elevated blood pressure. That's why OTC inhalers are off-limits if you have a heart condition or high blood pressure.

SAFER ALTERNATIVES

Whether your asthma flares once a day or once a year, asthma experts now recommend that you use one of the newer, safer prescription bronchodilators such as albuterol (Ventolin, Proventil), terbutaline (Brethaire), or metaproternol (Alupent). These adrenaline-like medications help relax the muscles surrounding the bronchioles within minutes.

Studies have shown that these medications are equal to or better than adrenaline for opening airways. Their effects last longer, and because they work directly on the lungs with less effect on the heart, there is less risk than with adrenaline. Among these medications, the state-of-the-art product is albuterol—it works within 15 minutes and lasts up to 6 hours.

You can swallow these bronchodilators in liquid form, but there's an advantage to puffing them through a hand-held, metered-dose inhaler. This canister device releases a premeasured dose of medication in a fine mist that can be delivered directly to the windpipe. Because less of the drug is absorbed into your bloodstream, you're less likely to experience shakiness or nausea. (You may feel *slightly* jittery after using an inhaler, but if you have major jitters or heart palpitations, you should contact your doctor.)

PRE-EXERCISE PRECAUTION

Besides arresting an asthma attack in progress, the new bronchodilators might help prevent an exercise-induced attack, allowing you to stay in the game without being sidelined with wheezing. "A rush of cold, unhumidified air into the lungs as occurs during strenuous exercise can trigger the contraction of muscles in the airway," explains Dr. Weinstein. "Puffing these bronchodilators 20 minutes before exercising may block the asthma response."

But the new bronchodilators aren't perfect—you may still find yourself wheezing again a few hours after taking them. And like epinephrine, they can overstimulate your heart if you take them too often. So if these newer bronchodilators aren't giving you what the commercials like to call "lasting relief," doctors might want to add a low dose of another, older bronchodilator called theophylline to your regimen.

Theophylline comes in liquid, tablet, and capsule form. It relaxes the muscles surrounding the air tubes, and it may also help clear mucus. The short-acting form of the drug (such as Slo-Phyllin) is for rapid relief from an infrequent asthma attack that may fail to respond to your other medication. Long-acting theophylline (Slo-Bid, Theo-Dur) takes a longer time to kick in but lasts longer—8 to 12 hours. It's ideal for overnight use to block the typical 4:00 A.M. asthma attack.

How much theophylline should you take? It's a tough question. Everyone reacts differently to the drug; you and your doctor have to work out a dosage level that works for you—and blood levels of the drug must be monitored carefully. Too much theophylline can cause nausea, headaches, and other side effects. In a few cases, deaths have resulted from incorrect dosage levels, especially in children with flu or other viral illness where theophylline levels in the body can increase dramatically. Theopylline effects can also vary with the use of certain drugs such as erythromycin. Coordination with your doctor is essential.

If your asthma does not respond to inhaled adrenergic or theophylline bronchodilators, you may need preventive medication such as an inhaled steroid to reduce airway inflammation or cromolyn sodium (Intal) to make the airways less reactive.

Check with your doctor if you have questions about any asthma medications. *See also* **atropine; coffee; inhalers; steroids**

buchu (BOO-koo) Members of the Hottentot tribe of South Africa regard the dried leaves from the buchu plant as a cure for diseases of the kidney, urinary tract, and prostate.

When buchu crossed into the New World in the middle of the last century, physicians began recommending the herb for a number of ailments—most commonly to combat inflammation and infection of the bladder, urethra, and kidneys. You can still find buchu teas sold for kidney and bladder infections in some health food stores.

Can buchu really beat urinary infections? "No one has studied this herb, so we don't really know," says Daniel Mowrey, Ph.D., director of the American Phytotherapy Research Laboratory in Salt Lake City. Perhaps buchu's therapeutic reputation stems from diosphenol, a volatile oil that acts as a diuretic, stimulating urination, says Dr. Mowrey. Diosphenol goes through your system unchanged. But on its way out, the urine turns slightly antiseptic, he says.

Buchu's germ-killing action is believed to be very mild, however. And physicians now have more effective drugs such as antibiotics to clean out infections. "It's really a step backward to use this old-time remedy," says Ara Der Marderosian, Ph.D., professor of pharmacognosy and medicinal chemistry at the Philadelphia College of Pharmacy and Science.

C

caffeine In an age when the words "caffeine free" on a label have become almost a badge of distinction, it's not surprising that many people consider this substance to be more of a foe than a friend. But caffeine has therapeutic properties that may surprise you.

For starters, it can help asthma sufferers in a pinch. Drug makers profit from its ability to help relieve common aches and pains. Studies suggest caffeine may even be of help to men trying to cut calories and dieters of either gender who've trimmed down and want to stay that way.

Caffeine is one of a group of organic compounds called methylxanthines that occurs naturally in more than 60 species of plants. You're most likely to consume it in coffee, tea, soft drinks, and chocolate. But don't rule out over-the-counter and prescription drugs or baked goods, where it's sometimes used as a flavoring agent.

Caffeine is most noted for its powerful stimulant effect on the body. It is so potent that it is medically classified as a drug. It's quick, too. It storms its way into the bloodstream within minutes and begins to take effect immediately. Once in, it scrambles to block the brain chemical adenosine from settling in special receptors meant for adenosine alone. With the sedative adenosine locked out, the neurons can keep on firing merrily, restoring the alertness you felt before fatigue or boredom set in. Caffeine's power peaks within 30 minutes to 1 hour, the point at which it typically achieves its maximum concentration in the blood.

Caffeine's ability to boost alertness is no secret to the makers of popular over-the-counter stimulants like No Doz, which will give you a concentrated 100-milligram dose of caffeine (the same as a cup of coffee), or Vivarin, which will jolt you with 200 milligrams.

More Than a Stimulant

Caffeine added to analgesics like aspirin enhances their pain-relieving ability, an effect noted by researchers in a review of 30 clinical studies involving 10,000 patients. It is particularly effective teamed with ergotamine in medications designed for sufferers of migraine headaches.

Chemically, caffeine resembles the asthma drug theophylline. In fact, some asthma sufferers use coffee or cola to relax their bronchial passages if they feel an attack coming on and no theophylline is available. (Three strong 6-ounce cups of coffee may work in a pinch. But don't use it as a regular medication replacement: Caffeine is only 40 percent as potent as theophylline.)

If you're a man trying to lose weight, you might also try a few diet colas or cups of black coffee to take the edge off your appetite. A study at Laval University in Quebec found that men who ingested caffeine a half hour before mealtime ate nearly 22 percent fewer calories than those who didn't. Unfortunately, caffeine didn't have the same effect on women.

If you've just lost weight, a moderate amount of caffeine may help boost your sluggish metabolism, according to a Harvard University study. That might help prevent weight rebound. A single dose of 100 milligrams of caffeine (the equivalent of one cup of coffee or two cans of cola) increased the resting metabolic rate of the "newly thin" by 3 to 4 percent over 150 minutes. When given a 100-milligram caffeine tablet every 2 hours for 12 hours, their metabolism increased 8 percent—a boost that translates to an extra 75 to 100 calories burned a day. This was the first study to show that moderate amounts of caffeine can pep up metabolism over an extended period of time.

Just don't overdo it. Of course, individuals vary in their response to caffeine. In general, however, more than 300 milligrams a day in those who are not accustomed to caffeine may can cause the caffeine jitters: increased heart rate, insomnia, nervousness, headaches, irritability, diarrhea, and frequent urination. To keep your total under 300, limit your daily consumption to no more than three cups of regular brewed coffee, four cups of tea, or four cans of soda—or less, depending upon your intake of other sources of caffeine. *See also* **coffee**

calamine lotion   "There's an old saying: If a rash is wet, dry it; if it's dry, wet it," says Arthur H. Kibbe, Ph.D., director of scientific affairs for the American Pharmaceutical Association. In the case of poison ivy, the rash is often so wet, it's weeping.

Calamine lotion can help dry those tears. In fact, this common over-the-counter treatment for poison ivy is also a soothing medicine for a number of other weepy, itchy skin eruptions.

The lotion gets its distinctive pink color from a tiny amount of ferric oxide (which adds nothing to the therapeutic effect). But people don't wear calamine lotion because they want to be covered with pink dots. They wear it for the zinc oxide it contains. That's the ingredient that dries irritated skin.

Zinc oxide actually draws fluid from the type of tiny skin blisters you get with poison ivy. You'll still have the rash, but it will be tame instead of raging. "Calamine lotion is not a cure, but it does dry the rash and relieve the itching," says Dr. Kibbe.

Calamine lotion is very safe and

effective, as long as it's used externally. (Internally, it's a poison.) It can be applied as often as necessary, with no side effects. But if calamine doesn't start to dry up your rash in a day or two, you should see your doctor.

A VERSATILE REMEDY

Even if you manage to steer clear of the poison ivy patch, you'll be glad to have calamine lotion packed among the camping gear.

Perhaps you feel a pimple coming on. In a pinch, calamine lotion can absorb excess skin oil and nip that blotch in the bud, according to Thomas Goodman, Jr., M.D., assistant professor of dermatology at the University of Tennessee Center for Health Sciences in Memphis.

Just before turning in for the night, wash and dry your face and hold an ice cube on the bump for a minute or so. (Cold reduces inflammation of the really red ones). Then apply the calamine lotion. Wash it off in the morning. A few nights of this routine, says Dr. Goodman, and that angry red bump may be barely noticeable.

Calamine lotion can also help take the itch out of fly and mosquito bites, says Claude Frazier, M.D., a North Carolina allergist.

Even if you are not a fan of the great outdoors, however, you should keep a bottle of calamine lotion handy. It can be a welcome soother for super-itchy conditions such as chickenpox or its grown-up cousin, shingles. The latter condition is caused by the same virus that causes childhood chickenpox. Only now, the pain seems worse than

you ever remember having as a kid. As the virus attacks a nerve, you feel a burning sensation. Several days later, red blisters erupt from the pain site. And then the itching sets in.

Calamine lotion can help hasten the drying of shingles sores and relieve the maddening itch at the same time, says James Nordlund, M.D., chairman of the Department of Dermatology at the University of Cincinnati.

To boost the effectiveness of calamine lotion for shingles, poison ivy, bug bites, or other itchy blisters, you can ask your pharmacist, with your doctor's written consent, to whip up a special calamine mixture with alcohol and phenol. The ingredients for this special mixture, according to Dr. Nordlund, are 20 percent rubbing alcohol (a good antiseptic), 1 percent phenol (to fight the itching), 1 percent menthol (for cooling), and 78 percent calamine lotion. If you find that the calamine mixture is too strong and causes a mild irritation, you can dilute the preparation with water.

"My patients find that this mixture makes them feel terrific. The itching and burning is gone for 2 to 3 hours at a time," says Dr. Nordlund. He recommends continuing to apply this calamine concoction until the blisters crust over.

calcium.　*See* **nutritional therapy**

calcium channel blockers　For many of the approximately 58 million Americans with hypertension, drugs called calcium channel blockers can help them lower their high blood pressure to safer levels. People with angina pain, heartbeat irregularities, and migraine headaches also are benefiting from this relatively new class of drugs.

The calcium channel blockers include drugs such as diltiazem, nifedipine, and verapamil. Here's how they work.

Normally, the muscles surrounding the blood vessels contract when calcium passes through special channels in each cell. But people with hypertension don't *want* their blood vessels to contract because that raises their blood pressure. Calcium channel blockers, as the name suggests, prevent calcium from getting inside, which allows the muscle walls to relax and expand. That makes the blood pressure go down, says David R. Rudy, M.D., professor and chairman of family medicine at the University of Health Sciences at the Chicago Medical School.

When blood vessels dilate (open wider), it's easier for blood to flow through the body, Dr. Rudy explains. This translates into less work for the heart. And because calcium channel blockers also decrease the *force* of the heartbeat, this further lowers the pressure.

In addition, the heart muscle gets more blood. This helps relieve angina—chest pains that occur when the heart doesn't get enough oxygen. Finally, calcium channel blockers cause blood vessels in the brain to expand, which may help prevent some types of migraine headaches.

"Migraine appears to have two phases—a constriction phase followed by dilation," Dr. Rudy says. "The calcium channel blockers prevent the whole sequence of events. If you prevent the constriction of the blood vessels, you may not get the headache that follows."

Not all doctors agree that calcium channel blockers are the best bet for treating migraines. In fact, some people actually get headaches when they take them. However, the headaches usually go away after a few days of taking the drugs, Dr. Rudy says. If you do suffer from migraines, ask your doctor what he or she thinks about these drugs.

HEARTBEAT HELPER

Calcium channel blockers commonly are used to correct irregular heartbeats, called arrhythmias. There are many types of arrhythmias, some of which may be life-threatening. Calcium channel blockers slow the passage of nerve signals through the heart muscle, which helps regulate the heartbeat.

In some experimental studies, calcium channel blockers have been shown to reduce atherogenesis, a process in which artery-clogging plaque is deposited in the coronary arteries. Because atherogenesis is a major factor in heart disease, this finding may be especially important for people—such as those with high blood pressure—who already are at risk for heart attacks.

Calcium channel blockers also may relax the muscles of the esophagus and lower intestine. Some researchers have suggested these drugs might be used for relieving esophageal spasms and irritable bowel syndrome.

Before calcium channel blockers came along, conditions such as angina and hypertension were often treated with a class of drugs called beta blockers, Dr. Rudy says. The beta blockers, however, can cause fatigue, depression, and in some cases, a dangerous tightening of the airways. The calcium channel blockers, however, don't cause any of these problems.

"Finally—and this might be the most important thing for some people—the use of beta blockers may result in a worsening of serum cholesterol levels," Dr. Rudy says, and increases of 15 to 20 percent aren't uncommon. Calcium channel blockers don't affect cholesterol at all, he says.

This doesn't mean that calcium channel blockers are free of side effects. In some cases, people's blood pressure drops *too* low, causing dizziness, nausea, and vomiting. Nor are these drugs safe for people with serious heart problems. "That's one of the caveats about calcium channel blockers," Dr. Rudy says. "If your heart is in danger of not contracting enough for its own good, these drugs certainly can worsen the situation." *See also* **antihypertensives; beta blockers**

canola oil.   *See* **monounsaturated oils**

capsaicin.   *See* **peppers, hot**

caraway   To fans of rye bread, the tiny brown caraway seed is zest in the slice of life. It's also the perfect topping for everything from ham to sauerkraut, pork chops to potatoes. And it flavors certain liqueurs and can be made into tea.

Here's something else: Caraway can relieve indigestion.

Because it is a carminative, caraway soothes digestion by helping expel gas, explains Varro E. Tyler, Ph.D., professor of pharmacognosy at Purdue University. "My old pharmacy professor used to refer to carminatives as something that gave you a good burp, and I guess that's still a pretty good definition," he says.

Caraway isn't a seed at all. It's a fruit. And while it won't provide handfuls of vitamins and minerals, a pinch of the seeds can help settle the stomach and relieve flatulence.

How much do you need? One to 2 grams, or in teaspoon terms, about ¼ to ½ teaspoon, Dr. Tyler says.

You can munch on the seeds to get the desired effect, Dr. Tyler says, or eat them in foods. Or the seeds may be ground and the powder used to make tea. Because it's the volatile oil in the seeds that gives you the desired effect, eating the seeds themselves gives you the greatest amount of the oil, he explains.

Caraway shares its soothing effects with some of its spice siblings, including peppermint, fennel seed, cinnamon, and clove. "They all act in about the same way," Dr. Tyler states. "So really, the selection is a matter of which taste you like and which is more pleasing to you." *See also* **cloves; fennel; peppermint**

castor oil   People haven't always trusted nature to take care of their bowel movements. When constipated, they forced themselves to gag down a few ounces of castor oil. More punishment than medicine, the nasty-tasting stuff did the trick—rather too well, say today's experts.

"Castor oil stimulates more contraction [in the intestine] than is necessary," says R. Thomas Holzbach, M.D., head of the Cleveland Clinic Foundation's gastroenterology research unit. "The active component is ricinoleic acid, which causes a watery diarrhea."

Taken regularly, castor oil may cause "lazy bowel" syndrome, in which the large intestine contracts *only* when stimulated by this too-tough laxative. Once they've lost the capacity for natural bowel movements, people actually can get hooked on castor oil.

Constipation usually stems from physical or dietary problems, such as too little fiber. It's better to treat the underlying problem, doctors say, than simply to pull the plug. When a laxative *is* required—before some diagnostic tests, for example—castor oil probably should be the last choice.

TORTUROUS TRADITION

In folk medicine, castor oil—which is derived from the fatty beans of the castor oil plant—was used for many conditions, says Richard S. Gubner, M.D., medical director of Safety Harbor Spa and Fitness Center in Clearwater, Florida.

"When you look back 100 years, you'll find castor oil was a common prescription, not only for constipation but to induce labor," Dr. Gubner says. But no matter what it was swallowed for, "it was just plain unpleasant," he adds.

Used *externally*, castor oil is a bit easier to tolerate. An emollient, it helps lubricate dry skin when added to bathwater. (Of course, bath oils are much less expensive.) Castor oil also helps soften corns and calluses.

While some people still use castor oil despite its unpleasant taste and texture, there's little use for it in modern medicine, Dr. Holzbach says. "There are other agents that are much more agreeable." *See also* **laxatives**

catnip   In laboratory studies, scientists have noticed that chicks given catnip take more catnaps. And among humans, catnip has considerable reputation as a sedative, especially when the dried, minty-flavored leaves and flowering tops are brewed into a hot tea and taken at bedtime. One of the active components in catnip resembles a chemical in valerian, another aromatic herb used for its calming properties.

Herbal authorities say a cup of catnip tea may also soothe the digestive tract or quell menstrual cramps,

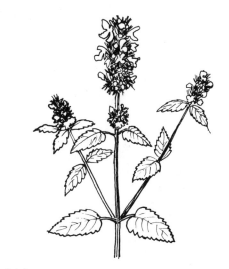

Catnip

presumably due to its antispasmodic properties.

Catnip has also been used as a folk remedy for a long list of other ailments, but evidence that it works is hard to come by. These include amenorrhea (cessation of menstrual periods), anemia, bronchitis, colds, colic, convulsions, diarrhea, fever, flatulence, headaches, hives, nightmares, runny nose, scurvy, and toothache. "There's not enough evidence to justify using catnip for those ailments," says James A. Duke, Ph.D., a botanist and toxicology specialist with the U.S. Department of Agriculture in Beltsville, Maryland.

PUTTING A LID ON CATNIP

Catnip grows wild in many parts of the United States. You can also buy the herb in most health food stores. To make catnip tea, stir about ⅓ ounce (a wad about the size of a golf ball) into a pot of hot water. (That's about 2 teaspoons per cup.) Dr. Duke says he likes to add some bee balm and lemon balm for flavor. Let it steep for 10 minutes or so before you drink it.

According to Dr. Duke, catnip tea is even safer than coffee—most people can drink up to three cups a day without side effects.

cauterization In the old Saturday afternoon Westerns, there always was one scene in which the cowboys, hard at work on the range, sat around a campfire that positively bristled with red-hot branding irons. Their cows, as you might expect, looked on nervously.

Ranchers still use hot steel, not just to mark their herds but to stanch the flow of blood from open wounds, says Lisa Encinias of the Sharp Ranch in Corona, New Mexico. That may sound pretty awful (from the bovine point of view), but cauterization does work, and it works on people, too, says dermatologist Bruce Bart, M.D., of the Hennepin County Medical Center in Minneapolis.

Cauterization is the destruction of tissue by heat, electricity, or chemicals. Commonly used to remove skin growths, cauteries also close blood vessels and sterilize surgical incisions. Doctors are a bit more sophisticated than ranch hands, though, so don't look for hot pokers under the examination table!

The electro-cautery unit is built like a soldering iron. Often used by surgeons, its hot tip cuts right through skin and tissue. The electro-desiccator zaps wartlike growths with electricity. "A little spark jumps from the tip of your instrument to the patient—the patient is the [electrical] ground," Dr. Bart explains. Lasers are the newest cauteries, cutting tissue and sealing blood vessels with blinding speed. In fact, lasers can actually "weld" severed blood vessels back together.

Intractable nosebleeds may be stanched with cauteries. Tattoos, blasted with laser light, quickly turn to ash and disappear. There's little risk of infection, Dr. Bart says, because cauteries sterilize as they cut. In addition, laser cauteries seal nerve endings as well as blood vessels. That means less pain.

Don't let all this talk of lasers, electricity, and hot probes scare you

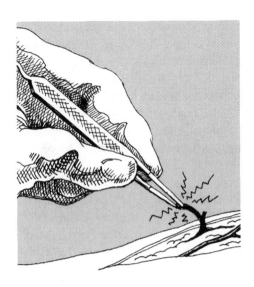

Cauterizing blood vessel

away. Many cauterization procedures are nearly painless, Dr. Bart says. "If you turned the cautery up high enough, you'd get some pain, but when it's used under low voltage, you get very little discomfort," he says. *See also* **laser surgery**

chamomile (KAM-uh-mile *or* KAM-uh-meel) Many of us first heard of chamomile at a tender age, thanks to Beatrix Potter's *The Tale of Peter Rabbit.* Following Peter's ordeal in—and subsequent escape from—Mr. McGregor's garden, his mother gave the hapless rabbit chamomile tea. And although we hadn't the foggiest notion what this brew was, we got the point: Chamomile settled the poor bunny's upset stomach, soothed his aching head, and calmed his frazzled nerves.

Herbalists have long attributed those calming, sooothing, settling properties—and more—to this daisy-flowered, apple-scented herb. The ancient Egyptians used it to treat fever, and folk healers throughout the ages have turned to chamomile to relieve pain and colic, heal wounds and burns, promote sleep, and combat fungus.

Even today, it's valued as a minor-complaint cure-all in Europe, where it's used to aid digestion, treat menstrual cramps, and soothe various inflammations. The Germans have a phrase for it, *alles zutraut,* meaning "capable of anything."

REDUCES INFLAMMATION

Although much of the evidence for chamomile is anecdotal, some scientific verification does exist. According to Varro E. Tyler, Ph.D., a plant-drug specialist and professor at Purdue University, German studies have shown that at least two of the major components of chamomile extract can reduce inflammation in skin and mucous membranes (mouth, nose, and elsewhere) caused by infection or injury. There's some evidence that one of its main components may help protect against stomach ulcers. And ingredients in chamomile extract have been shown to combat some common bacterial and fungal infections in animals.

At Roswell Park Memorial Institute in Buffalo, New York, a few cancer patients are using a chamomile extract to prevent an unpleasant side effect of chemotherapy: irritation of the mouth and salivary glands, which allows infections to start. In informal studies, swishing the extract in the mouth has prevented infection, but more rigorous testing is under way.

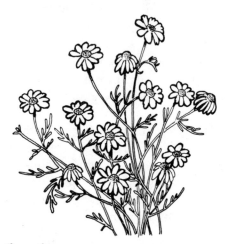

Chamomile

mile is considered one of the safest herbal remedies around, it can cause an allergic reaction in sensitive individuals. If you are allergic to ragweed, aster, or chrysanthemums, you may have a reaction to even one cup of chamomile tea. Hives, hay fever, and asthma have been reported in susceptible persons.

charcoal, activated   In 1831, a French pharmacist with a flair for drama stood before his colleagues at the French Academy of Medicine and quaffed a lethal dose of strychnine.

In Europe, chemically standardized extracts of chamomile are widely available in throat sprays, ointments, creams, lotions, and inhalants. In the United States, chamomile is mostly found in tea form.

It's easy to grow your own chamomile for use in tea. You may choose either German chamomile (a tall annual) or Roman chamomile (a low perennial), although the German variety is more common. Pick entire flowers and dry them in a cool, shady area. To make tea, steep 1 to 2 teaspoons of pulverized dried flower heads in 1 cup of hot water for 10 to 15 minutes. Dr. Tyler suggests drinking the tea three or four times a day for stomach or menstrual cramps. To ease canker sores, swish the tea in your mouth for 3 minutes. For irritated skin, mound moistened flower heads directly on the skin. Be aware that boiling the flowers evaporates some of the volatile oil that gives the herb its strength.

One caution: Although chamo-

No, it wasn't about tenure, and Monsieur Touery survived. He simply wanted to demonstrate that charcoal, which he gulped simultaneously with the strychnine, is an effective treatment for poisonings. Today, doctors in emergency rooms and poison centers still use a specially processed, or activated, charcoal to treat poisonings and overdoses.

Like the briquettes you burn for backyard barbecues, activated charcoal is pure carbon. Unlike regular charcoal, however, activated charcoal has extremely large surface areas—as much as 1,000 square meters *per gram*—that readily absorb (lock onto) toxins from the stomach and intestine and usher them out of the body.

"If you look at activated charcoal under the microscope, you'll see it has lots of little tubes with holes in them—there's lots of room for poisons to come in contact with it," says Jeffrey Brent, M.D., assistant medical director of Rocky Mountain Poison Center in Denver. "Activated charcoal binds the toxin as it's passing through the intestine, and it doesn't let it get back into the blood."

ALL-PURPOSE ANTIDOTE

Charcoal is used for most types of poisonings, Dr. Brent says. "People swallow virtually everything you can imagine—any chemical you can buy in the hardware store or chemical shop. It's just unbelievable the diversity of things people come into contact with and ingest."

Activated charcoal isn't the only treatment for poisonings. Syrup of ipecac, often used at home to induce vomiting, may also be effective. In fact, doctors may begin treatment with syrup of ipecac, then follow it with activated charcoal an hour later, says Joseph A. Barone, Pharm.D., chairman of pharmacy practice at Rutgers University and pharmacy clinician at Robert Wood Johnson University Hospital in Piscataway, New Jersey. Vomiting generally removes about a third of the stomach's hazardous contents, while activated charcoal picks up the remains.

Of course, giving activated charcoal to someone who feels nauseous isn't always pleasant—for the doctor, that is. "Drinking activated charcoal is like drinking dirt suspended in water," Dr. Barone says. "If you've already made someone vomit, and then make them drink suspended dirt, you'll be *wearing* some of the charcoal—unless you stand back real quick."

Outside of emergency rooms, activated charcoal has been used to filter water, eliminate foot odors, and wick toxins from insect bites. More com-

monly, people use products such as Charcoal Plus or Charcocaps to relieve gas pains. "Charcoal is taken to break up gas pockets in the intestine—it's like throwing sand on the bubbles," Dr. Barone says. *See also* **emetics**

chelation therapy   (kee-LAY-shun) The word *chelate* comes from the Greek word *chele,* which means "to claw" or grab, much in the way a lobster would. Chelation is the process where a man-made amino acid grabs or latches on to a variety of unwanted toxic metallic substances such as lead, mercury, and iron, as well as calcium, that have been deposited in the body.

Patients who undergo chelation therapy receive a slow intravenous drip of the amino acid—known as a chelator—which lasts approximately 3 hours. The new compound formed when the amino acid grabs hold of the unwanted substances is then excreted through the urine. By comparing the urine before and after chelation, physicians can determine just how much of the unwanted substances is being eliminated. The chelation is typically done two to three times a week for approximately two to three months, depending on the diagnosis and severity of disease.

Chelation therapy has successfully been used for conditions such as lead poisoning and Cooley's anemia, a rare condition in which repeated transfusions have overloaded the body with iron. There are different kinds of chelators, but one of the most effective appears to be EDTA (ethylene diamine tetraacetic acid).

HEART OF THE CONTROVERSY

Back in the 1940s, physicians began giving EDTA to battery factory workers who had lead poisoning. What they unexpectedly discovered was after patients received chelation therapy to eliminate lead, those with atherosclerosis (a condition in which vessels and arteries have plaque buildup that can cause heart attacks) showed dramatic improvement in blood circulation, breathing, and so forth—suggesting their clogged arteries had opened.

But for the last three decades, members of the medical community have locked horns over the idea that EDTA chelation therapy might help reverse atherosclerosis. No one argues that the drug is effective for treating digitalis poisoning, hypercalcemia (too much calcium in the blood), and certain types of heavy metal poisoning; the Food and Drug Administration (FDA) has approved it for these applications. Further, in 1991, the FDA approved a new oral chelating agent for the treatment of severe lead poisoning. But most chelation proponents insist the drug is not effective for treating heart patients.

Physicians who do use EDTA for atherosclerosis insist that calcium is reduced inside the cell in the blood vessels and arteries and is removed from them (though not "grabbed" in the same way that, say, lead or iron is) at the spots where fatty deposits and other minerals are deposited.

One of the results, chelationists say, is that plaque buildup can be reduced and circulation in the arteries in the legs and coronary vessels supplying the heart improved.

When doctors at Tulane University Medical Center, for example, analyzed 2,870 Brazilian atherosclerotic patients who were treated intravenously with EDTA, they found a major improvement in symptoms related to heart disease in 77 percent of all patients. In the case of patients with various vascular diseases linked to heart problems, the news was even better: 91 percent showed marked improvement after chelation.

"This [study] supports a conclusion that intravenous chelation therapy with [EDTA] is safe and effective in the treatment of patients with chronic degenerative diseases, especially atherosclerotic cardiovascular disease," concluded James P. Carter, M.D., professor and head of the nutrition section at Tulane University School of Public Health and Tropical Medicine.

An FDA-approved long-term study at three major Army hospitals to determine the effects of EDTA on plaque buildup in the leg arteries of people with atherosclerosis is also under way.

POSSIBLE DANGERS

Critics of chelation therapy, however, point to early studies that linked EDTA to kidney damage. More recently they have suggested it may contribute to bone-weakening osteoporosis and might even cause fatal complications.

Practitioners do acknowlege that in the early years of chelation, the appropriate dosage level had not yet been determined. Some patients were given too high a dose of EDTA too quickly.

Most medical doctors and scientists in the United States are still skeptical about treating heart patients with EDTA. The American Medical Association, the American Heart Association, and the National Institutes of Health advise that until there's scientific evidence that EDTA is effective against artery disease, patients would be better off with proven measures: low-fat diets, exercise and other lifestyle changes, and in some cases, bypass surgery.

chemical peels On the surface, her body is a sleek and sexy dark brown. But just beneath the surface of her tanned skin, the 30-year-old blonde is already beginning to pay the price of all those hours of sunbathing by the pool.

"In ten years, she's going to look like an old bag," says David Morrow, M.D., dermatologic plastic surgeon and director of the Morrow Skin Institute in Rancho Mirage, California. "Her skin aging processes are going to be accelerated because of that sun exposure. She'll develop lines, spots, and wrinkles that are going to look ugly. And she has an increased risk for skin cancer."

But Dr. Morrow and other surgeons say they can use acids and other chemicals to peel away wrinkles, remove age spots, and lower skin cancer risk.

New Skin for Old

When used properly, the chemicals burn through the upper layers of the skin, clearing away old, damaged tissue while promoting regeneration of new, fresh, healthy skin.

Sometimes, though, the chemicals can destroy pigment cells, causing some sections of skin to permanently lose their natural color. The peels can also cause scarring and infections. And they also aren't the best treatment for all skin abnormalities. A manual skin sanding procedure called dermabrasion, for example, is a more effective way of removing acne scars, plastic surgeons say.

But for many people, chemical peels are a safe way to eliminate unwanted signs of aging and damaged skin. About 14,000 people undergo this form of plastic surgery each year, according to the American Society of Plastic and Reconstructive Surgeons. In comparison, about 17,000 people receive dermabrasion treatments and another 49,000 have face-lifts each year.

For years, chemical peels were almost exclusively done on the face. But now some surgeons such as Dr. Morrow are using peels to rejuvenate skin on other parts of the body.

Likely candidates for chemical peels range from the truck driver who dangled his left arm out the window for years to the former sun worshiper who now avoids strapless dresses and short skirts because she has brown blotches on her chest and legs, Dr. Morrow says.

Picking Your Peel

"There isn't just one type of chemical peel and there isn't one type of chemical. There are many chemicals and we need to use them in different ways, depending on the part of the body we're dealing with," he says.

Phenol and trichloroacetic acid (also called TCA) are two of the most common chemicals used during peels. Both are used in varying concentrations.

Phenol, the stronger of the two chemicals, is used to burn out deeply embedded wrinkles.

Phenol peels are usually done in a surgical setting equipped with electrocardiogram monitoring equipment. The patient often is sedated. The surgeon applies the phenol on small sections of the face or body with a cotton swab. The solution is put on slowly to prevent rapid absorption into the bloodstream, which in rare cases can cause heartbeat irregularities. When the surgeon finishes applying the phenol, he covers the face with either ointment or tape. The operation can take up to 3 hours.

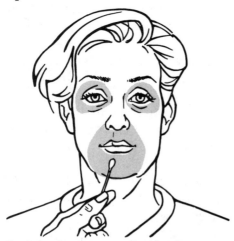

Chemical peel treatment around mouth and eyes

If tape is used, the patient won't look too good when it's removed after about two days. "You can look pretty swollen for one to three weeks," says Mark Mandel, M.D., a Los Angeles plastic surgeon and author of *Sculpture: A Man's Guide to Cosmetic Surgery.*

"It's not something you can do over the weekend and be back at work on Monday," agrees Thomas Baker, M.D., a Miami plastic surgeon.

Itching, pain, and insomnia are common side effects of a phenol peel. They usually are treated with hydrocortisone creams and powerful painkillers such as Demerol. The skin is likely to remain red or pink for up to three months. Most patients, however, begin to feel and look better within a week, Dr. Baker says. Most can wear makeup after ten days.

Despite the discomfort, phenol peels produce excellent results that can last up to 15 years. TCA peels, on the other hand, are more superficial and usually need to be done more frequently.

But TCA does have its advantages, Dr. Mandel says. First, it's cheaper—because it can be done without anesthesia. Second, the effects of TCA are less painful and less noticeable than with phenol. In fact, a person who undergoes a TCA peel often can return to work the next day.

"With TCA, you still have some redness and swelling, but you look like you went to the beach for 6 hours and forgot to put on sunscreen," he says. "A lot of people who have phenol peels hide out for the first couple of weeks. With TCA, you may not want to go out to a major social event the next day, but you look okay."

TCA also is a better choice than phenol for non-Caucasian people, because it is less likely to affect skin color. Unlike phenol, it is available in varying strengths. TCA peels, because they burn less severely than phenol, can be redone as little as six weeks after the initial treatment. Phenol patients must wait several months before having another chemical peel.

But before you rush out to have a skin peel done, Dr. Morrow suggests that you consult with a dermatologist to be advised of all options available to treat your problem.

chemotherapy (kee-mo-THER-a-pee) Medical science has come up with more than 40 chemotherapy drugs— agents that interfere with the growth and spread of cancer cells. Dozens of others are either in development or up for review by the Food and Drug Administration. Thanks to chemotherapy, several formerly fatal types of cancer are now considered curable. (See "Cancers That Respond to Chemotherapy" on page 140.)

Whether or not chemotherapy is prescribed for a particular patient depends on the size and type of tumor, where it's located, whether it's spread to the lymph nodes, and whether it's likely to spread further or recur. For systemic types of cancer, like Hodgkin's lymphoma, for example, chemotherapy is the first and foremost line of attack. What drugs are prescribed, how much, how often, and for how long depends on many factors. When warranted, treatment usually starts within six weeks after surgery and continues for about six months.

Injected into the bloodstream via an IV tube or taken by mouth, chemotherapy drugs flood the system, squelching distant, often undetectable cancer cells. The goal is to either increase the chance for cure or, if cure is not possible, delay symptoms for as long as possible.

REDUCING SIDE EFFECTS

Invariably, chemotherapy damages normal cells along with tumor cells. Many chemotherapy drugs suppress bone marrow function (increasing the risk of bleeding) and kill off white blood cells (increasing the risk of infection). Other common side effects include nausea, vomiting, and hair loss. Doctors are devising ways to reduce these side effects. And the results look promising. Research shows that injecting growth factors into bone marrow to clone extra white blood cells, for example, may enable doctors to use more of a drug with fewer side effects and less damage to healthy tissue, improving chemotherapy's chances for success with even advanced cancer.

"Nearly all of chemotherapy's side effects are reversible," says Greg Curt, M.D., at the National Cancer Institute. "Excellent antinausea medications exist, which can be taken 5 or 6 hours before treatment or during treatment.

"Other tricks for minimizing toxic effects include infusing a drug over a period of 30 minutes instead of 5," says Dr. Curt. "That avoids sudden, high peaks in blood levels without sacrificing effectiveness." To minimize damage to bone marrow, doctors can monitor the white blood cell count and cut the dose long enough to give blood cells time to recover.

Cancers That Respond to Chemotherapy

As indicated by this partial list, chemotherapy fights different kinds of tumors with varying degrees of success.

Curable in Advanced Stages by Chemotherapy

Acute lymphocytic leukemia
Acute myelogenous leukemia
Burkitt's lymphoma
Diffuse large-cell lymphoma
Follicular mixed lymphoma
Hodgkin's disease
Lymphoblastic lymphoma
Ovarian cancer
Small-cell cancer of the lung

**Curable by Chemotherapy
Used with a Primary Treatment**

Breast cancer
Colorectal cancer

**Responsive to Chemotherapy
in Advanced States but Not Curable**

Bladder cancer
Breast cancer
Cervical carcinoma
Endometrial cancer
Gastric carcinoma
Head and neck cancer
Prostate cancer

SOURCE: Adapted from *Cancer: Principles and Practice of Oncology,* vol. 1, 3rd ed. (Philadelphia: J. B. Lippincott Co., 1989).

"Hair loss disturbs chemotherapy patients the most," says Dr. Curt. "But when treatment stops, hair grows back."

According to Dr. Curt, the best place to get chemotherapy is an outpatient clinic run by a cancer specialist, and the best person to give it is a nurse who specializes in the task. "These are powerful drugs, which, unless administered carefully, can do real damage." *See also* **antiemetics; growth factors; radiation therapy; retinoids**

cherries In the four decades since Ludwig W. Blau, Ph.D., wrote an article in a Texas medical journal that credited cherries with ending his gout attack, many people have claimed that eating the fruit relieves this painful form of inflammatory arthritis.

"My husband had gout for years and took medication that made him ill. I read about cherries and decided to try it," a Fort Lauderdale, Florida, woman wrote in a recent letter to *Prevention* magazine. "I served him cherries every day, and he never needed another dose of medication."

Another *Prevention* reader from Lubbock, Texas, who had gout in a swollen and tender finger for months, claimed that eating cherries helped relieve her symptoms in just ten days.

While such stories may help keep the folk remedy alive, most doctors feel it should be a dead issue. They've found nothing to explain the healing power of cherries.

NO SCIENTIFIC EVIDENCE

"I know of no evidence at all that supports that idea," says John Renner, M.D., president of the Consumer Health Information Research Institute in Kansas City, Missouri. In fact, no viable scientific studies of cherries and gout have been conducted, Dr. Renner says.

Sanford Roth, M.D., medical director of the Arthritis Center in Phoenix, Arizona, agrees. "I have no reason to believe that cherries really should make a difference," he says. He does admit, however, that he has had

gout patients who have claimed that cherries eased their pain. But he believes that those patients were influenced by the placebo effect. In other words, cherries worked for them because they *believed* that they would.

Dr. Renner has another theory. He thinks that cherries simply replace foods you would otherwise eat—like those containing purines, substances that contribute to the accumulation of uric acid in the body. In some people, excessive uric acid collects in the joints and forms crystals that cause gout's pain.

Seafood, poultry, whole grain cereals, spinach, red meat, and mushrooms are among the foods high in purines. Traditionally, the only treatment for gout was eliminating purine-containing foods from a diet. Unfortunately, a purine-free diet is difficult to follow. "There's practically nothing you can eat while you're on it," says Ronenn Roubenoff, M.D., a rheumatologist at Tufts University in Boston. "We now have medications so good that it really isn't necessary to restrict diet to that point."

Dr. Roth agrees. Two drugs, Allopurinol and Benemid, effectively eliminate gout attacks, he says. However, the patient needs to take the drugs for several months, and both have side effects such as skin rash, headache, and nausea.

"They're not effective during a gout attack. In fact, those drugs can make the attack worse. But they can prevent you from having the attack in the first place," Dr. Roth says.

But Dr. Roth also doesn't completely reject the notion that a folk remedy may help some people. "There is always the potential that something unconventional will work," he says.

If you do decide to try eating cherries to relieve your gout, check with your doctor first and don't forsake other aspects of your treatment program. Where to start? People who have done it claim that fresh, frozen, and canned cherries—even cherry juice concentrate—have all worked.

chicken soup   Got a miserable cold? Have some chicken soup! You'll feel better.

Traditionally recommended by Jewish moms for the home treatment of upper respiratory ailments, chicken soup does seem to have some medicinal properties. Several years ago, doctors at Mount Sinai Medical Center in Miami Beach, Florida, carefully measured chicken soup's effects on nasal secretions in healthy adults. The results? Hot chicken soup sped the flow of mucus through stuffy nasal passages faster than hot water alone—possibly due to the soup's taste and pungent aroma.

Marvin Sackner, M.D., who was involved in the study, speculates that chicken soup could be beneficial when you have a severe head cold. By making your nose run, it shortens the amount of time cold germs spend inside your nose, giving the virus less time to be fruitful and multiply.

Although this was a one-of-a-kind study, Dr. Sackner says the results are still valid. (Other hot beverages, like

tea, may do the same thing, but no one has studied them.)

And of course, chicken soup lovingly prepared by someone who cares about you contains another active ingredient, TLC, which can't help but make you feel better.

In any case, Dr. Sackner recommends "chicken soup and more chicken soup" for anyone with an upper respiratory infection.

Chinese herbs   What distinguishes Chinese herbs like gingko, Dong quoi, ma-haung, and countless more from other herbs is not just their origin but the way they're used. According to traditional Chinese medicine, disease is viewed as an imbalance of two opposing energies, yin and yang, in the major organ systems. Herbs are used to restore the balance of these forces and are matched according to how each herb works on the major systems.

"Traditional Chinese herbal remedies are primarily used to treat a person's constitution or nature, rather than the symptoms or disease," says Subhuti Dharmananda, Ph.D., director of the Insititute for Traditional Medicine and Preventive Health Care in Portland, Oregon.

As the Chinese herbalists see it, your illness, for example, might be the result of a deficiency of energy (called chi). In that case, to treat it, you would be told to take a chi tonifier (energy builder) herb such as ginseng and a number of other herbs that have some lesser action on your symptoms.

In this way, Chinese herbs help

your body heal itself, according to Qingcai Zhang, M.D., primary researcher at the Oriental Healing Arts Institute in Long Beach, California.

In contrast, says Dr. Zhang, the typical Western way to treat an illness would be to take a drug that would swiftly squelch your symptoms. The only problem is, the drug could leave you feeling like you've been hit with a gong.

"Chinese herbal remedies are more subtle and work more gently because the whole herb is used and not just extract," says Dr. Zhang. Other constituents in the herb balance out harmful effects, he says.

What's more, Chinese herbs are rarely used singularly. Rather, they are combined with other herbs (up to 15 in some cases) that are carefully selected for their synergistic effect on the body. The combination of the herbs is said to help reinforce positive effects and neutralize harmful effects.

In the United States, Chinese herbs are sometimes used in a Western way: singularly and according to their reputed health benefit for a specific disease or symptom.

That could be a mistake, some experts say. "Chinese herbal remedies can't be followed like a cookbook," says Charles Lo, M.D., who has a preventive health practice in Oak Park, Illinois, and is one of the few Western-trained doctors using Chinese herbs. "You need to understand the action of herbs and match them to your symptoms and particular constitution," he says.

TESTING NEEDED

How do we know that these herbs work?

"You can simply look at thousands of years of testing on real, live people," says Dr. Zhang.

Unfortunately, only a few of the hundreds of Chinese herbs have undergone the kind of rigorous, scientific tests required in order for a treatment to be considered effective in modern medicine. "To pass such a scientific test, you would need to isolate the active ingredient," says Dr. Lo. "And taking only the extract would ruin the natural balance and create the potential for side effects." What's needed is a new system to scientifically study whole herbs and formulas.

Until more Chinese herbs go through these tests, however, Western-trained physicians will not be convinced about their usefulness, says Sheldon Saul Hendler, M.D., Ph.D., assistant clinical professor of medicine at the University of California at San Diego and author of *The Doctors' Vitamin and Mineral Encyclopedia.*

Researchers in Europe, China, Russia, and Japan have begun studying Chinese herbs for everything from antiaging therapies to cancer treatments. And a few U.S. doctors and researchers are starting to take note.

"This research is in its earliest stages and is usually confined to test tubes and animals," says Dr. Hendler. "Yet the Chinese herbs are offering some interesting clues to chronic diseases that have so far stumped modern medicine."

Take licorice, for example. This sweet-tasting herb is included in half of the Chinese formulas to improve the taste of other herbs and to "harmonize" their effects. Licorice is a well-known sore throat soother, and a licorice extract has been found to be protective against ulcers. There is also new evidence indicating that glycyrrhizin (an extract of licorice root) has an anti-inflammatory effect. Further, some researchers claim that this extract can inhibit the human immunodeficiency virus (HIV) responsible for AIDS.

Other herbs, astragalus and ligustrum, are being used in China to help cancer patients protect their immune systems from the effects of chemotherapy and radiation. In the United States, preliminary tests conducted by investigators at the University of Texas demonstrated that an extract of astragalus helped restore the immune defenses in test-tube cells taken from cancer patients.

Leaves from the ancient ginkgo tree have been used for centuries to treat chest complaints and to strenghten the heart and lungs. Now research is suggesting that ginkgo extract may help humans live longer, healthier lives, says Dr. Hendler. German researchers have shown, for instance, that ginkgo extract can increase the oxygen supply to brain tissue in the elderly. A British study found that ginkgolide B, the possible active therapeutic agent in gingko, seems to interfere with platelet-activating factor, a chemical in the body that appears to play a role in asthma and other medical conditions.

Still another Chinese remedy, Dong quoi, seems to be "a treasure trove of pharmacologic chemicals," says Dr. Hendler. Substances isolated from Dong quoi have demonstrated anti-inflammatory, analgesic, antiseptic, and bactericidal properties, he says.

HERBAL CAUTIONS

Chinese herbs now available in the United States are not standardized in formulation. That means the potency can vary from product to product. "It's likely you'll get an herbal tea or tablet that has skimped on high-quality herbs," says Dr. Lo. "It may be too weak to do you any good."

On the other hand, lack of standardization means that you might sometimes get a super-potent herb. What's more, many of the herbal "tonics" may not be traditional Chinese formulas composed of herbs that supposedly neutralize any toxic effects.

Taking some Chinese herbs "straight" could be downright dangerous. Ma-huang (which contains the adrenalin-like decongestant ingredients ephedrine and pseudoephedrine) and ginseng both may increase blood pressure in some people when taken in large doses.

Dr. Lo advises that you avoid the stronger, pure extracts of herbs. He suggests seeking out a practitioner trained in traditional Chinese medicine who can help you with correct dosages, based on your own physical makeup.

"If you have high blood pressure

or you are pregnant or nursing, you should not use Chinese herbs without consulting a doctor," says Dr. Lo. And certainly if you are taking a drug for any medical condition, you shouldn't abandon it. *See also* **ginseng**

chiropractic Derived from the Greek words *cheiro practikos*, the term *chiropractic* means "done by hand." Doctors of chiropractic (D.C.'s) treat disease and pain by manipulating the spinal column and joints, a technique commonly referred to as "an adjustment." You can actually hear a "crack," although the noise is not made by your bones but by the air moving around your bones. Sometimes chiropractors combine an adjustment with other treatments, such as heat, ice, physical therapy, exercise, or nutrition.

Chiropractors are not medical doctors; they are not trained or licensed to prescribe drugs or perform surgery. But they believe that for many conditions involving bones and joints, chiropractic is a viable alternative to drugs and surgery.

Although spinal manipulation was practiced by the ancients, chiropractic as we know it was founded by a self-taught healer named Daniel David Palmer in Davenport, Iowa, in 1895. Palmer believed that the nervous system controlled the body and that disease was caused by what he called "subluxations," or misalignments, in the spinal column. Palmer also believed that adjusting the spine could take pressure off the nerves and cure all sorts of diseases (including infections, diabetes, and epilepsy).

"Chiropractic is totally different from conventional medicine," says Milton Fried, M.D., D.C., of Atlanta, who is a medical doctor and a chiropractor. "Conventional doctors treat the disease; chiropractors treat the person. By restoring balance in the body, chiropractic allows the body to heal itself."

Chiropractic, however, has had its share of controversy. In fact, during the 1960s and 1970s, the American Medical Association (AMA) called chiropractic an "unscientific cult" and actively discouraged its members from referring patients to chiropractors, even for musculoskeletal problems like back pain, which chiropractors are highly effective at treating. Charges were filed against the AMA (and other professional organizations that joined their campaign), and in September 1987 the U.S. District Court prohibited the AMA from interfering with chiropractors and their practices.

HELPS BACK PAIN

Medical skepticism aside, chiropractic seems to work well for some problems and not so well (or not at all) for others. A study reported in the *British Medical Journal* supports the use of chiropractic for low back pain caused by injury, not disease. People treated with chiropractic fared better than others who were treated with physiotherapy as hospital outpatients. And they continued to feel better for two years. In fact, some chiropractors (including

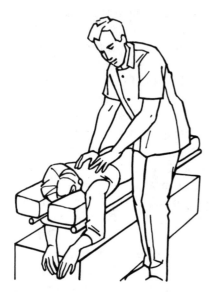

Chiropractic adjustment

chiropractic orthopedists) specialize in treating orthopedic problems, including whiplash or work-related back injuries.

"For low back pain, chiropractic adjustments are more likely to produce an immediate reduction in pain than bed rest or massage," says Kenneth Edington, D.C., past president of the National Association of Chiropractic Medicine, an organization that monitors the scientific accuracy of chiropractic care research.

Many chiropractors also claim they can relieve a host of conditions. Certain kinds of headaches, respiratory disorders, allergies, neuralgias (nerve pain), digestive disturbances, and fatigue are among them. But further scientific research is needed. Meanwhile, medical doctors insist that chiropractic is ineffective in treating common ailments such as high blood pressure, heart disease, stroke, cancer, diabetes, and infectious disease.

SATISFIED CUSTOMERS

Chiropractors have many satisfied patients who claim to have found relief. Chiropractors are licensed in all 50 states, and chiropractic care is reimbursable through Medicare, Medicaid, workers' compensation, and private health insurance plans.

Some people even choose chiropractors as their primary care physicians. This is not necessarily inappropriate— if the chiropractor knows his or her limitations, says Dr. Fried. "A good chiropractor is trained to know when to refer you to an M.D. for treatment," he says.

As far as safety is concerned, Dr. Fried says, "chiropractors don't necessarily use force to manipulate the spine, and patients needn't fear a chiropractor will break a bone. Chiropractors have a good track record."

chlorophyll   Some things truly do fit into the "without it, life as we know it would be impossible" category. Consider chlorophyll, for instance. This green pigment in leaves enables plants to change sunlight into edible starches, sugar, and cellulose.

Chlorophyll has a long and fascinating history of medicinal use, especially among the Swiss and Germans. Because it cannot be patented, chlorophyll offers little promise of profit for its marketers. "Unfortunately, there does not seem to have been much health-related incentive to do research in this area," admits Alvin B. Segelman, Ph.D., formerly chairman and associate professor in the Department of Pharmacognosy at Rutgers University and now vice-president for research and development at Nature's Sunshine Products, Inc., in Spanish Fork, Utah. The company specializes in herb-based health-related products.

ODOR FIGHTER

A form of chlorophyll called chlorophyllin copper complex is approved by the Food and Drug Administration (FDA) as a safe and effective deodorizing compound. This product, sold in tablet form, is given to incontinent patients in nursing homes to neutralize the odor of urine and feces. The tablets are also used by people who've had a colostomy or ileostomy (surgical openings on the abdomen for the purpose of evacuating the bowels). They can be taken orally (the usual dosage is one or two 100-milligram tablets a day) or placed directly into the collection bag.

Just how chlorophyllin copper deodorizes isn't known. It may bind directly to the offensive molecules, just as activated charcoal does. Or it may somehow change the mechanism of odor-causing microorganisms.

Some people with no odor problems take chlorophyllin copper because they think it neutralizes toxins in the bowel. But there is no proof chlorophyll has any protective effects in the bowel or anywhere else in the body, Dr. Segelman says. Unlike some other plant pigments, such as carotinoids (which give carrots and other orange or yellow vegetables their characteristic hue), no studies suggest that dietary chlorophyll acts to help prevent cancer.

Chlorophyllin copper is also FDA-approved for use in a few wound-healing salves. It seems to have an antibacterial effect. Some studies done in Russia suggest it may speed protein synthesis and cell regeneration. In one study, a salve containing chlorophyllin copper and an enzyme called papain was found to be particularly helpful in treating slow-healing wounds, especially bedsores. "No good U.S. studies have examined claims that chlorophyll can speed healing, and chlorophyllin copper creams are not widely used," Dr. Segelman says.

People use chlorophyll-containing products and eat chlorophyll-rich foods for a variety of unsubstantiated health reasons, Dr. Segelman says. Any green plant is rich in chlorophyll. Chlorophyll products are often made from alfalfa grass or algaes such as *chlorella,* both rich sources.

Chemical derivatives of chlorophyll have been tried in an experimental cancer treatment called photodynamic therapy, a treatment that kills sensitized cancer cells with light. But these chlorophyll derivatives have proven to be less effective than some other substances used for the same purpose, says Thomas Dougherty, Ph.D., head of the Division of Radiation Biology at Roswell Park Memorial Institute in Buffalo, New York.

cholesterol-lowering drugs You've given up double cheeseburgers. You've eaten enough oat bran to feed a circus. You've dropped so much weight that you've got to keep yanking up your pants. And you continue to walk at least 3 brisk miles a day. Yet the doctor tells you that you still have miles to go to bring your blood cholesterol down to a healthy level. Perhaps it's time to start thinking about medication.

Cholesterol is that fatty goo that gums up your arteries and can lead to a heart attack. In large part, the amount of cholesterol in your blood depends on what you eat (fat is bad, lean is good), your body weight (less is better), and how much exercise you get (never is bad, a few times a week is good). But for some, living the lean life just proves too demanding. For others, no matter how Spartan a diet and exercise program they follow, their blood cholesterol levels *still* ring a warning bell.

For those to whom genetics dealt a bad hand, and for those who just can't make the right lifestyle changes, medications may zap cholesterol and reduce the risk of heart disease. The American Heart Association reports that for every 1 percent drop in total blood cholesterol, the risk of coronary heart disease falls 2 to 3 percent. Take a glance at the table on the opposite page. With some quick arithmetic, you can see that these medications may greatly reduce your chances of

succumbing to America's most active killer.

NOT FOR EVERYONE

Approximately 3.5 million Americans take cholesterol-lowering drugs. Perhaps twice as many more *should be* taking them. But that's not to say that these medications are for everyone, says Basil Rifkind, M.D., an authority on cholesterol and heart disease with the National Heart, Lung, and Blood Institute of the National Institutes of Health.

Despite cholesterol's dangers, doctors tend to be cautious when prescribing cholesterol-lowering drugs. In fact, with very few exceptions (those whose cholesterol levels are up in the stratosphere), drug therapy is typically chosen only as a *secondary* line of attack.

"The *first* thing I do with patients is convince them to lose weight and modify their diet. This will often be enough to take their cholesterol levels out of the danger zone," says Margo A. Denke, M.D., assistant professor at the University of Texas Southwestern Medical School's Center for Human Nutrition in Dallas. In fact, adopting a low-fat diet alone will often reduce cholesterol levels by 10 to 15 percent. With weight reduction, you can typically knock off another 5 to 7 percent.

A diet and weight-reduction plan should start to chisel down your cholesterol within four to six weeks—"but you need at least three to six months to see if it's really going to work," says Dr. Denke. That's how long it takes to modify your diet consistently to affect cholesterol levels—and to see how well

EFFECTIVENESS OF CHOLESTEROL-LOWERING DRUGS

Drug	Expected Drop in Total Blood Cholesterol (%)
Bile acid sequestrants (cholestyramine, colestipol)	10–15
Gemfibrozil	10
Lovastatin	20–35
Nicotinic acid	10–15
Probucol	10–15

you can adjust to a life devoid of cheesecake and eggs Benedict.

If these cholesterol-lowering strategies don't work, *then* your doctor may wish to write out a prescription. Government health experts say you're a good candidate for drug therapy if—despite dietary therapy—your level of LDL cholesterol (the bad kind) is 190 milligrams per deciliter of blood or higher. If you already have heart disease or any other factors that put you at risk of heart attack (like high blood pressure, for instance), the threshold point for drug therapy may be lower.

SURVEY THE OPTIONS

If you and your doctor decide that cholesterol-lowering medications are for you, there still remains a big decision: Which drug?

Choosing between the various medications is tough. "There is no such thing as a best drug—each drug has to be matched properly to the patient," says Dr. Denke. Some drugs cause nausea, stomach upsets, and constipation in some patients. Another may cause hot, tingly sensations known as flushing. Aside from the question of side effects, different drugs have different potencies and different costs.

"A lot of times, you'll have different options, which might include a single drug or a combination of drugs," says Dr. Denke. Finding the right drug or combination may take some time. "You try one for a couple of months, then another. It's a trial to compare and contrast and find the best method," she says. Obviously, such a trial calls for close cooperation between you and your doctor.

The drugs of first choice over the past few years have been a class of medications called bile acid sequestrants, such as cholestyramine and colestipol. Nicotinic acid, a B vitamin (prescribed as a drug in much higher doses than you'll find in supplements on your supermarket shelf), is also very commonly used. But a fast-rising star, lo-vastatin, has become the most popular cholesterol-lowering drug on the market today, says Dr. Rifkind.

Cholestyramine and nicotinic acid both have been shown to lower the risk of coronary heart disease, and their long-term safety is well established. Nicotinic acid is the preferred drug for patients who, in addition to high cholesterol, also have high levels of triglycerides (another fatty substance in the blood). But these drugs are often difficult to take, and they sometimes bring unwelcome side effects. Too often, bile acid sequestrants produce gastro-intestinal problems, and nicotinic acid causes flushing, itching, and hives.

The new drug, lovastatin, has minimal side effects—patients often say that they feel like they're not taking any drug at all. It is also proving itself the champ at lowering cholesterol. In one large study of people with moderately high cholesterol levels, doctors found that lovastatin lowered nasty LDL cholesterol 24 to 40 percent. In addition, lovastatin is easy to take—you just pop a pill (as opposed to some other medications, like cholestyramine, which come in hard-to-swallow powder form). Still, "some fear lovastatin might have serious toxic effects—although we're gradually being reassured as to its safety," says Dr. Rifkind.

Two other drugs on the market are gemfibrozil, which is often better at lowering triglycerides than cholesterol, and probucol. Both are relatively easy to take but may cause gastrointestinal upset.

STAY THE COURSE

As different as various cholesterol-lowering drugs are, they also have certain things in common. None of these medications, for example, offers a quick cure. "These medications are not like other drugs where you might take a limited dose for two weeks to fight an infection. Taking drugs to lower cholesterol is most often a lifelong commitment," says Dr. Denke.

She advises you to make that commitment before you start. "I've had many patients who take these drugs for a while, and their cholesterol levels do well, so they decide to stop the medication. As soon as they do, their cholesterol levels go right back up," she says. "It's like having brown hair and dyeing it blond. If you stop dyeing it, the roots will always grow out the old color."

Another unhappy truth about these drugs is that they do not give you a license to gobble up barbecued ribs and triple shakes at will. Cholesterol-lowering drugs are much more effective if coupled with a low-fat diet, says Dr. Rifkind. Keeping your diet lean will also allow you to minimize your dosage (and so minimize potential side effects).

One study in the *Journal of the American Medical Association* clearly shows the one-two punch of a low-fat diet combined with medication. People with high cholesterol were split into groups—some ate lots of fat, others ate little fat, still others combined their controlled diets with medication.

Compared to the low-fat diet alone, those on a low-fat diet *and* lovastatin had greater reductions in total cholesterol (23 percent vs. 17 percent) and LDL cholesterol (30 percent vs. 23 percent). The combination of the two allowed 80 percent of all participants in this group to drop their LDL cholesterol levels below the danger zone. Of those taking medication while continuing to eat fatty foods, less than 50 percent met that goal.

One final note: Regardless of your medication, you need to carefully follow your doctor's orders and take your medication regularly, says Dr. Denke. Many of the medications, including the bile acid sequestrants, are most effective if taken along with your largest meal. Nicotinic acid should always be taken with food to minimize the side effects. And lovastatin is usually taken with supper—preferably a *lean* supper.

chromium. *See* **nutritional therapy**

chymopapain (kye-mo-pah-PAY-in) Mr. Bachrach was walking to the store, not a care in the world, when a flash of green caught his eye. There on the sidewalk was a crisp dollar bill—and no one in sight, either. He smiled at his good fortune, bent down, and . . . "Ouch!" he cried.

Sorry, Mr. Bachrach. That buck just cost you a slipped disk—and maybe an operation.

Fortunately, back surgery isn't his only choice. A shot of chymopapain—an enzyme extracted from the papaya

plant—often cleans up herniated disks just as neatly as surgery, and with less trauma and fewer complications.

When chymopapain was approved by the Food and Drug Administration in the early 1980s, "it was like opening Pandora's box," remembers Herbert Alexander, M.D., chief of orthopedic surgery at Oakland Naval Hospital in Oakland, California. "In a little less than six months, 6,500 surgeons were trained in the use of chymopapain."

When you get a herniated (slipped) disk, the gelatinous material inside sometimes oozes out and presses against nearby nerves, sending dreadful, radiating pains through one or both legs, a condition called sciatica. In addition, muscles in the lower back may go into spasm, which produces lower back pain.

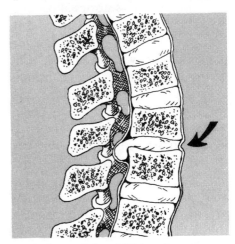

Spinal column with slipped disk (arrow)

PRESSURE EASED

In a procedure called chemonucleolysis, your surgeon injects chymopapain dead-center into the herniated disk. Chymopapain dissolves the disk, thus relieving painful pressure on the nerves.

People who receive a chymopapain injection spend less time in the hospital than people who have surgery, Dr. Alexander says. What's more, the injection leaves only a needle prick— there's not a 6-inch incision in the small of your back to slow you down.

"With surgery, you have a mortality rate that is two to three times higher than with chemonucleolysis," says Dr. Alexander. "And the overall complication rate is nine times higher."

Why would doctors even consider surgery when there's a treatment that's as noninvasive as chemonucleolysis?

Despite the excitement chymopapain generated when it first arrived in orthopedic and neurosurgical circles, it fell from grace as stories about paralysis, hemorrhage, and fatal allergic reactions made the rounds. Doctors quickly put away the needle and took up the scalpel again. Dr. Alexander says complications are rare these days, but the taint remains. Nationally, chymopapain probably is used only a few hundred times a month, he says.

Dr. Alexander hopes all of that will change, now that doctors understand the risks of the treatment and how to avoid them. And Dr. Alexander thinks chymopapain *should* be used first. When he looked at the progress of 100 people who had been treated for herniated disks—about half had conventional diskectomies, the remainder received chymopapain injections—he found the initial success rate for both groups hovered near 80 percent. However, the people who didn't benefit from chymopapain were still able to benefit from surgery at a later date. The initial surgical failures, on the other hand, had used up their options. And the benefits don't end there.

FASTER RECOVERY

People tend to recover more quickly from chemonucleolysis than they do from surgery, says Jim Dexter, a physical therapist at the University of New Mexico Hospital in Albuquerque. The more you move in the days after an operation determines, to some extent, the range of motion you'll have later.

"We can be more aggressive with the chymopapain patients than we can with people who have had diskectomies," he says. "It's important, early on, to get them moving."

As everyone with sciatica and back pain knows, long-term relief often is an elusive goal. It's not unheard of for people to have chemonucleolysis, surgery, *and* physical therapy without eliminating their pain once and for all. "If back surgery were a drug, the FDA never would have approved it," Dexter says.

Dr. Alexander agrees that back problems sometimes are tough to resolve. Chymopapain, which is less traumatic than surgery, and cheaper, is a reasonable place to start, he says.

"It's the final conservative measure prior to surgery," he says. "Chemonucleolysis is just a needle in the back to dissolve the disk; we don't destroy the architecture back there."

clay In ancient Persia, swallowing clay tablets was considered *the* antidote for nausea and vomiting. African medicine men used clay in potions to treat dysentery and problems associated with pregnancy. Here in America, we take Kaopectate, which contains a clay-derived ingredient, to stop diarrhea.

And some people still eat clay, continuing a practice that is many thousands of years old—and common to every continent but Antarctica. The practice, called geophagy, is most common among pregnant women but certainly not limited to them, says Donald Vermeer, Ph.D., a George Washington University professor of geography and regional science who is a leading expert on the subject.

No, he says, people don't eat clay straight out of the ground. Usually, it's dried in the sun or an oven, or smoked. Clay eaters consume a few ounces a day, on average, and commonly after meals. His investigation shows that pregnant women who eat clay do it based on custom—and sometimes because of cravings—rather than out of desire to alleviate discomfort.

That's not to say clay is without benefits. But the benefits may differ, depending on the clay's mineral composition. Dr. Vermeer analyzed one kind, for example, and found it high in calcium. He also found that the clay used by medicine men in the African village of Uzalla contained compounds closely resembling those in antidiarrheal products.

This type of clay, called eko, works by adsorption, Dr. Vermeer says. It pulls toxins to the surface, flushes them out of the system, and helps to smooth the walls of the gastrointestinal tract.

"Of course, too much clay will choke the motion of the gut, encouraging constipation," he says. On very rare occasions, doctors have had to open the gut and remove clay plugs.

MASKS AND MUD BATHS

The use of clay as medicine isn't limited to the inside of the body. It's also a prime ingredient in certain facial masks, and it may be present in the "mud" of some mud bath spas. The mud cures that people seek at Dr. Wilkinson's Hot Springs in Calistoga, California, for instance, contain volcanic ash or a clay called bentonite. In the case of the baths, general manager Mark Wilkinson attributes healing benefits to their heat—104°F. (For this reason, mud baths are not recommended for pregnant women or people with heart conditions.)

Topical mud application may do more harm than good, warns Kentucky dermatologist Joseph Bark, M.D., chairman of dermatology at St. Joseph's Hospital in Lexington, Kentucky. "We advise against mud and gel masks because they leave small particulate matter—little chemical corks, if you will—inside the oil glands."

A thinner application of specially modified clay, from a spray called Ivy Block, may prevent poison ivy itch. The manufacturer says the clay latches onto the poison ivy oils so they can't penetrate the skin. Laboratory studies show the product, which is awaiting

Food and Drug Administration approval, to be highly effective for people who are only mildly to moderately reactive to poison ivy. For people who are "exquisitely sensitive," Ivy Block may not prevent a reaction, but it can minimize it, says Tony Schulz, technical director of United Catalysts, the firm that makes Ivy Block. *See also* **Kaopectate**

cloves Their spicy smell may remind you of Easter hams, hot mulled cider, or linen-closet pomanders. Cloves are used for more than seasoning or scent, though. Oil distilled from these tropical evergreen flower buds has long been used to fight pain and infection, especially in Indonesia.

The most well known active ingredient in clove oil, eugenol, is a potent anesthetic. In the United States, a solution of 85 to 87 percent eugenol is approved by the Food and Drug Administration for use in toothache drops. You should follow the package directions carefully and not use these drops for more than seven days in a row, says Thomas Gossel, Ph.D., chairman of the Department of Clinical Pharmacy at Ohio Northern University in Ada. The oil is so potent, in fact, that it can kill a tooth's nerve if it's applied full strength. That's why it should not be used on a tooth that only hurts intermittently, says Dr. Gossel: "Pain that is not constant may mean your tooth nerve can be salvaged." If you use clove oil toothache drops and irritation persists or fever and inflammation develop, discontinue the drops and see your dentist or doctor, Dr. Gossel cautions.

Eugenol is also mixed with zinc oxide for use as a temporary filling. It is an ingredient in Noxzema Medicated Skin Cream and Lavoris mouthwash.

Clove oil also apparently has the ability to kill many fungi and bacteria, according to one of many reports supporting its traditional use as a treatment for intestinal gas and similar digestive ailments, says Varro E. Tyler, Ph.D., professor of pharmocognosy at Purdue University.

But that doesn't necessarily mean you should be taking it for any of those conditions, warns Dr. Tyler. It is very irritating and should be used with caution. Like many essential oils, in large amounts clove oil is toxic. Clove and clove oil should be used in medicinal amounts only with supervision by a doctor experienced in their use.

coffee Take a good, deep breath. Ahh! What can be nicer than waking up to the aroma of freshly brewed coffee? Coffee drinkers like it so much, in fact, they imbibe on average more than 3 cups every day. That's the equivalent of 1.75 cups for every man, woman, and child over the age of ten in the United States.

No wonder we're so perky!

Despite coffee's stimulating reputation, however, it's more than an eye-opener. A complex beverage containing some 2,000 compounds, coffee can boost endurance, ease headaches, and relieve asthma. Black magic? Let's see.

As you know, coffee's kick comes from caffeine. Caffeine is a chemical relative of theophylline, a potent bronchodilator often used by people with asthma. Italian researchers, after interviews with 72,284 people, concluded that people who drank one cup of coffee a day reduced their risk of asthma by 5 percent; those who drank two or more cups a day lowered their risk more than 20 percent.

Coffee is best known for its morning (and afternoon, evening, and midnight) jump-starts. "During the wee hours of the morning, coffee can help people stay awake and perform better on routine tasks," says William R. Lovallo, Ph.D., associate professor of psychiatry and behavior sciences at the University of Oklahoma and associate research career scientist at the Oklahoma City Veterans Affairs hospital.

If you're already awake and rested, coffee won't further boost your mental performance, Dr. Lovallo says. However, it may boost your *athletic* performance.

"Coffee or caffeine can liberate free fatty acids, which can assist in long-term endurance exercise, like marathon running," he says.

Does that mean you should shake hands with Mr. Coffee before you head for the spa? Not necessarily, Dr. Lovallo says. In the first place, some people don't like coffee. For others, it may cause problems. "If your doctor has told you to reduce your risk for high blood pressure, you might not want to drink two or three cups of coffee," Dr. Lovallo says. Coffee can actually increase blood pressure during exercise.

Joan Miller, Ph.D., a clinical psychologist in Marietta, Georgia, is also reluctant to give coffee an unqualified

thumbs-up. Some people find that drinking coffee eases their migraine headaches, says Dr. Miller. The caffeine in coffee reduces the swelling of cerebral blood vessels during a migraine attack. "But people may get rebound migraine or tension headaches from caffiene *withdrawal*," says Dr. Miller. "So I never recommend caffeinated coffee."

BLOOD-THINNING EFFECT

A cup a day may keep the heart surgeon away. Researchers at the University of Cincinnati Medical Center found coffee extracts, mixed in human and rabbit blood, inhibit the aggregation of clot-producing cells, called platelets. In effect, coffee "thins" the blood and reduces the risk for heart attacks, says M. T. R. Subbiah, Ph.D., a scientist who conducted the study.

Here's something else to think about while you sip your evening espresso. Researchers at the University of Michigan Medical School discovered that coffee drinkers 60 years and older were more sexually active than nondrinkers of the same age. It's not certain why (or if) coffee ignites the libido; the Michigan study may have more to do with coffee drinker's attitudes than with coffee. So enjoy your brew, but don't gulp a dozen cups at bedtime!

Over the years, coffee has been tentatively linked with all sorts of health problems, from colon cancer and elevated cholesterol to cardiovascular disease. However, researchers from Boston University School of Medicine have concluded that coffee does not contribute to large bowel cancer and that heavy coffee consumption—five or more cups a day—actually may *reduce* the risk of colon cancer.

Coffee simply is full of contradictions, Dr. Lovallo says. "There may be some coffee extracts that can inhibit platelet aggregation—that might be valuable for reducing heart attacks. On the other hand, there are some studies that indicate heavy consumption [of coffee] may increase the risk for heart attacks."

Dr. Lovallo's advice? If you don't already drink coffee, you may not want to start. Coffee is a beverage, not a prescription. If you *do* drink coffee, enjoy your morning cup; taken in moderation, it's a great way to start the day. *See also* **caffeine**

cognitive therapy   Meet Sally and Sue. Sally sees half a glass of water and calls it half-empty. Sue sees the same glass and calls it half-full. To Sally, problems at work are constant sources of aggravation, every failure is a blow to her self-esteem, and a drizzly weekend turns her into a pit bull on a strained leash. To Sue, problems at work are challenges, every failure is a learning experience, and a rainy weekend is a magnificent opportunity to munch popcorn by the fire.

Their worlds may be identical in every *physical* sense, but Sally and Sue live in two very different *mental* worlds. Sue's is obviously a happier place. She may have been born an optimist—or she may have gone through cognitive therapy.

Cognitive therapy doesn't aim to change the physical reality of your world but rather to change the way you *perceive* it. To some, the term refers to a specific kind of psychological therapy developed by researchers at the University of Pennsylvania. More often, it refers to any of a number of therapies that share this principle: How you *think* about your experiences (rather than the experiences themselves) determines how you react emotionally.

FAST AND EFFECTIVE

This simple concept, this tying together of thoughts and emotions, has virtually revolutionized the field of psychology. In the past few decades, changing people's uncomfortable emotions by changing their thoughts has grown from a radical theory to a well-established practice. Since this practice is designed to fine-tune one's concept of reality—not change the channel—cognitive therapy is *not* the therapy of choice for the most profound psychological problems, such as schizophrenia. It *is* an effective therapy for problems such as anxiety, phobias, panic attacks, and—especially—depression.

In fact, cognitive therapy may now be the prevailing psychotherapy when it comes to tackling all but the most soul-crunching kinds of depression, says Richard L. Wessler, Ph.D., chairman of the psychology department at Pace University in Westchester, New York. "It's definitely better than classical Freudian analysis," he says.

The reason for cognitive therapy's popularity? It *works*—and it works fast. Feeling down lately? Cognitive therapy may turn your frown to a smile in as few as five to ten sessions, says

Joseph T. Martorano, M.D., a psychiatrist in private practice in New York City and author of *Beyond Negative Thinking.*

In areas other than depression, cognitive therapy has also been put to the test and has come through shining. In one study at the University of Pennsylvania, 17 persons prone to panic attacks markedly reduced the frequency and severity of their attacks after short-term cognitive therapy. (And those gains were still evident a year after the therapy.) In one British study, of 11 patients plagued with raging jealousy, all but one shed their green-eyed monster after cognitive therapy. (One chap came to realize that every strange car parked opposite his house did not mean that his wife was having an affair.)

A CHANGE OF TUNE

Each school of cognitive therapy has its own strategy for zapping bad thoughts. Should you go to Dr. Martorano, he might ask you to first "identify your negative thoughts as they are expressed in words." You must know how your negative script reads before you can change it, he says. Then, you might be asked to keep a journal, taking careful notes as your nasty inner voice chatters away.

Your next step may be to identify whose voice you're actually hearing. Is it Mom's? Dad's? Aunt Wanda's? What's the tone? Is it carping? Judgmental? How does the voice make you *feel*?

Once you've tuned into your mental recording, you'll be ready for the *coup de grace* of cognitive therapy: Exterminating that heinous little voice. For instance, if it says, "I'm *never* going to be able to land a job (sigh); I'm a failure," Dr. Martorano might suggest you replace that negative notion with something upbeat—"These are rough times, and it may take a while before I get a job; but I will." Hopefully, before you know it, you'll be sounding, thinking, and *feeling* more like Sue and less like Sally.

How can you join this revolution in therapy? First, talk to your family physician, says Dr. Wessler. Mixed-up feelings are sometimes linked to bad body chemistry. Your doctor should be able to tell if this is the case. He may also know of a crack cognitive therapist. For more referrals, check with your local university or the Center for Cognitive Therapy at the University of Pennsylvania (133 South 36th Street, Room 602, Philadelphia, PA 19104).

As with any kind of therapy, finding a good therapist "is a little bit like dating—you should shop around," says Gary Emery, Ph.D., director of the Los Angeles Center for Cognitive Therapy. "Call. Make an appointment. Go and talk. See if you click." *See also* **behavior therapy**

Coke syrup When memories of childhood skitter through our thoughts, one of the warmer images many of us still embrace is that of Mom ... and all the special attention she gave us when we were ill.

One touch of her TLC came in the form of a sweet, thick liquid she gave us to drink in order to settle our tummy: Coke syrup.

It always seemed to work. Or did it? Although generations of parents, kids, and even some doctors swear by Coke syrup's stomach-soothing properties, there's a strong possibility that this remedy for nausea is little more than an unproven folk medicine.

Labeled Coca-Cola Syrup, this old-fashioned cure for an upset stomach is still sold in most pharmacies today. Yet its reputation reaches back to the late 19th century, when Georgia pharmacist and entrepreneur John S. Pemberton—who concocted home remedies like little liver pills and Indian Queen hair dye—combined the African kola nut with the extract of coca leaves. The thick syrup seemed to give folks lots of energy, partly due to the cocaine in the coca, which has since been removed.

Coca-Cola Syrup was also marketed as an "ideal brain tonic," touted to increase IQs plus treat just about everything, including jangled nerves, headaches, hysteria, and yes, nausea. Was there anything to this reputation?

"In terms of science, there really is no evidence to suggest it actually works," says psychologist and psychopharmacologist Daniel Mowrey, Ph.D., director of the American Phytotherapy Research Laboratory in Salt Lake City, Utah. "Not only is there no scientific proof it works, but doctors who have tried it out on their patients are pretty well split down the middle in terms of its effectiveness. It seems to work sometimes, and sometimes it doesn't."

Dr. Mowrey speculates that the secret in the formula may have to do with the heavy amount of sugar in the syrup. "In other words," he explains, "I don't think Diet Coke would have the same effect."

Though he's skeptical about the syrup's ability to soothe, Dr. Mowrey won't dismiss the possibility that because people *think* it will make then feel better, it will.

"Let's face it," he says, "Any time Mother says, 'Here, take this. It'll make you feel better,' you're gonna believe it. You know, Mom is not going to let you down. And who wouldn't feel better when she's showering you with all that TLC?"

cold remedies Scientists have not yet invented an antiviral agent that can wipe out all the viruses that cause the common cold. "The cold is not just one disease, so there will probably never be a single vaccine or cure," says Jack Gwaltney, M.D., professor of internal medicine and head of epidemiology at the University of Virginia in Charlottesville.

But you've got deadlines to meet and places to go—you don't have a week to wait while your body's natural, internal defenses battle and ultimately destroy the enemy virus. Besides, you've had enough of looking like Rudolph the red-nosed reindeer, coughing like Rover, and feeling like something the cat dragged in.

Drug manufacturers know just how you feel and have developed special all-in-one products to relieve your misery: They're called combination cold remedies, and they're designed to wipe out several symptoms with one capsule.

These symptom destroyers contain two or more of the following: an antihistamine (to dry up your runny nose), a decongestant (to open up your stuffy nose), an antitussive (to quell your cough), and a pain reliever (to ease your aches).

If you want to use the combination products, you do so with the government's blessing, as long as your symptoms match up specifically with the listed ingredients.

The Food and Drug Administration (FDA) has tentatively rated the combination cold remedies "safe and effective for use on multiple cold symptoms." (The FDA expects a final regulation ruling within the next few years).

They based this favorable rating on studies of the individual active ingredients. These studies showed that each ingredient was safe and effective for treating a specific symptom. The FDA also reviewed studies of combination drugs submitted by the manufacturers and found there were few adverse reactions. However, whether combos really work or not has not been widely studied, notes Robert Donohoe, M.D., reviewer and former medical officer with the FDA.

HIT OR MISS?

What do other doctors have to say about the combination products? Many believe these cold remedies (also called shotgun remedies because they attempt to hit all the symptoms) don't always work so well.

For starters, when you buy a cold product with several active ingredients, you may be paying for drugs you don't need. You're stuck with a fixed formu-lation—there's no way to adjust the doses of the ingredients to match your particular symptoms. The dose of one drug may be too puny to relieve your severely congested nose, for instance.

While currently available combos may give you too much or too little of a certain drug, you could also be getting a drug ingredient that is just plain useless for your symptoms.

"If you just have a cough, you need a cough medicine and not a product that also includes a decongestant designed to help a stuffy nose," says Dr. Gwaltney.

What's more, if you use the shotgun and develop a side effect, you may not know which drug ingredient hit you, adds Helen Krause, M.D., assistant clinical professor of otolaryngology at the University of Pittsburgh.

Other experts are bothered by the inclusion of aspirin in some combination products. A mild fever is rarely a bother and higher fevers (over 102°) may be an indication that you have a bacterial infection and should see a doctor, says John Cormier, Pharm.D., associate professor and associate dean of the College of Pharmacy at the Medical University of South Carolina in Charleston: "Masking a fever with aspirin could be a mistake."

Giving aspirin to kids or teens who have a fever can be downright dangerous. Aspirin has been associated with Reye syndrome, a potentially fatal disease that afflicts young people.

"The idea of a combination 'cocktail' is a good one," says Dr. Gwaltney. "But the products currently available don't offer effective ingredient levels of some components."

The best advice for choosing cold remedies is to make your medicines match your symptoms, says Dr. Gwaltney. If you only have a stuffy nose, for example, you might choose a decongestant nasal spray.

"Targeting individual symptoms may mean you have to juggle a lot of bottles, but that's the best route until scientists develop an effective combination product," reminds Dr. Gwaltney. *See also* **antihistamines; cough medicines; decongestants; painkillers; sore throat remedies**

cold therapy Also called cryotherapy, cold therapy is now the frontline first-aid remedy for treating everything from sprains and muscle spasms to bruises and insect bites. Itchy skin, arthritis flare-ups, and minor burns are also prime targets for a soothing chill. No wonder applying some form of cold is all in a day's work for athletic trainers, physical therapists, nurses, and paramedics. The function of all forms of cold is the same: to put the freeze on swelling and promote healing.

When you bruise a muscle or injure a ligament or joint, blood vessels are ruptured, and blood spills into surrounding tissues. That causes swelling. The more swelling that occurs, the less you will be able to move. And when you can't move, muscles lose their tone and start to waste away. Joints become stiff. Healing is impaired.

Placing cold against the injury site constricts blood vessels, reducing the amount of blood passing into the tissues. Swelling subsides and movement is regained. Cold also helps reduce the body's release of histamines—substances that cause inflammation.

POWERFUL PAINKILLER

With swelling and inflammation under control, pain melts away. In fact, cold can be such a powerful natural painkiller that the need for painkilling drugs is reduced, according to William Mitchell, M.D., staff physician for the Brookline Sports Medicine Clinic in Brookline, Massachusetts.

In a study conducted at the Southern California Center for Sports Medicine in Long Beach, a group of patients who had been operated on for knee injuries had electric cooling blankets placed on either side of their surgical wounds. The results? Those who were treated with the cooling blankets required less than half the amount of pain medication as patients who did not receive cold therapy. In addition, those given cold therapy were up and walking quicker and moving more freely than their counterparts.

Other doctors have found that patients who place cold packs on arthritic joints at intervals throughout the day seem to have less pain and may rely less on pain medication.

Most likely, cold freezes out pain in more ways than one, says Dr. Mitchell. As cold reduces swelling, pressure on sensitive nerve endings is reduced. Cold may also act as a counterirritant, blocking the transmission of pain sensations to the brain.

If you're experiencing an acute muscle injury, curling up with a bag of ice may be the last thing you want to consider. But it should be the first. "To avoid the shock of the initial cold sensation, place a hot moist towel over the area first, then place a cold pack over the towel. In 5 to 10 minutes the area will gradually become cold and the pain will begin to dissolve," says Margo McCaffery, R.N., pain consultant and coauthor of *Pain: Clinical Manual for Nursing Practice.*

In fact, many people find they prefer a cold pack over a hot water bottle for relieving low back pain, arthritis, and other conditions.

That's not surprising, says Irene Von Estorff, M.D., assistant professor of rehabilitation medicine at New York Hospital–Cornell University Medical Center. Cold is not just a pain reliever—it can rival heat's *healing* properties as well. The standard recommendation for treating an acute injury or inflammation has been to apply cold for one to three days to reduce swelling. Heat is then suggested to dilate (widen) the blood vessels and send a healing rush of fresh blood and nutrients to the sore area. But, over time, cold may produce these same effects all by itself, says Dr. Von Estorff: "Initially, cold constricts the blood vessels, but eventually a reflex action occurs. The vessels dilate and the area is flooded with fresh blood." The bottom line: "If cold gives you relief, continue to use it," she says.

CHOOSE YOUR CHILL

Which of the many available cold agents you select will depend on personal preference, as well as which part of your body needs treatment. (One warning: If you have impaired circulation or diabetes, consult your doctor before using ice or extreme cold.)

For dermatitis or poison ivy, a cold, wet cloth can help dry out oozy, itchy skin, and the coolness can quell the inflammation, according to John Romano, M.D., clinical assistant professor of medicine (dermatology) at New York Hospital–Cornell University Medical Center. A moist compress can also help soothe a bee sting by constricting the blood vessels so that less venom circulates. Cold milk can be more soothing than water. Put an ice cube in a glass of milk, dip in a washcloth, wring it out, and cover your skin for 20 minutes, Dr. Romano suggests.

A dip in a bucket of cold water (about 65°F) for 20 minutes can bring relief to hot, swollen joints of the hands or feet. It's also recommended for tension headaches and back pain. Here's another dunking tip: Plunging burned fingertips into cold water can be less painful than holding them under running water or applying ice. Remove your fingers from the water after 4 minutes to avoid frostbite. And never immerse your whole body in icy cold water. That can be dangerous, even fatal.

Commercial cold packs are flexible, reusable, and a lot more sanitary than placing a cold steak on your black eye. Gel-filled packs remain malleable when you freeze them, so the pack conforms to any body part, from foot to forehead. In a study conducted by Seymour Diamond, M.D., at the Diamond Headache Clinic in Chicago,

71 percent of headache patients who used a gel pack reported it helped reduce head pain.

ICE ADVICE

A bag of frozen peas (banged on the counter to make it malleable) can be a handy first-aid remedy. Or crush some ice, put it in a plastic bag, wrap it in a thin cloth, and place it on the injured area. For a hamstring injury, use an ice burrito—slip ice chips inside a towel, then wrap it around your leg. A wet towel dipped in ice chips will provide even more accelerated cooling.

If you are reasonably thin, you should expect to feel relief in about 10 minutes after applying ice. If you have more fat insulating you, give the ice about 20 minutes to dull the pain. Don't exceed 20 minutes, three or four times each day, advises Dr. Mitchell. You could cause vascular damage to the skin (frostbite), especially in knee and elbow joints, where there is little fat to act as a protective barrier.

You can expect your skin to turn slightly red from applying ice. "If it turns white, you've gone too far. Remove the ice pack and rewrap it with more protective toweling," says McCaffery. If your injury is too tender to touch, you may get relief from icing the area just above or below the pain, he suggests.

Never use those blue-tinted chemical blocks intended for use inside ice buckets or coolers directly on your skin—you could get frostbite.

If you have a sprain or strain, follow the standard RICE first-aid recipe, used by many physical therapists and other health professionals, in its entirety. *Rest* (if you increase vigorous activity too soon or while an area is numb, you risk further injury), *Ice* the area, *Compress* the area with an Ace bandage to further reduce swelling, and *Elevate* your injured limb. Gentle range-of-motion exercises can also augment the effects of cryotherapy.

A 5- to 10-minute ice massage—combined with gentle stretching—is an effective prescription for relieving tendinitis, tennis elbow, and superficial muscle strain, says Glen Halvorson, M.D., medical director of Sport Training and Rehabilitation of Tempe/Tucson, Arizona. Dr. Halvorson recommends two or three massage/stretching sessions daily. Although relief may last only a half hour initially, it can last up to 4 hours with regular daily treatments.

Fill a paper cup, freeze it, and peel back the sides to make an ice pop massager. Freeze an ice cream stick in the middle of your ice pop and you have a means to massage your own back spasm without a partner.

Sometimes applying ice to specific points on the body can bring relief of pain in other areas. If you have a headache or toothache, for example, you might try an ice massage by rubbing the webbing in the V-shaped area between your thumb and forefinger. In studies conducted by Roland Melzack, M.D., Ph.D., of the psychology department at McGill University in Montreal, intense dental pain was reduced by 50 percent or more by rubbing an ice cube into the V-shaped area where the bones of the thumb and forefinger meet. *See also* **hydrotherapy; RICE**

color therapy You're trying to lose weight but all you can think about is food, so you focus your eyes on a cardboard square the color of bubble gum and soon the urge to splurge passes.

No, this isn't just another wacky weight-loss method. In fact, color therapy is part of the weight-control program at the Health, Weight, and Stress Center at Johns Hopkins Medical University in Baltimore. At this prestigious center, the color pink is taken as seriously as diet and exercise.

REVVED UP BY RED

Color as a therapeutic tool is not new. For centuries, people have believed that the subtle vibratory energies of various colors can affect the body and mind in several ways. Red, orange, and yellow, it's been said, excite the nervous system; blue and green are calming; black is depressing. These theories appear to have at least some basis in truth. Consider that when London officials decided to paint their black bridges a shade of blue, bridge-related suicides reportedly decreased by nearly half. When a famous American restaurant chain added a lively orange to its blue decor, diners' appetites soared.

Some doctors have reported that viewing blue and green can relieve migraine pain. And many dentists paint their offices blue to reduce "drill dread." But most of the bona fide medical studies have been done with colored

lighting rather than colored *pigment* (paints and dyes), says Scott Hassom, Ed.D., associate professor and director of research at Texas Women's University in Houston.

In his own research, Dr. Hasson found that focusing on a red light increased electrical activity in the muscles, while staring at a blue light had a calming effect that resulted in decreased hand grip force. At least one well-established treatment depends on the body's chemical response to light of a certain color or wavelength: When newborns with jaundice are exposed to blue light, the condition disappears. And some optometrists are now using various colored lights to help treat vision problems.

Experts remain in the dark concerning exactly how color affects the body. But they have some theories. "We believe that light enters through the eyes or skin and travels along neurological pathways to the hypothalamus and pineal glands, which control all our physical and psychological functions," explains Harry Wohlfarth, Ph.D., professor emeritus, University of Alberta, and president of the International Academy of Color Sciences. "Different wavelength frequencies appear to have different effects."

IN THE PINK

A few of the studies linking colored pigments with health focused on the color pink. Alexander G. Schauss, Ph.D., director of the American Institute of Biosocial Research in Tacoma, Washington, found that when aggressive inmates at correctional institutions stared at a cardboard plate of a precise shade of pink, called Baker-Miller pink or bubble gum pink, they relaxed and the risk of violence was reduced.

In Canada, researchers observed a definite calming effect on mental patients sequestered in a pink room for 20 minutes. "We believe that staring at pink shuts down the adrenal production," says Dr. Wohlfarth.

That apparent tranquilizing effect on nerves is why bubble gum pink is part of the Health, Weight, and Stress Clinic program at Johns Hopkins. While studying 1,700 subjects over a four-year period, clinic director Maria Simonson, Sc.D., Ph.D., found that 32 percent of nervous snackers who ate a balanced diet and used bubble gum pink as a relaxation tool lost weight. Only 27 percent of those who used diet and relaxation without pink had equal results. "It appears that bubble gum pink relieves anxiety and stress-related nibbling," says Dr. Simonson.

Other studies have shown that people who focus for 10 minutes on a series of colored cards experience different physiological changes depending on the color they view, says Dr. Wohlfarth. Blood pressure, pulse, and respiration are increased most significantly when viewing yellow, orange, and red in that order. And blood pressure, pulse, and respiration are lowest when viewing black, followed by blue and green.

This doesn't mean you should toss out your hypertension medication and stare at a blackboard. But the emerging research in light and color therapy could lead to new and stronger evidence that hues may affect health in more ways than one. In the meantime, says Dr. Simonson, "it can't hurt to consider color choices more carefully, and it could help you stay healthy." *See also* **light therapy**

comfrey   Like many a fallen idol, comfrey has suffered a decline in its fortunes of late. In its heyday—dating back to at least 400 B.C. and continuing to the late 1970s—comfrey was revered as practically a one-herb pharmacy. Herbalists touted comfrey tea for everything from stomach ulcers, respiratory ailments, and whooping cough to hemorrhoids, gout, and gangrene.

Comfrey's fall from grace began around 1978. That's when a study found that rats eating a diet containing dried comfrey roots and leaves developed liver tumors after six months. On the human front, one woman who consumed large quantities of both comfrey tea and capsules for several months suffered serious liver damage, as did a young boy whose parents gave him comfrey tea for chronic intestinal problems.

The culprit seems to be certain chemical compounds (pyrrolizidine alkaloids) in comfrey roots and leaves. Taken internally, they become toxic and produce the nasty, slowly cumulative effects. Indeed, this lag time between the start of comfrey use and the onset of symptoms may explain why doctors and herbalists have traditionally been hard-pressed to pinpoint the herb as the guilty party.

SAFE FOR EXTERNAL USE

On the brighter side is the news that when used *externally,* as a poultice or compress, comfrey seems to pose no hazard. When applied to the skin, its toxic compounds are neither absorbed by the body nor processed by the liver.

Long before the days of modern medicine, cloths soaked in comfrey paste—which dries as hard as plaster— were wrapped around broken bones to fashion crude casts. That may account for the herb's old-fashioned name of "knitbone."

This herb has also been used for more than 2,500 years to help relieve inflammation and reduce swelling. Credit for these healing properties probably belongs to allantoin, a chemical in the plant that promotes cell growth.

To use comfrey externally on bruises and sprains, sprinkle some of the powdered root on thoroughly washed skin, and cover with a moist compress.

computer therapy   You drag yourself into the doctor's office with a fever and a sore throat. "Open your mouth and say 'aaaah,'" intones the computerized robot in the white coat. Two steely red eyes probe your mouth as cold synthetic fingers press gently against your glands. "Looks like you have an infection," it says, reaching for a needle. "Bend over, please."

Science fiction?

Pure science fiction. But the use of computers in the health professions is very real—just not this sophisticated yet, says Marc Schwartz, M.D., a New Haven, Connecticut, expert in both computers and health. From the high-tech CAT scan—which allows doctors to study your organs without scalpels—to the electronic microscope— which moves in response to a surgeon's voice so that his hands remain free— computers are coming to replace the comparatively simple tools once found in the doctor's little black bag. But they are not replacing the doctor himself. Not yet.

In one area of health care, however, computers are making inroads as competent medical assistants. That area is in the treatment of psychological problems, particularly depression and addictive behaviors like smoking. Come meet "Morton" and "TED"—two modern mechanical therapeutic marvels.

TELL IT TO MORTON

"Some of my colleagues are about to shoot me. At meetings they glare at me," says Paulette M. Selmi, Ph.D., a psychologist in private practice and director of psychology at Desert Vista Hospital in Mesa, Arizona. Why the glares from other psychologists? "They think I'm looking to put them out of business," says Dr. Selmi. Actually, it's Morton who concerns them. Morton is a computer program she designed.

Morton reached celebrity status among therapists when it made print in the *American Journal of Psychiatry.* A study by Dr. Selmi looked at 36 people who were feeling down. Some were given six therapy sessions with a flesh-and-bones therapist. Others were treated to an equal number of sessions with metal-and-microchips Morton. Both Morton and its human counterpart used a style of therapy called cognitive-behavioral, known to be potent in beating depression.

How does Morton work? During your first session, it might flash on the screen something like, "Hello, Judy, my name is Morton. I hear you've been kind of depressed lately. Is that true?" Every question is followed by several possible responses. You answer by pushing the right selection on the keyboard. "Well, how long have you been depressed?" asks Morton. "Was there anything particular going on in your life at that time?"

How good a therapist is Morton? In this one study, Morton showed itself "as effective in the treatment of mild to moderately depressed outpatients as a therapist . . . ," concluded Dr. Selmi and her associates. But Dr. Selmi asserts that she is *not* looking to put therapists out of work. "I don't see the computer as a replacement for human beings. I see it as a tool that may assist the therapist and reduce costs for the patient."

Despite Morton's stunning performance, computers lack the flexibility and intuition of human therapists. And they certainly shouldn't be a primary form of therapy for most people, particularly seriously disturbed ones, says Dr. Selmi. "I *don't* think these pro-grams should be marketed in your local Radio Shack," she says. Morton and other computer programs like it are still experimental. So, at least for now, you *won't* find them on sale at the mall.

TED LENDS A HAND

TED is the joint creation of Dr. Schwartz, a psychologist, and a computer scientist. TED works in Connecticut but is accessible to people anywhere in the United States who are looking to kick the cigarette habit. TED is a firm but friendly IBM computer that gives therapy over the telephone.

Call TED up and tell it you want to quit smoking (you "talk" to TED by pushing buttons on your touch-tone phone). TED will help you set up a program. It will monitor your progress. It will congratulate you if you succeed and help you if you fail. "People who use TED don't use it as a normal computer. They personify it. They develop a relationship with TED, and that relationship becomes influential," says Dr. Schwartz. "We've had people say they won't hang up on TED because they don't want to hurt 'his' feelings."

Many who work with TED make progress. "About 70 percent of smokers who set a goal to quit by a certain date do quit. At the end of six months, the success rate is still about 25 percent. That's double or greater the rate of success for people trying to quit on their own," says Dr. Schwartz. In the future, he and his colleagues hope to adapt TED to also help callers deal with stress and overeating. For more information, contact It's Your Call,

26 Trumbull Street, New Haven, CT 06511.

coronary bypass Being stretched out on a table and hooked up to tubes and wires probably isn't your idea of fun. A coronary bypass operation is serious stuff. It should be used only when the heart is in immediate danger of suffocation, or after all other efforts to clear your coronary arteries have failed.

The heart needs oxygen, and oxygen is carried by blood. But when cholesterol and other substances pile up in one or more of the arteries around your heart, blood can't get through. The result is often angina pain, or worse, a heart attack. Bypass surgery may be a more attractive alternative.

What is it? A vein, usually plucked from your thigh or calf, although sometimes from your chest, is sewn into the arteries of the heart in places where the blood flow has stopped. As if the doctor placed a tiny "Detour—turn here" sign at that point, the blood flows in one end of the newly attached vein and out the other. Circulation is restored and your happy heart can breathe again.

That's a simple definition, but the operation itself is anything but simple. It usually requires two surgeons, an anesthesiologist, a team of nurses, and the use of a "heart/lung" machine to keep your blood circulating while your heart's tied up in surgery. The operation generally takes 3 to 6 hours, although this can vary greatly. After the surgery you'll be in the hospital recovering for at least a week, maybe a few days more.

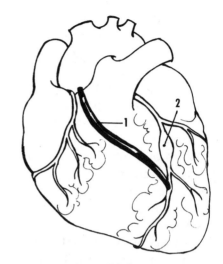

Bypass (1) around area of blockage (2) in coronary artery

To Bypass or Not?

In the past several years a number of simpler alternatives to bypass surgery have had good results in clearing clogged arteries. The most popular alternative is angioplasty, a procedure where a small balloon is inserted into the artery and expanded to compress plaque and widen the vessel.

So why would anyone in his right mind want to submit to a bypass? Because in some cases, angioplasty and other techniques simply won't work, or won't work as well, says Howard S. Bush, M.D., a cardiologist at Fort Lauderdale's Cleveland Clinic. Some arteries, for instance, get so packed full of fatty sludge that doctors can't push a balloon through. In other cases, a patient may have plaque buildups at several sites, again making a bypass the best option, says Dr. Bush.

Patients who have undergone angioplasty or other declogging techniques are also prone to "restenosis." That's when the arteries fill up with plaque again. With angioplasty the chances are about 30 percent that your arteries will start to reclog within three to six months after the procedure. With bypass surgery, however, early restenosis is much less common.

When the saphena vein from the leg is used to create the bypass, about 50 percent of all patients will still have clean passage in their bypassed arteries after seven to ten years. When the internal mammary artery from the chest is used (which isn't always possible because it's smaller than the saphena vein), the success rate after ten years climbs to 95 percent, says Dr. Bush.

What's the danger involved in a bypass? Nationally, there's about a 1 in 20 chance that once a patient closes his eyes on the operating table, he'll never open them again. Oddly, that's a higher number than a few years ago. Surgeons say it's because more people are getting angioplasties—leaving only the highest-risk patients to face the scalpel. If you're scheduled for a nonemergency bypass, and you're otherwise in good physical condition, the odds of a fatal outcome drop to about 1 in 30.

Clearly, the decision whether to have a bypass, or bypass a bypass in favor of other treatments, is one you'll need to make with your cardiologist.

THE PATIENT'S ROLE

Should you have a bypass, there's much more for you to do than go to sleep and leave your fate to the doctors. Doctors need a patient's help, says Nicholas Kouchoukos, M.D., professor of surgery at Washington University School of Medicine and chief of surgery at The Jewish Hospital, both in St. Louis.

Chances are, your lifestyle prior to your operation had something to do with the mess in your arteries. Following bypass surgery, it's more important than ever to adhere to a heart-smart lifestyle. This means eating a diet low in fat, watching your weight and blood pressure, keeping your stress in check, and "absolute cessation of smoking," says Dr. Kouchoukos. Once you're feeling up to it, it's also important to get started in an exercise program (with the guidance of your doctor).

Take good care of yourself, do what your doctor says, and you could be back in the full swing of things within six weeks to two months, says Dr. Kouchoukos. *See also* **angioplasty; atherectomy**

corrective lenses   Do corrective lenses really work? Let's put it this way. For millions of people who would otherwise be legally blind without these vision aids, as well as millions more with less serious vision defects, seeing is believing.

"Corrective lenses include the gamut of man-made lenses that are used to correct refractive errors in the human eye, as well as other deficiencies in vision," says James Sheedy, O.D., Ph.D., of the School of Optometry at the University of California at Berkeley. He stresses the word "correct," noting that lenses cannot be classified as cures for vision defects.

Most lenses work on the same

principle. They selectively bend (refract) incoming light rays to compensate for defects in the eye's own natural focusing system. The result is clear vision—a sharp image falling on the retina at the back of the eye.

Myopia and More

Corrective lenses work well to relieve myopia, or nearsightedness—a condition that causes distant objects to appear blurry, says Dr. Sheedy. Myopia usually occurs before the age of 8 and frequently worsens until a person reaches 20. Then, in some cases, it levels off and stops deteriorating. In fact, nature may atone for this defect when a person reaches old age, allowing some nearsighted people to read without the bifocals their contemporaries must wear.

Corrective lenses also help compensate for hyperopia, or farsightedness—a condition in which people see far objects better than they do near objects, says Dr. Sheedy.

Another common condition helped by lenses is presbyopia, the inability to read print. "By the age of 45, we lose the ability to see clearly and comfortably at a normal reading distance," says Dr. Sheedy.

Some people overcome this disability by purchasing glasses for reading in addition to their normal glasses, says Dr. Sheedy. Others opt for bifocals—a pairing of two sets of lenses with two different functions. Bifocals are designed to allow distant objects to be focused on through the upper part and near objects to be focused on through the lower part of each lens.

In addition, older people who are beyond middle age may need a third lens that helps them focus at an intermediate range. These are known as trifocals.

Those who wear contact lenses sometimes get the same effect they would from bifocals by wearing one contact for close reading and another for everyday tasks. This innovation is known as "monovision."

However, "learning to use only one eye at a time is an act that must be mastered, and not everyone can do this easily," says George W. Weinstein, M.D., chairman of the Department of Ophthalmology at West Virginia University in Morgantown. But "for those who eschew the use of glasses, monovision can be a useful device," he notes.

Corrective lenses may also help people with blurred and imperfect vision that is a result of astigmatism. Astigmatism is a condition of the eye in which "one meridian or axis of the cornea is steeper than the other," says Peter R. Laibson, M.D., a member of the American Academy of Ophthalmology and director of the cornea service at Wills Eye Hospital in Philadelphia. In other words, there is an irregularity of the cornea, he says.

Finally, corrective lenses also are sometimes useful in treating esotropia, or "cross-eye," says Dr. Sheedy. Certain lenses "help the eyes straighten up" and work together in many cases, thereby reducing the discomfort level, he says.

Eyewear Options

There are three main types of corrective lenses: eyeglasses, contact lenses, and intraocular lenses.

Eyeglasses, or spectacles, are the most common sight for sore eyes. The advantage of eyeglasses is that people "can obtain a more precise correction of vision," says Dr. Sheedy. "Depending on the individual, for many people we can obtain sharper vision with spectacles than we can with contact lenses," he notes.

Contact lenses are popular with people who like the advantage of having improved vision without having the look that the school bully used to call "four eyes." In addition, you "don't have the bothersome edges of the eyeglass frame in your field of view," says Dr. Sheedy.

Contact lenses can be soft or hard, says Janet S. Sunness, M.D., a researcher at Johns Hopkins Hospital's Wilmer Institute. "Soft lenses are generally more comfortable and they allow better oxygenation of the cornea," she says. They are a disadvantage for people with abnormally shaped corneas, however,

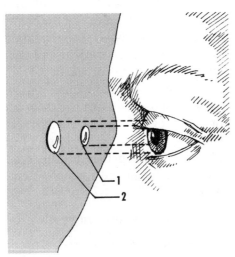

Contact lenses compared: (1) rigid gas-permeable lens (2) soft lens

because they cannot adequately correct astigmatism, she cautions.

In addition, with soft lenses "the vision may not be quite as sharp," says Dr. Weinstein.

Hard lenses are less comfortable, but many people feel they get a sharper image with them, says Dr. Sunness.

Still other people can wear either style equally well. "For many people there is no problem regarding either sharpness of vision or comfort" with either hard or soft lenses, Dr. Weinstein says.

A third option, gas-permeable lenses, combines some of the benefits of both hard and soft lenses. Like hard lenses, they are rigid and durable. But like soft lenses, they let more oxygen pass through to the cornea. Although easier to adjust to than hard lenses, gas-permeable lenses are usually not as comfortable as soft lenses.

Contacts can be worn anywhere from a day to a week, depending on the type. A hard contact lens "can be worn for 5 minutes or all day," says Dr. Laibson. "It comes out at night and is placed back in the eye the next day."

Soft contact lenses, which contain anywhere from 30 to 75 percent water, range from daily-wear types to extended-wear types that can be worn for up to a week without removing them. There also are disposable soft contacts that are worn for a week, thrown away, and replaced with another set.

"Most physicians recommend daily-wear soft contacts because those are the safest," says Dr. Laibson. "Compared to extended-wear lenses, even the disposable ones, there is significantly less chance of infection if you wear daily lenses, remove them at night, clean them, and put them back the next day," he says.

Except for disposable types, all contacts must be sterilized. "Manufacturers who make lenses recommend different ways to clean them," he says. "Some use heat; some use chemical disinfection."

Whatever the method, sterilization is important. "If you don't clean the lenses, protein, mucus, and lipid deposits build up on the surface," says Dr. Laibson. "These can trap bacteria, fungi, and acanthamoeba [a protozoa] that grow on the surface of the cornea," he says. Sterilization kills the lot of these bad-news bugs.

The final lens category—much less common than either eyeglasses or contacts—is intraocular lenses. "These are lens implants that the surgeon puts into the eye after cataract surgery," says Dr. Sheedy.

THE RIGHT PRESCRIPTION

Two different professionals are qualified to prescribe corrective lenses. The optometrist uses eye charts and instruments to assess a person's vision but is not allowed to treat eye diseases or injuries. A physician—known as an ophthalmologist or eye specialist—*can* treat them, as well as perform surgery for cataracts and other eye conditions and, of course, test vision.

After the optometrist or ophthalmologist determines what to recommend to improve a person's vision, a prescription is written, says Dr. Sheedy.

If the patient opts for eyeglasses, an optical laboratory can then grind the lenses from premanufactured blanks and shape them to fit into whatever frame is chosen.

The procedure for manufacturing contact lenses depends upon whether they are hard or soft.

"Hard lenses typically are made by putting a small piece of plastic on a lathe and then grinding and polishing the surface to the exact curvature desired," says Dr. Sheedy.

Soft lenses can be made in a variety of ways. Some are cut in a dry state and then water is added, says Dr. Sheedy. Others are placed on a rotating machine and spuncast to the right curvature.

cortisone   We hear a lot about anabolic steroids, the performance-boosting hormones used (and abused) by some young athletes. Less well known are the corticosteroids, hormones that help the body maintain healthy levels of blood sugars and mineral salts.

Cortisone is a natural derivative of hydrocortisone, one of many corticosteroids produced in our adrenal glands. You might take cortisone if, for example, your adrenal gland goes out of whack and stops producing its own supply of hydrocortisone. More commonly, cortisone, an anti-inflammatory drug, is prescribed to reduce all types of swelling. If you have asthma, for instance, a cortisone-loaded inhaler may help clear airway inflammation. If you've hurt your back, twisted your ankle, or gone to bed with an arthritis flare-up, cortisone can take some of that swelling right down.

Cortisone is one hard-working drug.

Unfortunately, it has some hard-working side effects, too. Briefly, cortisone has been linked with gastric ulcers, osteoporosis, and runaway infections. It may stunt growth in children. It even has been linked with psychosis. Make no mistake: Cortisone has the potential to cause all sorts of problems.

No, don't toss your prescription in the trash. Occasional injections of cortisone, or small daily oral doses, are still considered quite safe for most people.

RAPID RELIEF

We'll talk more in a bit about side effects. For now, let's just say that cortisone really slams the brakes on inflammation. Injected into a swollen joint, it stops just about every aspect of your body's inflammatory response. When you need relief from swelling *now*, cortisone will do the trick.

Like aspirin, cortisone inhibits your body's production of prostaglandins, compounds responsible for triggering pain and inflammation when you get hurt. Cortisone even permeates your joint linings, which prevents inflammation-causing cells from getting in.

Athletes long have known about the fast-acting benefits of cortisone. Injected right where the hurt is, cortisone may save days—or weeks—of bench time. Cortisone won't heal you, of course, but it relieves enough of the swelling for you to begin moving again. That's why injured athletes, eager for physical therapy, often rely on cortisone shots to get them started more quickly.

Cortisone works as well for rheumatoid arthritis as it does for athletic injuries. Once you reduce the swelling around a joint, you'll find a wider range of motion—with a lot less pain—at your disposal.

In the past, doctors often preferred cortisone injections. They could put the drug right where they wanted it and minimize the side effects. But cortisone seems to work however you take it. Small daily doses, taken orally, appear to relieve the chronic pain of rheumatoid arthritis as well as injections, while perhaps reducing the risk of side effects.

Cortisone also may be combined with bronchodilators to ward off pending asthma attacks. In fact, if a life-threatening asthma attack already is under way, doctors may give massive doses of cortisone to get you breathing again.

You've probably seen nonprescription cortisone ointments in your drugstore. Applied with a fingertip, cortisone helps relieve poison ivy itching and swelling, as well as other skin irritations. Taken rectally, cortisone will help suppress hemorrhoids and some bowel inflammations.

POSSIBLE DANGERS

When cortisone is taken in *maintenance* doses—20 to 30 milligrams a day—it doesn't appear to cause many problems. But large doses of cortisone, often required for serious inflammation, present some serious risks. That's why doctors often advise people to try aspirin, ibuprofen, or some other non-steroidal anti-inflammatory drug before turning to steroids.

Here are some side effects commonly linked with cortisone: sodium retention, high blood pressure, muscle weakness, osteoporosis, peptic ulcer, impaired wound healing, and the masking of signs of serious infection.

Cortisone, taken for a long time, may shut down your body's natural hormone production. When treatment stops, therefore, your well might run dry. (Adrenal function generally returns, but it often takes careful management—and a long time.)

Cortisone also suppresses your immune system. Sometimes that's good—if you suffer from one of the many diseases related to the immune system, such as rhumatoid arthritis or inflammatory bowel disease, for example. On the other hand, a depressed immune system gives all kinds of infection the chance to make your life miserable.

Another thing to remember is that your body actually *needs* some inflammation—it's part of the healing process. Stop the inflammation by taking cortisone, and you may stop some of the healing.

As you can see, cortisone is a mixed bag. Yes, it's strong medicine—medicine with some potentially serious side effects. Clearly, you don't want cortisone for minor aches and pains. Sometimes, however, you want a really tough anti-inflammatory drug. When you do, cortisone might be the right choice.

See also **anti-inflammatories; hydrocortisone; prednisone; steroids**

cotton swabs Lend us an ear as we move to this dictionary entry. Of course, we mean that only in a metaphoric sense—*not* a physical one. That's because even though cotton swabs are to ear cleaning what Tammy Faye Bakker is to mascara, the association is an unfortunate one.

"Grandma was right when she said you shouldn't stick anything smaller than your elbow in your ear," says David Fairbanks, M.D., spokesman for the American Academy of Otolaryngology and a practicing ear, nose, and throat specialist in Washington, D.C.

"Ear wax falls out of your ear naturally, thanks to gravity. When you stick small objects into your ear in an effort to remove that wax, what you're really doing is pushing it in deeper, so it can't migrate out—and that can cause problems. By small objects, I'm talking about twisted napkin corners, bobby pins, pencil erasers, and *especially* cotton swabs. A doctor can use swabs in your ears because he has special lighting and has been trained to do it without hurting you. But as a self-help tool, unless you're using them on the crevices or folds of your outer ear, which is okay, they're *not* made for your ears."

SOME SAFER USES

So then what are cotton swabs good for? Well, some folks use them to clean those hard-to-reach nooks and crannies of their car's dashboard. Others find them a valuable painting tool—again to reach spots a paintbrush can't. But anatomically speaking, you can pick up these soft sticks to:

Beautify your belly button . . . "Cotton swabs are perfect for cleaning out your belly button," says Dr. Fairbanks. "Dead skin, clothing lint, bacteria—all kinds of stuff—tend to accumulate in your belly button, and unless it's cleaned regularly, you can get a little infection. Just put a few drops of peroxide in there, let it fizz up, and clean it with a cotton swab."

. . . and yourself. What makeup wearer hasn't used cotton swabs to apply or remove eyeshadow or put on cold cream? White-faced circus clowns the world over, as well as more than a few women, swear by them.

Stomp out foot fungus. One of the ickiest aspects of athlete's foot and other foot foul-ups is . . . uuuuuugh, having to touch that nasty stuff between your toes. "Even the ointments for athlete's foot and other conditions can leave your hands very greasy, so you want to avoid that if you can," says Dr. Fairbanks. "A cotton swab is the perfect size for applying ointment or getting at whatever is between the toes."

Apply first aid. If you think Florence Nightingale was a softie, check out the tender touch of cotton against your bruising boo-boo. "Cotton swabs are excellent for applying medicine, whether it's first aid to a cut or scrape or for an ongoing condition like psoriasis. Using them can lower the chance of infection," Dr. Fairbanks continues. "Doctors have long used cotton-tip applicators for applying med-

icines and ointment—but back then, they were long wooden sticks with a ball of cotton on the end. In fact, they used to say that you could tell who was a careful and thorough doctor by the number of cotton-tip applicators in his wastebasket."

Swabs are especially handy for those hard-to-reach places. "Before there were antibiotics, mothers used swabs to apply iodine for a sore throat," he says. If you're using them to treat a scrape or minor cut, don't worry if strands of cotton get stuck in the wound. They'll fall out or shed when the scab is formed.

HELP FOR HALF-PINTS

Although cotton swabs are now mainly associated with cleaning ears, they were actually invented—way back in 1937—to help clean babies. "They were first called cotton buds and created primarily to clean the skin folds as well as the ears of babies," says Dave Swearingen, a spokesman for Johnson & Johnson. "Our company and a competitor (which markets Q-Tips) introduced them to the market within 45 days of each other. Both companies were working on the product without the other knowing about it; apparently, both saw the need for such a product in a growing market. I believe swabs were created because they were a safer and more efficient alternative to the old wooden sticks doctors used—and they were less likely to splinter and hurt someone."

cough medicines It begins with a tickle. Then there's some preparatory throat-clearing. Finally, after a dozen false starts, it comes: "Ack, ack, ack!" explodes your cough. "Ack, ack, ack!" Your chest hurts, your throat hurts, and you sound like Bill the Cat of comic-strip fame. Isn't there something that will stop that raucous cough?

It depends on the cough, says Barbara Phillips, M.D., associate professor of medicine at the University of Kentucky Medical Center in Lexington. If you're bringing up phlegm, you probably don't *want* to stop it. If it's a dry, racking, rattling cough, however, it might be time to take a cough suppressant.

HELPING PRODUCTIVE COUGHS

"If someone says, 'Doc, I've got this in my chest; I can feel it rattling, but I can't get it out,' that's when I might give expectorants," Dr. Phillips says. Expectorants and mucolytics make phlegm easier to cough up, primarily by thinning it. Guaifenesin, one of the more common expectorants, is the key ingredient in scores of cough remedies and cold medicines.

Another expectorant, Organidin (iodinated glycerol), has been found to ease the coughs associated with chronic asthma and bronchitis—conditions that afflict approximately 16 million Americans. According to one study, Organidin helped improve "cough symptoms, chest discomfort, mucus clearance, and patient well-being."

Some expectorants aren't found in the drugstore. Oven-hot foods, for example, stimulate mucus secretions and thin out pulmonary phlegm, which may explain the faith many people put in chicken soup. Spicy foods also break up congestion. A bowl of chili or a few drops of Tabasco mixed in a glass of water might help.

STOPPING DRY COUGHS

Few things are as unpleasant or as painful as persistent, hacking coughs. Coughs that come up dry as winter leaves. Coughs that leave you gasping for air. Coughs that may, during severe attacks, fracture ribs.

For nonproductive, out-of-control coughs, doctors may recommend cough suppressants such as codeine or dextromethorphan—drugs that block the brain's cough reflex. "I'm not going to let someone sit around and cough his head off when he's got a cough that's making him miserable, keeping him awake, and keeping him from eating," Dr. Phillips says.

Frequent drinks of water may relieve tickles that lead to dry coughs. Hot, moist air almost always helps, which is why people feel better when they take a hot, relaxing bath or soak up moisture in the steam room.

Just remember that coughing is a symptom, and people don't cough unless something else is wrong, Dr. Phillips says. "There are treatable medical conditions that cause coughing, such as asthma, postnasal drip, even heart failure."

Many dry coughs, for example, are caused by airway irritations. Throat and chest infections are common culprits, as are chemical fumes and air pollution. Rather than suppressing the coughing, it's better to eliminate—or avoid—what's causing the problems.

That's especially true for cigarettes, Dr. Phillips says. "Chronic cigarette smoking is the most common cause of productive coughs in this country. I'm not going to throw drugs at people who smoke cigarettes. I'm going to try to get them to quit." *See also* **eucalyptus; horehound**

CPR   The best lifesaving equipment you can find is free, readily available, and easy to operate. Simply using your mouth and your hands, you may be able to revive someone who is not breathing and whose heart is not beating. A procedure called CPR could keep the person alive until advanced life support arrives.

CPR is short for cardiopulmonary resuscitation, a basic life-support technique that involves using your hands to compress a victim's chest, reestablish heart action, and restore blood circulation. You use your mouth to blow air into the victim's lungs and restore breathing.

In a sense, CPR enables you to become the ultimate Good Samaritan. Anytime, anywhere, you may be able to save someone who has just drowned, suffocated, overdosed on drugs, or been involved in a highway accident.

The most likely occasion to use CPR, however, would be if someone in your household suddenly collapsed. According to the experts, 75 percent of sudden deaths result from unexpected cardiac arrest (heart stoppage) in a person's own home.

The top candidates for sudden death are people at risk for heart attack.

"If you live or work with someone with heart disease or who may be at risk for heart disease, it makes sense to learn CPR," says Larry Newell, Ph.D., senior associate for development for health and safety for the American National Red Cross.

Studies have shown that promptly performing CPR can double the victim's chances of surviving cardiac arrest.

HOW TO LEARN IT

The best way to learn CPR is to take a course sponsored by the American Red Cross or the American Heart Association. Such classes give you the opportunity to practice your newly learned skills on a mannequin under the supervision of trained instructors.

No one disputes that hands-on instruction is the most effective way to learn CPR. But if you can't possibly fit the full 4-hour certification course into your agenda, there are some shortcut alternatives. "Watching a CPR video or reading instructions can teach you enough skills to perform CPR and save a life," says Michael Eisenberg, M.D., professor of emergency medicine at the University of Washington in Seattle.

Currently, emergency medicine experts are trying to expose as many people as possible to CPR. Many workplaces and community centers now offer an abbreviated CPR course. And some public places, such as sports arenas, have installed prerecorded CPR-coaching audiotapes next to fire extinguishers. In case of an emergency, the rescuer puts on earphones and is talked through the CPR sequence while he is reviving the victim.

The more easily people can pick up CPR skills, the more lives can be saved, says Dr. Eisenberg. "I'd rather have a lot of people knowing a little about CPR than a few people knowing a lot," he says.

Experts are hoping that as CPR becomes more accessible, people will become more comfortable using the procedure. "Don't be afraid of intervening," says Robert Rosenthal, M.D., associate professor of emergency medicine at George Washington University. "Your skills don't have to be perfect," he says. In the case of a person who has no pulse, imperfect is better than nothing.

Because the technique, performed forcefully, does have the potential to crack a rib, the biggest danger is performing CPR unnecessarily on someone who is still breathing and has only fainted. "That's why it's so important to recognize when to use CPR," says Dr. Rosenthal. "But if the victim does not have a pulse, then obviously the benefits of revival outweigh the potential for injury."

Your major concern should be starting CPR immediately. The moment breathing and heartbeat stop, you have about 4 to 6 minutes before lack of oxygen begins to deteriorate the brain.

There is good evidence to show that if you start CPR within 4 minutes, the victim has a four times greater chance of surviving than if you start CPR *after* 4 minutes. "Speed is the key to survivability," says Dr. Rosenthal.

KNOW THE ABC'S

What's the first thing you should do if you come across someone who appears unresponsive? Yell for help. Then ask bystanders to dial 911 or the emergency operator. "Remember that CPR is only one in a series of emergency lifesaving procedures," says Dr. Newell. "The victim's chances of making it depend on the arrival of backup lifesaving systems that can actually restart the heart."

If there is no one around to call for emergency backup, you should perform CPR for 1 minute, stop, and dial 911 yourself. Return and resume the CPR sequence.

The following ABC's will help you remember the sequence of actions to take in an emergency.

Airways. After calling for help, roll the victim over on his back. Supporting the head and neck, open the airway while gently lifting up the chin with one hand and tilting the forehead back with the other.

Breathing. Rescue breathing should only be performed on someone who is absolutely not breathing. Bend your ear to the person's mouth. If you don't hear sounds of breathing, don't see the chest rise and fall, and don't feel the breath on your check, then prepare to perform rescue breathing.

Pinch the victim's nostrils with your thumb and index finger. Open your mouth, take a deep breath, and place your mouth tightly over the victim's mouth (mouth and nose for an infant or small child). Breathe into the victim's mouth two times. Watch for the victim's chest to rise. Repeat the breathing procedure, allowing the lungs to deflate between breaths.

Circulation. To determine if the heart is beating, find the pulse by placing your fingers in the groove between the Adam's apple and neck muscle. If there is no pulse, you will have to pump blood through the body yourself.

Kneel near the victim's chest. Move your fingers up the center of the chest to the notch where the ribs meet the breastbone. At this notch place the heel of your other hand two finger-widths above the fingers of first hand. Remove your fingers from the notch and place this hand on top of your other hand. Fingers should not touch the chest. With your elbows straight and your shoulders directly over your hands, press down quickly about 1½ to 2 inches. Allow the chest to return to normal position, keeping your hands on the chest. Pump rhythmically by counting out loud "one-and, two-and, three-and, . . ." Hold the chest compressed for the same length of time as the relaxation phase.

After every 15 compressions, take your hands off the chest and deliver two rescue breaths. Perform four complete cycles of 15 compressions and two breaths. Then, determine if the victim's pulse has returned. If there is a pulse but no breathing, take your hands off the chest, pinch the nostrils, and continue rescue breathing. If there is no pulse, repeat the 15 compressions and two breaths.

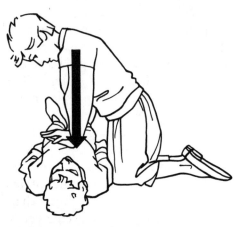

CPR chest compression technique

That's the condensed version of CPR. Remember, you can more effectively learn this technique and practice your skills by signing up for a CPR certification course. The more confidence you have in your CPR skills, the less likely you'll hesitate to use them in a real emergency.

cranberry juice Cranberry juice has been a favorite old-time remedy for ridding the body of bladder infections. According to popular theory, if you drink enough nectar from this tart-tasting, acidic crimson berry, the acid in your urine will wipe out the bacteria and that sharp, burning sensation when you urinate will disappear.

Acid *is* an enemy to *E. coli* bacteria, the bugs that cause urinary tract infections. Normally, these bacteria reside in the intestinal tract without causing trouble. But when they migrate to your urinary tract, they attach to bladder walls and cause inflammation. Hence, the stinging sensation when you go to the bathroom.

But does this cranberry juice home remedy really work in practice? Doctors are doubtful. "The role of cranberry juice as a urinary acidifier is poorly established," says Mark Soloway, M.D., a professor in the Department of Urology at the University of Tennessee Center for Health Sciences in Memphis. "The early studies are just not convincing."

If cranberry juice does raise the acidity of urine, it's not enough to keep bacteria at bay, Dr. Soloway says. In one study, researchers were able to show that drinking cranberry juice daily for three weeks stopped urinary infections in three-fourths of the patients. But for 61 percent of them, the infection returned just six weeks after they stopped drinking the juice.

The explanation for this temporary effect is simple, says Joseph Corriere, M.D., director of the Division of Urology at the University of Texas Medical School in Houston. "In the first 12 to 24 hours, your body begins to adjust by making buffers to check the higher acidity," he says. "As a result, the urinary tract becomes more hospitable for bacteria to breed again."

A BLOCKING EFFECT

There is some research to indicate that apart from its acidity, cranberry juice has the ability to block bacteria from clinging to the bladder walls.

"Bacteria have an outer capsule membrane with prongs that attach to the bladder wall," explains Michael J. Manyak, M.D., associate professor of urology at George Washington University. "Bacteria seem to adhere more easily in people with chronic bladder infections." So it makes sense that if bacteria could be prevented from latching onto the bladder wall, they could more easily be washed out by the fluids you drink.

In a study conducted at Youngstown State University in Ohio, 15 of 22 people showed this antiadherence effect in the urine 1 to 3 hours after drinking 15 ounces of cranberry cocktail (a mixture of cranberry juice, water, and sugar).

Doctors point out that this experiment shows only that after cranberry juice is consumed, bacteria don't adhere to bladder walls. "This study does not show that cranberry juice stops urinary tract infections," reminds Dr. Manyak.

If you have a bladder infection, doctors don't recommend turning to cranberry juice as a first line of defense. "You need an antibiotic to kill the bacteria," says Dr. Corriere. Sometimes all it takes is one dose of ampicillin, for example. "Ninety percent of bladder infections will clear up with one pill," he says.

Does this mean we should forget cranberry juice altogether? Maybe not. As a *preventive* measure, drinking lots of cranberry juice or any other fluid each day promotes frequent urination, says Dr. Manyak. The flood of fluids helps force out stray bacteria and prevent recurring infections.

Dr. Corriere agrees. "If cranberry

juice helps control your recurring bladder infections, then use it," he says. But plain water may work as well.

crying You don't remember your birth? Let's jog your memory: A pair of giant hands yanked you by the skull, you felt a snip at your belly button, and some monster flung you upside down to give you a swift whack on the tush. You responded in the only way you knew: You cried.

Certainly crying is part of the human condition. From the moment we're born, through the splinters, the scrapes, the school graduations, the weddings, the wars, and the waving goodbyes; through the hurt, the joy, the laughter, and the misery, we cry.

Why cry? "Crying is a way of relieving emotional stress," says William H. Frey II, Ph.D., research director of the Dry Eye and Tear Research Center at Minnesota's St. Paul Ramsey Medical Center. Actually, even when you're not crying, your eyes depend on tears, Dr. Frey says. Each blink spreads a tiny teardrop that bathes the surface of the eye and protects it from infection. When irritants like smoke, dust, or onion vapors are present, the faucet drips faster. And when frustrations build at work, a loved one dies, or other events cause your throat to tighten, the faucet opens up.

LET IT FLOW

How tears actually reduce stress is uncertain, but "our studies certainly show that people feel better after crying," says Dr. Frey, who summarized much of this research in his book, *Crying: The Mystery of Tears.* This expert's advice? "Allow yourself to cry when you're emotionally distressed and feel like crying—do not stop this natural process. It's perfectly all right to feel anger, sadness, or exasperation," he says.

If the thought of crying embarrasses you—stop blushing. You're in good company. Eighty-five percent of women and 50 percent of men, for example, report having cried at least once on the job, says Jeanne M. Plas, Ph.D., associate professor of psychology at Vanderbilt University, and coauthor of *Working Up a Storm: Anger, Anxiety, Joy, and Tears on the Job.*

Whether you're experiencing anger, anxiety, joy, or grief—go ahead and cry, because "these kinds of tears are probably cleansing and helpful," says Dr. Plas. The only time tears are *not* healthy, she warns, is when "they are a *substitute* for an ability to express emotions." It's important, says Dr. Plas, to communicate your feelings with others—even as you cry. "Many people believe you can't talk and cry at the same time—that's nonsense. It's like chewing bubble gum and walking—of course you can," she says.

STRESS DISSOLVER

With a wealth of research now pointing in the direction of a strong link between a healthy mind and a healthy body, it's easy to speculate that crying may be good preventive medicine. There hasn't been a lot of research into the connection between tears and disease. But one study, at the University of Pittsburgh, found that healthy persons are more likely to be criers than are those with ulcers and colitis, two diseases thought to be stress-related.

Dr. Frey theorizes that the healing activity of tears is chemical. That is, tears may remove chemicals that build up from emotional stress. In studies comparing emotional tears (brought on by tearjerker movies, such as *Brian's Song* and *The Champ*) to irritant tears (triggered by hunkering down over diced onions), Dr. Frey found that both contained certain chemicals thought to be related to stress. These included ACTH, a hormone recognized as a reliable indicator of stress, leucine-enkephalin, an endorphin thought to affect pain, and prolactin, a hormone released into the blood in response to stress.

So if you've been bottling up your tears for enough years to fill a riverbed, maybe it's time you got back in touch with your feelings, says Dr. Frey. If you sense that you can't do that on your own, "seek the help of a therapist—that's what they're there for," he says.

cryosurgery In little more than the time it takes to say "freeze!" cryosurgery can wipe out liver spots, hemorrhoids, warts, acne cysts, and any number of other skin nasties, including precancerous and cancerous growths. Cryosurgery uses extreme cold to destroy the diseased tissue. Eventually, the treated area blisters, separates itself from healthy tissue, and sloughs off.

The procedure is simple enough to be done in a doctor's office. It rarely requires anesthesia. The doctor applies a liquid (typically liquid nitrogen at $-321\,°F$) with either a cotton swab, a metal probe, or—more commonly—a spray canister to the area to be treated. If the growth is deep, the doctor will also freeze a "halo" of normal skin that is as wide around as the tumor is deep, to ensure that enough cold is applied to do the job. Cancerous growths may need to be frozen a second time, after the skin has thawed, says Gloria Graham, M.D., a North Carolina dermatologist and cryosurgeon.

Posttreatment care is simple, too. "First you'll see blisters. Just keep the area clean with soap and water," Dr. Graham advises. "You don't have to use a dressing, because the wound will dry out better if you expose it to the air. In about one week's time, a crust appears. Just let the wound heal under that crust."

If you are going to have cryosurgery done on your face, you may want to schedule it when you have no social obligations. The treated area tends to be unsightly until it has healed, says Dr. Graham.

Does cryosurgery hurt? If it is done without anesthesia, it can feel painfully cold for a few brief moments. Luckily, the discomfort doesn't last long. Dr. Graham says she once treated eight cancerous skin lesions on a patient in just a few minutes time. (Thawing time can add another 3 to 5 minutes.)

Side effects are few, but they can include loss of skin pigment, which may be more noticeable in dark-skinned people. Cold treatments potent enough to zap skin cancers can also destroy hair follicles, says Dr. Graham. In fact, some ophthalmologists capitalize on this effect by using cryosurgery to treat people whose eyelashes have grown in toward the cornea, scratching the eye.

SUN DAMAGE REPAIRED

Dr. Graham says she uses cryosurgery most often for people who get solar keratoses, those hard little growths that come from overexposure to the sun. "It takes 10 to 15 seconds to treat sun keratosis," she says. "The cure rate is 95 to 98 percent." Cryosurgery works well for another common condition, too: the small bumps that sometimes linger on the legs after insect bites.

And a recent study showed it to be more effective than laser surgery at eliminating brown liver spots, she says.

In a Swedish study, cryosurgery proved itself an excellent treatment for 121 people with a type of eyelid cancer called basal cell carcinoma. The cryosurgery successfully removed all of the small tumors, most of which were on the lower lid. There were no recurrences during the two-year follow-up period.

Cryosurgery has also been used to treat cervical dysplasia, a precancerous condition, and to bring at least temporary relief to the sufferers of bronchial cancer. But its primary role remains the treatment of skin complaints.

"I think it is simple, efficient, and cost-effective," says Dr. Graham.

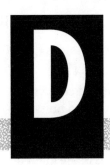

D & C   No gynecological operation is done more often than dilation and curettage, or D & C.

As the name suggests, it is a two-step procedure. First, a series of progressively larger rods, called dilators, are inserted—one at a time—to widen the narrow opening of the cervix. Then the doctor uses a spoon-shaped tool called a curette to scrape tissue from the upper layer of the uterine lining. Sometimes the doctor uses a low-suction device to vacuum the uterus instead of scraping it, a technique used to empty the uterus after a miscarriage and prevent infection.

But the most common reason for D & C's is to determine why a woman has abnormal uterine bleeding. Are there polyps, fibroids, an excessively thick uterine lining? Does the tissue show signs of endometrial cancer? These are conditions a D & C can diagnose.

Sometimes a D & C can even put an end to the abnormal bleeding, if polyps or an abnormally thick lining are to blame. That's because the scraping itself may restore the lining to normal, says Neil Jackson, M.D., direc-

tor of uro-gynecology at Women and Infants Hospital in Providence, Rhode Island.

The D & C can be done in the doctor's office, with just enough local anesthetic to numb the cervical area. Some women, especially those who have never been pregnant and are not sexually active, may require a general anesthetic to thoroughly relax the pelvic area. In that case, the operation is done in the hospital and requires a short stay.

The D & C procedure takes about 10 minutes. It's not unusual to experience mild cramps for an hour or two afterward. If it's done with a local anesthetic, the patient can usually be back at work within two days, Dr. Jackson says.

As with any surgery, there are potential complications. The three principal ones are perforation of the uterine cavity, hemorrhage, and infection, says Dr. Jackson, who is also a Brown University clinical associate professor of obstetrics and gynecology.

"It is a safe procedure," he says. "The complication rates are very low."

dandelion   It's been called a weed, a flower, and a salad green. People with infested lawns call it a darned nuisance. The Pennsylvania Dutch, on the other hand, say it makes a healthful spring tonic. Some herb experts praise it, while others simply mow it.

In short, there's much disagreement about one humble, ubiquitous plant: the dandelion.

"When the first dandelions come up in the early spring, you'll see people in the fields gathering them to make a hot salad," says Don Yoder, Ph.D., professor of folklife studies and American civilization at the University of Pennsylvania. "In fact, I eat them every year, and they're delicious."

Many people believe that these tough, hardy greens are not only salad fixings but medicine as well. Belonging to a group called the bitter plants, which includes yellowroot, gentian, and goldenseal, dandelion has been used as a laxative, liver tonic, and appetite stimulant. The milky fluid pressed from its root, leaves, and stem is even rumored to remove warts, although that may be stretching things, says James A. Duke, Ph.D., a botanist and toxicology specialist with the U.S. Department of Agriculture in Beltsville, Maryland.

"Wart cures are about as plentiful in folk medicine as snakebite cures, but I wouldn't say that dandelion milk has anything to do with a wart's disappearance," says Dr. Duke.

LIVER PROTECTOR?

He adds, however, that the dandelion's reputation for easing liver ailments may be justified. Researchers have suggested that a naturally occurring compound called lecithin may help prevent cirrhosis of the liver. Dandelion flowers, Dr. Duke says, contain nearly 30,000 parts per million of lecithin—almost twice the amount found in soybeans, a more widely known source.

In addition, dandelions also are rich in inulin, a slowly digested starch. Inulin—and, traditionally, dandelion—sometimes is recommended for people with diabetes who need to stabilize their blood sugar swings, says Dr. Duke.

Herbalists say that dandelion has both diuretic and laxative capabilities. For both uses, however, its effects appear quite mild, says Dr. Duke.

For the sniffles, however, a cup of dandelion tea, rich in vitamins C and A, might be helpful. "I would just grab a handful of dandelion, be it flowers, leaves, or root, and throw it in the pot, cover it with water, and boil it," says Dr. Duke.

When you simply have a hankering for dandelion salad, however, it's best to stick with the leaves, says Dr. Yoder. His method is to pluck the entire plant, shake off the loose dirt, cut off the root, and wash and drain the leaves. "Some people cook dandelion, but that's a mistake," Dr. Yoder insists. "It's better to mix something like a hot bacon dressing and pour it over the dandelion—it's very good."

decongestants   A stuffy nose is more than a nuisance. For starters, breathing through your mouth makes you look like a guppy. Your sense of smell is shot, your taste buds are kaput—even Mom's spicy-hot chili tastes flat. Plus, you have so much gunk clogging your nose that a truckload of tissues doesn't seem to help.

Fortunately, decongestant products can help unplug your nose and restore easier breathing.

Very likely, your trouble began when a microscopic cold virus or an allergen such as dust moved into your nose. This hostile newcomer caused quite a stir in the neighborhood. It irritated the delicate mucous membranes lining your nasal passages, causing the blood vessels to swell and fluid to accumulate in the surrounding tissue. As a result, your mucous membranes went into overtime producing gobs of mucus.

Trying to blow out the congestion only aggravates the problem. In fact, overeager nose blowing can force fluid into your sinuses—those hollow air spaces in the skull. Then, bacteria that are normally flushed out by free-flowing mucus may start to breed there. Before you know it, your stuffy nose has turned into a painful sinus infection.

"One of the best reasons for using a decongestant is to prevent simple nasal congestion from turning into sinusitis," says Neil Schachter, M.D., associate director of pulmonary medicine at Mount Sinai Medical Center in New York City.

Just as a traffic cop moves an obstruction blocking the flow of traffic, a decongestant helps shrink swollen blood vessels inside your nose, allowing air to travel in and out freely. A decongestant also halts excess mucus production that may be jamming your air passages. Swelling subsides, fluid drains, and you can breathe again.

SPRAYS ARE FASTER

You can take decongestants orally (by mouth) or topically (by spritzing them up your nose). Of the two, topical decongestants are the top choice of doctors.

To begin with, topicals ease breathing in minutes, compared to the hour it takes for medicine you swallow to wind its way through your system and finally unblock your nose.

Studies show that you can take a couple of squirts of oxymetazoline (the decongestant in many leading nose sprays) and presto: Your nose unclogs in 10 minutes and remains clear for up to 7 hours. With some products, such as Afrin, it's possible that one blast can last until bedtime.

Another advantage of nasal spray is that it puts the medicine directly where it's needed, says Jack Gwaltney, M.D., professor of internal medicine and head of epidemiology at the University of Virginia in Charlottesville.

Oral decongestants work like adrenaline: They stimulate the sympathetic nervous system. When the drug is absorbed into the bloodstream, it can make susceptible individuals feel jazzed up and cause blood vessels all over the body (not just in the nose) to constrict. That vessel-constricting action is what can boost blood pressure, raise heart rate, and elevate blood sugar.

Oral decongestants can be particularly hazardous if you already have high blood pressure.

One study conducted at the Vanderbilt Medical Center in Nashville, Tennessee, found a dramatic increase in blood pressure in patients with hypertension after taking the oral decongestant phenylpropanolamine hydrochloride. The researchers noted that decongestant doses given were identical to doses commonly found in over-the-counter cold medicines.

Clearly, if you need short-term relief for stuffiness, topicals are the better choice—especially if you have high blood pressure, heart or thyroid disease, prostate trouble, glaucoma, or diabetes, says Dr. Gwaltney.

Sprays are even better than drops or inhalers because they saturate larger portions of your nose while using less of the product. Plus, you'll swallow less of the medicine if it's in mist form.

CONGESTION SUGGESTION

To get the most benefit out of your nasal spray, squirt each nostril once, wait a few minutes and spray again, advises Branton Lachman, Pharm.D., clinical assistant professor at the University of Southern California School of Pharmacy in Los Angeles. "The first spritz clears some of the mucus and allows the second spray to penetrate more deeply so drainage is complete," he says.

Here's more good advice: Never share your nasal spray. The nose tip of the applicator may be loaded with germs that you can easily pass on to someone else. To guard against reinfecting yourself, wash the tip with mild soap after each use. Be sure to rinse it thoroughly, because the soap could irritate inflamed nasal passages.

Don't use your spray for more than three days. If you force your blood vessels to constrict longer than that time or use the spray too often, you may get "rebound congestion" and reach for more spray to get relief. Soon, you're hooked on the vicious rebound cycle. "The only way to break the rebound cycle is to quit cold turkey. Often, steroids are required to break the cycles. Or you can avoid it in the first place by stopping the sprays after three days and not exceeding the recommended dose," says Dr. Lachman.

If your nose is still stuffed up after three days of spraying (and you do not have hypertension or any of the disorders mentioned above and you're not taking medication for those conditions), a mild oral decongestant containing pseudoephedrine (such as Sudafed) may give you the extra drainage power you need.

"Despite their drawbacks, oral decongestants can reach remote areas in your nasal passages that sprays just can't reach," notes Dr. Lachman. They may also provide longer relief than some sprays.

Take your decongestant several hours before bed and follow label directions exactly. Limit alcohol while taking a decongestant; it could boost the drug's effects on your nervous system. Never take a decongestant without checking with your physician if you are taking monoamine oxidase (MAO) inhibitor drugs—the combination could be fatal.

See your doctor if you are still stuffy after a week of using an oral decongestant. *See also* **cold remedies**

dental floss For something that started out as a simple thread used to clean between the teeth, dental floss has come a long way. You can now choose from waxed or unwaxed, regular gauge or extra fine, thread or ribbon, looped or unlooped, plain or mint-flavored. But they're all designed to do the same thing: remove plaque, a soft, sticky, colorless goo that hardens on the teeth into calculus. Unchecked, plaque and calculus can jeopardize the health of your teeth and gums by causing periodontal disease.

Floss is an especially important component of a good oral hygiene program because it cleans between teeth and underneath the gumline, where your toothbrush can't reach. Even if you brush your teeth thoroughly after every meal, dentists say you still need to floss every day.

To get started, break off a piece of

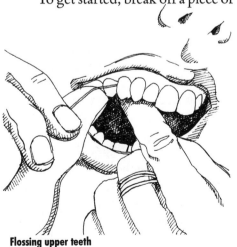

Flossing upper teeth

floss about 18 inches long. Lightly wrap most of the floss around the middle finger of one hand. Wrap the rest of the floss around the middle finger of the other hand. Holding the unraveled portion of the floss tightly between your thumbs and forefingers, insert it between the teeth and slide it gently to the gumline. Curve the floss into a C-shape and move it up and down against the side of each tooth. Use a new, clean section as the floss becomes frayed or soiled.

Proper flossing is an acquired skill. Your dentist or dental hygienist will be happy to coach you. Practice until you get the hang of it. (Floss threaders, floss picks, and other clever devices are available to make flossing less awkward.)

WHICH TO CHOOSE?

With a few exceptions, what kind of floss you use isn't as important as using it properly and frequently.

"Fine or waxed floss is helpful for people who have tight or crooked teeth," says Gary Maynard, D.D.S., clinical professor of periodontology at Virginia Commonwealth University School of Dentistry. "It doesn't shred as easily. On the other hand, if you have bridgework, dental implants, or wide spaces between your teeth and gums, larger floss can clean your teeth faster and more efficiently." Dr. Maynard recommends "three-in-one" type floss. The strands are precut into 25-inch lengths, with a stiffened end (to thread between your teeth), a middle section of yarnlike material (to "brush" between teeth), and an unwaxed section of regular floss. Compared to ordinary floss, the stiffened end of three-in-one floss is easier to thread through tight or hard-to-reach places, such as under fixed bridgework.

Looped floss threaders are another useful tool for flossing under bridgework and between crowns. Simply pull the first 4 or 5 inches of an 18-inch strand of floss through the nylon loop. Then pass the threader through the space under bridgework or between crowns and teeth.

As for the best time to floss—morning, noon, or night—Dr. Maynard says timing isn't critical. "Just make sure you do it around the same time every day—once every 24 hours—before plaque can harden."

dentistry, restorative They bite corn, munch apples, and crunch hard candy. They chew steaks and tear at taffy. Sometimes they even rip through boxes and envelopes. Our teeth get a rugged workout every day, so it's not surprising they need occasional repairs.

When dentists talk about restorative dentistry, they're referring to caps and crowns, fillings and bridges, implants and dentures—structural repairs that put the bite back into damaged teeth. Some procedures—filling a cavity, for example—have been around for more than a century. Others, such as dental implants, are just getting started.

Let's take a closer look at the most common procedures.

FILLINGS

As the name suggests, fillings are used to fill small holes, called cavities or dental caries, in the teeth. There are several reasons for having your teeth filled, says Henry W. Finger, D.D.S., president of the Academy of General Dentistry and former associate clinical professor of dental radiology at Temple University in Philadelphia. As you might expect, teeth with holes need some reinforcement or they might break. In addition, holes offer a hiding place for bacteria, which, given time, can cause nerve infections and abscesses and eventually could destroy the entire tooth.

Fillings traditionally have been made from amalgam, a durable mixture of silver, tin, and mercury. But amalgam fillings eventually shrink and pull away from the tooth, leading to what dentists call microleakage as bacteria move into the tiny cracks.

Many dentists now are using composite resins—plastic fillings that fit more tightly than amalgam, and with less shrinkage. Unlike amalgam fillings, which often require a lot of drilling to achieve a tight fit, the composite resins can be bonded to the tooth, creating a better seal. In addition, their color and texture nearly match the natural teeth, so they look better than metal fillings.

Both types of fillings, on average, will last about seven years, Dr. Finger says.

SEALANTS

These are applied to the teeth *before* cavities form. "On the chewing surface of the tooth, there are pits and fissures, which are where plaque collects," Dr. Finger says. "The sealant is a plastic material that actually seals these grooves so plaque cannot get in." Whereas unsealed teeth may host hundreds of thousands of cavity-causing bacteria, sealed teeth may stay bacteria free for years and often for a lifetime.

Children are especially vulnerable to pit-and-fissure cavities. When their teeth are regularly coated with sealants, however, they stand a good chance of growing up with zero cavities. That's good news for kids *and* dentists, Dr. Finger says. "When you don't have to give a needle to a 7-year-old child, everybody's much happier."

ROOT CANAL

This much-dreaded procedure scarcely lives up to its reputation, Dr. Finger says. In fact, root canal procedures rarely are any more painful—or complicated—than filling a cavity.

To understand what's involved, we have to look deep inside the tooth. Teeth, like trees, have roots that supply them with nutrients. Each tooth has at least one root, and some teeth have as many as five, Dr. Finger says. The roots—and accompanying nerves—are contained in channels, called root canals, that extend from the middle of the tooth to the jawbone below.

"If that nerve dies, either because of decay or trauma, you develop infections," Dr. Finger says. "The typical toothache is an infection in the root canal."

Dentists handle root canals much as they would a filling. First, they remove bacteria and debris—in this case, the decayed nerve. (Your tooth will do fine without it.) The canal, now hollow, is sterilized, then filled with a plastic filling. During a later appointment, the tooth is capped.

CAPS AND CROWNS

Technically, the crown of your tooth simply is the part above the gum line, while a cap is an artificial cover for the crown. But most of the time, Dr. Finger says, the terms are used interchangeably.

A tooth commonly is capped when it's too damaged to survive on its own. The cap simply slips over the entire tooth and takes the brunt of the pressure as the tooth goes about its duties. Amalgam isn't strong enough to bear the force of biting and chewing, so caps often are made from plastic, gold alloys, or porcelain, Dr. Finger says.

To install a cap, two sessions with the dentist generally are required. During the first visit, the dentist prepares the tooth and takes measurements for the cap. During the second appointment, the custom-made cap is cemented into place.

As with fillings, caps should last about seven years, although many will last a lifetime, Dr. Finger says.

DENTAL IMPLANTS

Many people, when they lose some of their natural teeth, don a set of dentures. But dentures never quite feel like the real thing. It can be a full-time job just to keep them from wobbling. As for eating apples or other hard foods—forget it!

Now there's a better way.

In a process called osseointegration, dentists surgically implant small titanium posts into the jawbone to serve as roots. After a few months, bone attaches to the metal, making a stout, permanent anchor. Prosthetic teeth, made from composite resins or other materials, are then attached to the posts.

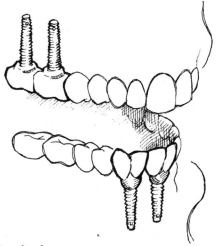

Dental implants

"There are now about 300,000 implant procedures performed yearly in the United States alone," Dr. Finger says. "Since the teeth are permanently attached to the posts, they're as stable as your own teeth. You can chew anything. It's definitely preferable to a removable bridge."

BRIDGES

Like implants, dental bridges simply hold artificial teeth—one or an entire set—in place. However, remaining teeth are used to support the replacement teeth, so artificial roots are not needed. That makes bridges less expensive.

Basically, there are two types of bridges: fixed and removable. The fixed bridge, often secured to healthy teeth, permanently holds false teeth in place. The removable bridge, on the other hand, is fitted with clamps. It can be popped out for cleaning, then snapped back into place. Less expensive than a fixed bridge, the removable bridge is somewhat less solid. It also tends to be more conspicuous.

"Obviously, the appearance of a removable bridge leaves a lot to be desired, because you can sometimes see the metal clamps," Dr. Finger says. He predicts that removable bridges will become less common as dental implants become more affordable.

BRACES

For generations of unsmiling children with crooked teeth, braces seemed little less than eternal punishments. They endured trapped food, taunts from their peers, and painful hours in the dentist's chair, all for that distant day when they, too, could smile without being called "metal mouth."

Today's braces are more comfortable and less conspicuous than the older stainless-steel catcher's masks. Nor are braces worn only by children, Dr. Finger says.

"Thanks to braces, people smile again, and feel good about themselves," he says. "And by providing the appropriate alignment, the teeth are made more self-cleaning. Very often, straight teeth can reduce people's risk for periodontal disease or decay."

Braces may be made from metal, clear plastic, ceramic, or, in some cases, sapphire, one of nature's hardest substances. Some braces actually fit on the *insides* of the teeth. They're invisi-

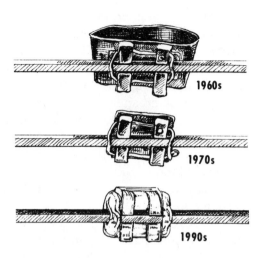

1960s

1970s

1990s

Orthodontic braces

ble to everyone but the dentist (and she won't tell).

COSMETIC HELP

As America's dental health improves, dentists will spend less time on structural problems and more time perfecting bright, sparkling smiles. "People say we're trying to put ourselves out of business with pit-and-fissure sealants, fluoride, and other preventive measures, but there are a lot of aesthetic and cosmetic types of dentistry that will be needed in the future," Dr. Finger says.

Crowns can not only repair a broken tooth but render it more attractive as well. In fact, today's porcelain crowns are nearly indistinguishable from adjoining teeth.

Veneers are extremely hard, thin strips of porcelain that are cemented to the front of a tooth. People with stained or chipped front teeth, for example, may cover the damage with veneers. Crowns also can conceal chips

and stains. More durable than veneers, they're also more expensive.

Somewhat less durable than veneers or crowns, a process called bonding actually builds up the tooth's surface with a tough, brush-on plastic. Not only can bonding conceal chips and stains, it can even reduce the gaps between teeth.

Bleaching is the least expensive option for hiding recalcitrant stains. Regularly applied by the dentist, bleaching substances have helped brighten many a smile.

THE FUTURE

Trips to the dentist, for most people, will become less frightening, Dr. Finger says. Lasers, common in many medical specialties, are appearing in dental offices, too. That's good news, because lasers eventually may be used to remove plaque, clean cavities, and make incisions—all with little pain and, in most cases, no need for anesthetics and needles. In fact, lasers may even make the dreaded drill obsolete—a hoped-for day indeed!

But the basics of good dental care—a healthy diet, daily flossing and brushing, and regular trips to the dentist—still count, Dr. Finger says. "The progression of dental disease, in adults, is very, very slow. If we can just convince people to brush and floss every day, and visit their dentist regularly, they won't have so many problems." *See also* **dental floss**

deodorants Unless you're a trapeze artist, a painter who does only ceilings, or a very unlucky bank robber, you probably know something about de-odorants, and more specifically, anti-perspirants. Unless you keep your arms over your head all day, you're going to need one.

"Walking around with your arms at your sides, as most people do, makes the armpits one of those areas—like the groin—that's closed in," says William L. Epstein, M.D., chairman emeritus and professor of dermatology at the University of California, San Francisco, School of Medicine and a longtime deodorant researcher. "That makes for an environment that sweat and odor-causing bacteria love to be in."

The problem is, when those two nasties get together, it tends to have a decidedly negative effect on the folks around you.

That's not to say your scent will be on the up-and-up if your arms are. "The odor from your armpits comes from a special kind of bacteria that grows in the glands of the armpits," says Dr. Epstein. "Many people think it's caused by excessive sweating, but it's not. Walk into a gym and you'll see that you don't have to sweat a lot to give off an odor. In fact, only about 20 percent of people have a sweating problem. But you've probably noticed that a lot more have an odor."

Which is why they use deodorants, to prevent that embarrassing sweating and kill the organisms that cause the odor. But such protection doesn't always come without a price. The very power these products have against smell and wetness can irritate and cause rashes in many people.

"The biggest problem with de-odorants is finding one that doesn't irritate," says Dr. Epstein. "What often happens is you'll buy one and after a while, it begins to irritate. So you switch to another brand and after a while, it also irritates you. So you switch back to the first one and it's fine. Finding the right deodorant often is a trial-and-error kind of thing. But no matter what you buy, most are pretty much the same thing."

That's because most if not all commercial brands have the same active ingredient: aluminum chlorohydrate—antibacterial salts that prevent sweating (because they're drying agents) while killing the organisms that cause the odor. But that's not all aluminum chlorohydrate–containing deodorants can do.

POISON IVY PROTECTION

Several years ago, Dr. Epstein was approached by the U.S. Forestry Service to come up with an inexpensive way to keep its rangers from contracting poison ivy. He found his answer in the same commercial deodorants you use. Dr. Epstein and his colleagues stumbled on the fact that the organic clay suspending agent in spray deodorants prevents the oils in poison ivy and oak from irritating the skin. "Deodorants contain around 2 to 3 percent clay, but 10 to 15 percent clay would work even better," says Dr. Epstein.

Deodorants have also been used to stop bleeding (wetness isn't the only thing aluminum salts help dry). "It works, but it's not recommended by dermatologists," says Dr. Epstein. Other proven, but not necessarily recommended, deodorant uses include preventing athlete's foot (a dry foot is a fungus-free foot) and killing the itch of insect stings. "Some people use deodorants for both of those purposes, and in theory, they work. But I don't think they work very well," says Dr. Epstein. "Besides, there are commercially sold products that do a better job and aren't much more expensive than a can of Right Guard."

HOMEMADE BRANDS

Those who are *really* pinching pennies probably already know that baking soda (sodium bicarbonate) is an effective odor killer and wetness preventer that's used by many as an inexpensive deodorant.

Sodium bicarbonate works by absorbing the odor. "However, don't be discouraged if this doesn't help you," says Dr. Epstein. "Sodium bicarbonate works fine for some people, but not others. And nobody knows why."

But there are other alternatives. Vinegar is another substance, for example, that cuts odor by boosting acidity. But you've got to smell pretty powerful to begin with to put vinegar — not exactly the sweetest-smelling stuff there is — under your arms.

Some people rub vitamin E ointments or opened capsules on their armpits. "This is *very* irritating and can cause bad rashes," Dr. Epstein says. "Besides, it's extremely expensive and it's not even clear if it works."

There are also expensive deodorant products that claim to last three or four days, but they are a waste of money

for most people, says Dr. Epstein. "If you've got a real sweating problem, they're not going to work for you. If you're like most people, you don't need them. Stick with the once-a-day brands; they're cheaper and just as effective."

desensitization. *See* **allergy shots; behavior therapy**

diabetes diet   Sometimes the best reasons for adhering to a diet have nothing to do with vanity.

If you have diabetes, for example, ignoring the dietary recommendations of your doctor or dietitian can — in the short run — lead to dehydration and diabetic coma, and — in the long run — increase your risk of obesity, blindness, kidney failure, high blood pressure, heart disease, and premature death.

"I would say the diet is the cornerstone of diabetes treatment," says Audrey Lally, a registered dietitian and certified diabetes educator at the Mayo Clinic in Scottsdale, Arizona.

The diet recommended for those with diabetes is a critical part of controlling their disease because it helps regulate the body's level of blood sugars. And that diet continues to evolve after centuries of guesswork and misunderstanding of how diabetes works.

About four million Americans have diabetes. There are two major types of this chronic and not yet curable disease. Type I, once called juvenile-onset diabetes, occurs when, for some unknown reason, the immune system attacks the pancreas and destroys the body's ability to make insulin. Insulin is a hormone that cells need to convert blood sugars into fuel. In addition to making diet modifications, people with this form of diabetes must take insulin injections.

Type II diabetes, on the other hand, usually occurs in adults. The peak years for onset are ages 50 to 60. After it strikes, the body is still able to produce insulin. But insulin isn't very effective at getting blood sugar into cells. Type II diabetics are able to control their disease with diet and exercise. But some patients with this form of the disease need to take oral diabetes medication or insulin shots.

"The resistance of cells to insulin in Type II is like a door with a rusty hinge. It can be opened and closed, but not too easily, so blood sugars can't get in as freely," says Richard Dolinar, M.D., a Phoenix endocrinologist and author of *Diabetes 101.*

Without insulin, cells can't absorb the blood sugars, and those sugars build up to dangerously high levels in the bloodstream, Dr. Dolinar explains.

"Our feeling is that when blood sugars get too high, you start seeing damage to major organs of the body such as the heart, eyes, and kidneys," he says. "We don't know if the high sugar itself does the damage or if the high sugar triggers a sequence of events leading to those problems."

But Dr. Dolinar and other doctors do know that those people with diabetes who keep their blood sugar under control are less likely to develop complications of the disease. And the best way to maintain control is diet.

ADVICE HAS CHANGED

Doctors have known since the time of Hippocrates that excessive amounts of dietary sugar, for example, are bad for diabetics, says David Johnson, M.D., an endocrinologist at the University of Arizona Health Sciences Center in Tucson.

In 1775, a British surgeon advocated that diabetics eat a diet that was devoid not only of sugar but of practically all carbohydrates. That recommendation, which became the hallmark of the diabetic diet, was followed for more than a century.

In the 1930s and 1940s, doctors recommended that diabetics eat a high-fat, low-carbohydrate diet that discouraged consumption of simple (refined) sugars such as candy, alcohol, starches such as breads and potatoes, and other carbohydrates such as fruits and vegetables. But many researchers now believe that that diet contributed to the high incidence of coronary heart disease among diabetics. In fact, studies indicate that coronary artery disease is 2.5 times more common among diabetics than among people who don't have the disease.

Today, doctors and dietitians believe that there is much more to carbohydrates and they should play a much larger role in a healthy diabetic diet than once suspected, Lally says. Researchers now know all forms of carbohydrate do not affect blood sugar levels in the same way.

Complex carbohydrates such as beans and whole grain breads are digested more slowly than simple carbohydrates such as honey, corn syrup, and molasses, Lally says. Because of that, complex carbohydrates are less likely to cause blood sugar to rise rapidly. Limiting simple carbohydrates is crucial in controlling diabetes.

Based on such research over the past decade, the American Diabetes Association now recommends a high-fiber, high-complex-carbohydrate, low-sodium, low-fat diet. The association suggests that a good diabetic diet consist of up to 55 to 60 percent carbohydrates, less than 30 percent fat, and the rest protein.

To simplify all that, the American Diabetes Association and the American Dietetic Association have developed exchange lists for foods in six broad categories—starch/bread, meat, vegetable, fruit, milk, and fat. Since servings of foods within each group have approximately the same amount of carbohydrates, proteins, and fats, they can be readily exchanged for one another. For example, a person could eat ⅓ cup of rice, one slice of bread, or ½ cup of pasta to fulfill the starch/bread portion of his or her daily need for starches.

The American Diabetes Association also recommends that up to 40 grams of dietary fiber, from sources such as fruits, vegetables, whole grains, and beans, be included in the diet each day. Research indicates that fiber slows the absorption of food and reduces the rate at which sugar enters the bloodstream.

For many people with diabetes whose blood sugar is under control,

table sugar and other sweets aren't totally frowned upon anymore. That's because modest amounts of sugars, when eaten with a full meal, aren't absorbed into the bloodstream as quickly as once thought, says Madelyn Wheeler, a registered dietitian and former American Diabetes Association vice-president. If you're trying to lose weight, however, you don't need the added calories from sweets.

Up to 5 percent of the recommended diet can come from refined sugar if eaten as part of meals, Lally says.

BONUS BENEFITS

A high-carbohydrate, high-fiber diet also helps diabetics lose weight. Obesity, often a consequence of diabetes, hinders insulin from doing its job and contributes to high cholesterol, Dr. Dolinar says.

Losing weight also can reduce the need for insulin, Lally says. Some of her patients with Type II diabetes who lost more than 50 pounds were able to stop using insulin and control their diabetes with a high-carbohydrate diet alone.

Many physicians also say the diabetic diet is a good diet for *all* people, not just those with diabetes.

"Rather than call it a diabetic diet, I think we should call it a healthy diet, because it's something that everyone should follow," Dr. Dolinar says.

If you have diabetes, doctors say that you shouldn't skip meals or eat too many large meals. That can cause unhealthy peaks and valleys in your blood sugar levels. Instead, Dr. Dolinar recommends that patients should eat several small meals daily. If they have insulin-dependent diabetes, they are advised to eat breakfast, lunch, and dinner, with three well-timed snacks between meals. If they have Type II diabetes, then three meals a day plus a late-night snack should help keep their blood sugar under control, he says. Be sure to check with your doctor, though, before making any changes in diet or medication.

digitalis (dihj-ih-TAL-iss) The name may sound like a hair tonic, but it actually refers to the fingerlike leaves of the foxglove plant from which this drug was first derived over 200 years ago. There are now two versions of the drug—digoxin and digitoxin—that are more chemically refined and that together have become the second most widely prescribed of all medications currently in use in the United States.

Their purpose: to boost the pumping power of the heart following a heart attack, to control heart rhythm disturbances, and to treat congestive heart failure, a condition in which fluid builds up in the body as a result of the heart's inability to adequately empty itself of blood.

The drugs work by improving the pumping action of the heart in two ways—first, by making more calcium available to cardiac muscle, thus improving a chemical-to-energy conversion responsible for the force of each beat; and second, by slowing the electrical impulses that make the heart contract, thus restoring irregular or quickened pulses to a normal pace.

POWERFUL MEDICINE

Of the two types of digitalis, digoxin is the more common. Digitoxin is usually prescribed only when a patient can't tolerate digoxin because of kidney disease. Because the therapeutic dose of both drugs is only one-third less than a dose that would be toxic, they must be monitored very closely for potentially harmful side effects—excessive fatigue, confusion, headaches, changes in vision, loss of appetite, nausea, vomiting, and diarrhea. Another negative side effect can be "heart block," a situation where the heart slows down *too* much.

Negative side effects of digitalis drugs are more likely to occur in the presence of low potassium levels. Since the drugs often are given in conjunction with diuretics, which can deplete the body of this important mineral, eating plenty of potassium-rich fruits and vegetables and/or taking a potassium supplement often is recommended for digitalis patients. Digitalis drugs also may react negatively with drugs such as antibiotics and antacids. Notify your doctor should you experience any negative effects from the drug.

Used properly under a physician's care, however, digitalis can be a relatively safe and extremely effective remedy for some potentially very serious heart problems.

dilation and curettage. *See* **D & C**

diuretics (die-yur-ET-icks) Commonly referred to as water pills, diuretics prompt your kidneys to flush more sodium and water from the body. Reduced salt and fluid lowers the volume of blood coursing through your arteries and veins, taking a burden off your heart.

Used since the 1950s, diuretics are a mainstay for controlling high blood pressure (and thereby preventing strokes and kidney failure). But lowering blood volume is also critical in congestive heart failure, a condition in which fluid backs up and accumulates in the lungs, legs, or elsewhere. Working on the intricate tubing that snakes within the kidneys, diuretics can flush away as much as 2 pounds or more of excess fluid a day, reducing edema (fluid buildup). As you might guess, people taking diuretics notice a substantial increase in urine flow.

3 WAYS TO FLUSH

When it comes to getting rid of excess fluid, diuretics get the job done. They fall into three basic categories.

Thiazide diuretics. This type, which includes chlorothiazide and chlorthalidone, is usually prescribed for high blood pressure. Thiazide diuretics have been shown to prevent strokes in people with high blood pressure.

On the minus side, thiazide diuretics may aggravate glucose intolerance, a potential problem in diabetics. They also tend to flush potassium—a vital mineral—out of the body, but this can be countered by eating potassium-rich foods (such as bananas), adding a potassium chloride supplement, and/or taking a potassium-sparing diuretic (see below).

At first, thiazide diuretics may make you feel unusually tired. But this side effect often disappears in time. Thiazide diuretics may also cause sexual problems—loss of desire, inability to sustain an erection, or decreased vaginal lubrication. Adjusting the dosage may help. Note, too, that thiazides may occasionally make you unusually sensitive to sunlight.

Loop diuretics. These drugs, including bumetanide, ethacrynic acid, and furosemide, are more potent than thiazides. They work on a portion of the kidney called the loop of Henle. When given intravenously, loop diuretics go to work in minutes, making them particularly useful for acute pulmonary edema (fluid buildup in the lungs), severe or hard-to-treat heart failure, or kidney failure.

Potassium-sparing diuretics. These diuretics, which include amiloride, spironolactone, and triamterene, do little to control blood pressure by themselves. They're primarily used to offset potassium losses triggered by thiazides.

Diuretics may be given as single therapy or combined with other drugs to enhance the effectiveness of all classes of blood pressure-lowering medication. *See also* **antihypertensives; beta blockers**

DMSO Few drugs have been worshiped—or condemned—as much as DMSO (dimethyl sulfoxide). Developed by a Russian scientist in 1866, it was not until 1947 that this substance began to spark any significant scientific interest. Chemists discovered that it was one whale of a solvent, capable of penetrating the human skin and entering the bloodstream so quickly that within minutes it could be smelled on the breath of anyone who touched it. In 1959, British researchers found that DMSO could protect red blood cells and other human tissue from freezing temperatures, and excitement over its medical applications grew from there. The drug soon had itself a word-of-mouth reputation as a miracle drug capable of treating sprains, strains, bruises, minor burns, and even arthritis, and was being used by tens of thousands of people.

So why the objections to DMSO? Years of testing by the Food and Drug Administration (FDA) have been able to earn the stuff approval as a treatment for one condition and one condition only: a rare bladder disorder known as interstitial cystitis, an inflammation of the walls of the bladder that occurs primarily in women over 40. None of the other claims for DMSO have been able to stand up to the FDA's scrutiny.

Testing of DMSO continues, however. It's being examined for potential benefits in the treatment of some forms of cancer, brain injuries, spinal injuries, stroke, and diseases of the autoimmune system and skin.

SAFETY ISSUES

Until these tests produce positive results sufficient to win FDA approval, however, most doctors caution strongly against its use. Even when used under medical supervision, DMSO can cause skin rashes and itching. It's also been associated with age problems such as blurred vision in people and cataracts in animals. Perhaps its greatest danger, however, stems from its power as a solvent: When applied to the skin, it penetrates into the bloodstream immediately, carrying with it any contaminant that may be on the skin or hands at the time the application is made. This can be especially dangerous because no standards of purity exist for most of the DMSO being sold. Several states allow industrial-grade DMSO to be sold over the counter as a solvent, but only DMSO purchased by prescription from a pharmacy can be assured to be contaminant free.

"No one should use DMSO without a doctor's prescription, and then only after asking to see the evidence that the substance is effective for the ailment in question," says Sheldon Saul Hendler, M.D., Ph.D., author of *The Doctor's Vitamin and Mineral Encyclopedia.* "The DMSO that is being sold in many stores and on the street . . . is almost never of the pure grade used in clinical trials, and contaminants pose a real risk."

Risky, too, is the garliclike stench put off by DMSO users. "I could clear a city bus in 30 seconds," one user has had the honesty to admit.

Dong quai.   *See* **Chinese herbs**

douching   Many women who want to eliminate vaginal odors or relieve itching and minor irritations still rely on this technique of flushing the vaginal canal with fluid.

But few doctors endorse regular douching. Studies suggest that the practice can increase a woman's risk of ectopic pregnancy and pelvic inflammatory disease (PID), a condition in which the uterus, fallopian tubes, and ovaries become inflamed.

"My own recommendation would be to bathe rather than douche," says Katherine Forrest, M.D., a California public health physician. (If vaginal odor can't be controlled by bathing, Dr. Forrest recommends having a doctor check for possible infection.) Examining the link between douching and PID, her team found a possible association, which received further confirmation in a University of Washington study of 100 municipal hospital patients with verified PID. That study found that women who douched three or more times a month were 3.6 times more likely to get PID than women who douched less than once a month.

The risk may be higher among women using some commercial douches than those using water or homemade vinegar-and-water solutions, Dr. Forrest notes.

No one knows exactly how douching might increase the risk for inflammatory disease. One theory is that douching may decrease the number of normal vaginal bacteria, so that disease-causing organisms can grow more readily. Another is that douching could flush vaginal and cervical microorganisms up into the uterine cavity.

IS USE JUSTIFIED?

These risks aside, the vagina is perfectly capable of cleaning itself, Dr. Forrest says. "As with any part of the body, there are white blood cells that scavenge dead cells. And the vaginal walls and cervix release lubricants that keep the vagina clean."

Are there any uses for douches? Some doctors recommend them on occasion for women suffering from a mild yeast infection. Manhattan, Kansas, gynecologist Rex Fischer, M.D., says they can help a woman who is using vaginal medication but experiencing heavy discharge. Eliminating the discharge can help the medicine work better, he says.

If you choose to douche, be gentle, says Dr. Forrest. "Most women probably put the douche nozzle up as far as they can and run fluid in as fast as they can. That will just increase their chances of getting the fluid—and possibly, problematic organisms—up into the cervix."

dream therapy   You don't need a leather couch and an analyst to learn from your dreams. Dream therapy experts say that with a little know-how, you can decode your dreams for greater self-knowledge and help in solving emotional problems, overcoming fears, and creating a healthier life.

In the self-help approach to dream therapy, also called "dream work," it's assumed that dreams have meanings that are relevant to problems in your current life. The function of dreaming, according to this view, is to make you more aware of feelings and information in your mind that you simply haven't recognized or thought of as important before. This is much broader than the traditional Sigmund Freud view that dreams represent repressed, unfulfilled childhood wishes.

Another difference: Some modern dream work experts believe that those wacky, weird images represent personal things only the dreamer can interpret; they are not fixed, universal symbols that require an advanced degree to decipher. "Insight comes from the dreamer, not the analyst," says Loma Flowers, M.D., director of the Delaney and Flowers Center for the Study of Dreams in San Francisco.

CAPTURING IMAGES

Do-it-yourself dream therapy starts by "catching" your dreams, a skill you can learn in a few days. This typically involves placing a notebook or, if you prefer, a voice-activated tape recorder by your bedside. Tell yourself before falling asleep that you will remember your dreams. Immediately upon awakening, lie still and try to "catch" fragments of your dream as they float into your consciousness. It's often possible to recapture an entire dream this way.

Once you've written out or recorded your dream, ask yourself a series of questions to get at the heart of its meaning. Consider each image and ask, "What does this image remind me of in my waking life?" Now ask yourself the same question about the plot.

For example, one woman, who had accompanied her husband on a business trip, dreamed about taking a timed test. Because the teacher wouldn't give her a booklet, she couldn't get started on the test. She was frustrated and worried that time would run out. She later interpreted the test as representing whether she and her husband—both busy people—could still find time

to have fun together. She also became aware of how much importance she had placed on that business trip as a recreational opportunity. She talked this over with her husband and they made plans to have fun together.

Use so-called dream dictionaries only as a source of ideas, experts advise. While it's true that there are common images and dream themes such as falling, flying, or being chased, the meaning of such themes and images differs from person to person and even from dream to dream. A dream about running, for example, could mean off and running, running away, or running into a snag. So look for the obvious as well as the abstract meaning represented in your images. Brainstorm about their meaning until you come up with an interpretation that seems to ring a bell with you.

Overall, the most important questions to ask yourself are: "How do the images and plot make me feel? Where in my current life are these same feelings being played out?" Based on this insight, you can then design alternative strategies to help you resolve this real-life situation.

If you need additional help uncovering the meaning of your dream, try making a drawing of it. Then give your drawing to another person to interpret. You might also try sharing your dream with a group.

Sometimes, when themes surface in a dream that are particularly complicated or that we are reluctant to deal with, it's easy to deceive ourselves or to overlook certain important aspects of the dream. "Dreams tell us the truth about ourselves; they don't lie," says Montegue Ullman, M.D., clinical professor emeritus of psychiatry at Albert Einstein College of Medicine in New York City and author of *Working with Dreams.* "Sharing your dreams with a group can keep you honest."

SHARING DREAMS

If you have an area of life where you seem to be stuck and haven't a clue as to how to free yourself, an ancient technique called "dream incubation" could give you some ideas. Before falling asleep, you simply think about the area where you have a concern and ask your dreaming brain to present you with a clear dream about the issue. Be persistent. "With a little practice," Dr. Flowers says, "you are likely to have a dream that brings the issue to the surface in a way that leads to resolution."

One man used dream incubation to help him solve his high blood pressure problem. Before falling asleep, he asked his dreaming mind what was going on in his life to drive up his blood pressure. That night, he had a dream about all the stresses in his life. The dream information led him to explore these issues one by one and apply appropriate stress-management techniques. He was eventually able to cut his medication in half.

Want a way to squelch recurrent, troublesome dreams once and for all? Try rewriting them. If you keep dreaming of being chased, rewrite the ending of your dream so that you turn around and confront your pursuer.

Then reflect on this creative solution before dozing off and see what happens. The ultimate goal of dream writing is not to give all your dreams happy endings but to heighten your awareness of choices in your waking life.

Can dream-shaping techniques like incubation, rewriting, and creative dreaming lead to a healthier, more effective lifestyle? Possibly. In her ongoing dream work studies with recently divorced people, Rosalind Cartwright, Ph.D., director of the Sleep Disorder Service at Rush-Presbyterian Hospital in Chicago, found that those people who incorporated creative solutions in their dreams also coped better in stressful, real-life situations.

Once you have become adept at sleeping on your solutions, you may be ready for an advanced form of creative dreaming known as lucid dreaming. In a lucid dream, you are aware that you are dreaming *while* you are dreaming. According to some dream researchers, the advantage of this technique is that it enables you to confront a problem or threat while you are dreaming, instead of having to reconstruct your dream and search for solutions later on. It may take weeks until you are able to actually have a lucid dream, but it starts with telling yourself at bedtime, "Tonight I want to recognize I'm dreaming."

But no matter what technique you use, don't expect dreams to solve all your problems. "Dreams can give you information, but it's up to you to act on this information in your waking life," says Dr. Flowers.

E

echinacea (ek-ih-NAY-see-uh) A purple coneflower doesn't sound like much of a force to be reckoned with, but the Plains Indians and other early Americans considered this plant to be potent medicine. They used it for headaches, toothaches, sore throats, enlarged glands, mumps, measles, smallpox, snakebites, and as an all-around antiseptic. And researchers today think they may have been onto something.

Better known as echinacea, this lovely perennial resembles a black-eyed Susan. But its decorative qualities are outstripped by its potential for healing. In repeated experiments, extracts of echinacea have been shown to stimulate the human immune system. According to Varro E. Tyler, Ph.D., professor of pharmacognosy at Purdue University, an extract of echinacea may even be effective in warding off colds.

INFECTION FIGHTER

Before the introduction of sulfa drugs in the 1930s, commercially refined echinacea was an extremely popular anti-infective agent. Although more powerful antibiotics are available now,

echinacea may still have value as an immune-system booster. Whereas most antibiotics kill off both good and bad bacteria, echinacea is believed to have a gentler mode of action. It seems to work by stimulating the respiratory system, the lymphatic system, and white blood cells in the circulatory system. Echinacea appears to be very safe: Dr. Tyler has heard no report of toxicity or side effects associated with its use.

Folk medicine has ascribed numerous benefits to the use of echinacea. Scientific evidence continues to accumulate in support of some of these anti-infective and wound-healing claims. A study from West Germany published in the *Journal of the National Cancer Institute* reports on experiments with a highly purified extract of *Echinacea purpurea*. The extract was found to stimulate macrophages (infection-fighting white blood cells) against several types of microorganisms and tumor cells. In a Polish study, echinacea was proven to have an inhibitory effect on organisms that cause vaginal yeast infections.

HOW IT'S USED

The most practical way you can use echinacea, according to Dr. Tyler, is to ward off an oncoming cold. When you start to get the sniffles, drink a mixture of about 20 drops of the extract in about 2 to 3 ounces of water. You can drink this concoction two to four times per day. The taste is apt to be initially sweet, then bitter. And don't worry if echinacea causes a tingling sensation on the tongue; that's normal.

Herbalists also recommend echinacea tea or extract diluted in water as a mouthwash to soothe gum pain. And they say that echinacea preparations can be applied to cuts, burns, psoriasis, cold sores, and eczema.

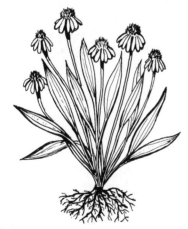

Echinacea

The active ingredients of the plant are in the root and are most effective in liquid-extract form. If you buy echinacea in a health food store, make sure it contains *Echinacea angustifolia* or *Echinacea purpurea*. Certain other, cheaper herbs often masquerade as echinacea. They not only would be ineffective but might cause unforeseen adverse reactions.

EDTA.   *See* **chelation therapy**

eicosapentaenoic acid (EPA).   *See* **fish oil**

electroconvulsive therapy   Popularly known as shock treatment, electroconvulsive therapy (ECT) is a controversial procedure to treat depression that appears to be making a comeback. A growing number of psychiatrists are enthusiastic about its potential to alleviate severe episodes of depression and mania that have not responded to other forms of treatment.

In this therapy, electrodes are placed on one or both sides of the head and an electric current—barely enough to light a 100-watt bulb for a few seconds—is delivered through them. The patient has a brief, controlled seizure. Within a minute or two after the seizure, the patient regains consciousness.

Between 30,000 and 50,000 people undergo ECT each year in the United States. Proponents say that it is safer than it ever was, because of certain modifications. For instance, just before therapy begins, the patient receives an anesthetic and a muscle relaxant to induce sleep and prevent injury from the electrically induced convulsion. The patient is also given oxygen during the procedure to guard against oxygen deprivation of the brain.

The American Psychiatric Association has recently provided clinical guidelines for the use of ECT. Treatments are typically administered about three times a week for two or three weeks. Patients rarely undergo more than twelve treatments.

No one is exactly sure how ECT works, but according to one theory, the procedure alters chemicals in the brain that control depression. Those chemicals are altered by the seizure activity, not by the electricity, says Richard D. Weiner, M.D., Ph.D., chairperson of the American Psychiatric Association's ECT Task Force. The electric current merely functions as a safe way in which to bring about a controlled seizure.

While ECT has fewer side effects than many drug therapies, it isn't totally benign. Patients often lose memory of the period immediately before and after the procedure. Most lapses are temporary. Evidence shows that using electrodes on only one side of the head is associated with fewer incidents of memory loss.

electrolytes There are about 50 trillion cells in the human body, and each one needs electricity to get things done. No, you don't need an extension cord—the power plant is inside.

The tiny electrical charges your body needs are provided by minerals—sodium, potassium, magnesium, and others—called electrolytes. Dissolved in fluids, electrolytes separate into electrically charged particles called ions, which produce the power your body needs to contract muscles, transmit nerve impulses, and maintain the appropriate fluid levels.

Most of the time, your body gets all the electrolytes it needs from the foods you eat: potassium from bananas, sodium from steak, and so on. Sometimes, however, your electrolyte balance goes out of whack. If your sodium levels abruptly rise, for example, so might your blood pressure. If you get too much potassium, on the other hand, heart problems can result.

In modern societies where processed food intake is high, many people take in far more salt than their body actually needs. Not only do the kidneys work overtime to eliminate the surplus, but blood pressure rises to speed things along. That's why people who already have high blood pressure, and thus are at higher risk for strokes and heart attacks, are advised to cut their salt intake *way* back.

People who suffer from severe diarrhea or vomiting—during a bout with cholera, for example—sometimes develop electrolyte imbalances that, if left untreated, can be fatal. "If you have massive diarrhea over a long period, then you're going to be low in almost all the electrolytes because they're not staying in the gut long enough to be absorbed," says one physiologist.

Electrolyte therapy is the first treatment step. In emergencies, solutions rich in sodium and other electrolytes may be supplied intravenously to rush fluids to dehydrated cells. Without this therapy, experts say, the mortality rate can sometimes exceed 50 percent. When the electrolytes are replenished quickly, on the other hand, the mortality rate may be kept below 1 percent.

People who take diuretics that flush fluids out of the system also are prone to electrolyte imbalances, particularly shortages of potassium, which can cause weakness, confusion, and in some instances, abnormal heart rhythms. That's why doctors often advise people who take diuretics to take potassium supplements as well.

BOOST FOR ATHLETES

Of course, it's important to maintain the proper electrolyte balance even if you aren't sick. During strenuous exercise, for example, people need to replace the electrolytes lost in perspiration. Without such replenishment, fatigue and weakness set in, and performance goes down. Some athletes say flavored sports drinks, rich in electrolytes, are superior to water for replacing lost fluids.

In a 12-week study, volunteers at the Letterman Army Institute of Research in San Francisco exercised hard, on treadmills and bicycles, for 4 hours each day. Some of the volunteers drank water, while others drank commercial beverages rich in electrolytes. The volunteers who imbibed extra electrolytes did, in fact, perform slightly better than their water-only cohorts. However, they also drank *more* of the sports drinks. The researchers suggest that "the major benefit of these products was to improve fluid balances by stimulating voluntary intakes."

Experts agree that, for most people, a well-balanced diet and frequent water intake will provide all the sodium, calcium, potassium, and magnesium they need to stay healthy and perform at their best. *See also* **banana**

electrotherapy Human faith in an "electrical cure" dates back at least as far as A.D. 46. According to a scribe alive then, electric eels were a popular treatment for headaches and gout. Eels are out of fashion among medical practitioners today, but they've been superseded by a number of more sophisticated electrical healing devices that are being used to help alleviate pain, temporarily banish body odor, zap hemorrhoids, and control tension headaches. Here's how they work.

Transcutaneous electrical nerve stimulation (TENS). Via electrodes placed on the skin, TENS applies a controlled amount of low-frequency voltage to the nerves. The device has been shown to alleviate acute episodes of pain and various kinds of chronic pain, including lower back pain and neuralgia that lingers after a shingles flare-up.

TENS has also been used to short-circuit tension headaches caused by shoulder-area stiffness. Fifty patients at a California clinic were given portable TENS units to use twice a day, for 10 minutes at a time. Electric currents from the device were able to relax muscle spasms in the neck and upper back. Within six months, all of the TENS users were nearly headache free.

Cranial electrotherapy stimulation. This technique uses high-frequency, low-voltage current to block headache pain. It can do the trick in as little as 20 minutes, according to a study at the Headache Unit of Montefiore Medical Center in the Bronx. One hundred people participated in the six-week study. Those who used the devices for 20 minutes reported that their pain decreased by an average of 35 percent. About 3 percent of the people who tried the procedure reported slight skin irritation.

Electrical muscle stimulation (EMS). EMS can help maintain muscle mass and tone when injuries, surgery, or confinement to a cast prevent use of the muscle. It is also used to treat muscle palsy, sprains, strains, and spasms. The technology has been in use for more than 50 years and is more popular than ever, says Joseph Kahn, Ph.D., a physical therapist who teaches the technique at Touro College on Long Island and at the State University of New York at Stony Brook.

The stimulators deliver a dose of current so low "it won't light a flashlight," says Dr. Kahn. Patients feel a pleasant tingle from the current, which causes muscle contraction.

In a British study, 7 men in full-length casts used portable EMS units at home to stimulate their thigh muscles. They administered treatment for 1 hour each day. After six weeks, muscle protein continued to be produced in their broken leg at the same rate as in their healthy leg. By comparison, 14 men who did not receive EMS lost 17 percent of their muscle mass while their legs were in a cast.

Electric sweat-control devices. These deliver low levels of electric current to temporarily plug sweat glands. University studies show that the devices can stop excessive sweating for up to six weeks. Side effects are relatively minor: temporary blistering, mild redness, and tingling.

These devices proved effective in a New York University Medical Center study of 18 people who suffered from excessively sweaty palms. After three treatments per week for three weeks, 15 of the 18 reported normal levels of hand perspiration. Lewis Stolman, M.D., author of the study, found that patients were able to maintain a more normal rate of perspiration by giving themselves home treatments every one to four weeks.

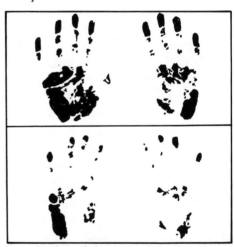

Sweaty handprints before (top) and after (bottom) electrotherapy

Electrotherapy for hemorrhoids. Using an electrical probe and low-power current, this device zaps offending tissue. You can have the procedure done in your doctor's office, with very little discomfort. "It has been very successful," says Nevada physician Daniel Norman, M.D.

In a study of 42 patients who received this treatment at the University of Nevada, all were symptom free in an average of two to three visits. There were no complications. After a three-year follow-up, there were no recurrences among patients with mild hemmorhoids and a recurrence rate of 15 to 25 percent among those with more severe hemorrhoids, Dr. Norman says. *See also* **acupuncture**

elimination diet Is there an intruder sneaking around in your body, invading your sinuses, loosening your bowels, and holding your achy muscles and joints hostage? If so, he could be the cause of other unexplained allergic symptoms as well, such as headaches, hives, and itchy, watery eyes. How did this hoodlum get under your skin? Right through the front door. The villain could be one of the foods you eat every day.

If these symptoms sound familiar, you may have a food allergy. Luckily, you can play detective and solve the mystery of your chronic symptoms. One by one you can rule out all the possible suspects until you find exactly which food is vandalizing your delicate inner wiring. That's where the elimination diet comes in.

"Following an elimination diet means avoiding specific foods—often called 'suspects'—for the purpose of diagnosing or treating food allergy," explains Eileen Rhude Yoder, Ph.D., founder of the International Food Allergy Association and author of *Allergy Free Cooking: How to Survive the Elimination Diet and Eat Happily*

Ever After. Which foods should you suspect? According to Dr. Yoder, the most common food allergens are milk and milk products, eggs, wheat, corn, soy, peanuts, peas, citrus fruits, chocolate, beef, chicken, and pork.

A FAIR TRIAL

Here's how the diet works. For about one week you don't eat any of the suspect foods. If your symptoms persist despite strict avoidance, then food may not be the culprit after all. If you start to feel better, however, or your symptoms disappear altogether, then you are on the right track.

The elimination diet can't really pinpoint the allergen, however, until you move on to the "challenge phase." If you decide to start with corn, for example, slowly reintroduce it to your diet on Day 1. After that you can eat full servings of the stuff in its various guises, continuing for about three more days. Corn on the cob. Corn flakes. Popcorn. Corn oil. Then move on, trying one suspect food at a time for about four days each. Wait and see what happens. If your old, familiar symptoms reappear after you try a particular food, you've caught your culprit!

Some people, including many children, for example, have very severe reactions to specific foods in the challenge phase. For that reason, try this technique only under the supervision of a certified allergist who can help monitor your reaction to each food you reintroduce.

By allowing you to pinpoint the problem food or foods with the challenge phase, the elimination diet can help you manage your food allergy, allowing you to live virtually symptom free. You simply bar the foods you're allergic to from your diet and learn to substitute other, nonallergenic foods.

But don't overindulge in other foods just because you're not allergic to them. "It is possible to develop new allergies through repeated exposure to foods that didn't bother you before," Dr. Yoder cautions. So once you figure out what you *can't* eat, the key for what you *can* eat is rotation—alternating permitted foods so that you are not eating the same types of items day after day.

SUPERMARKET SLEUTHING

Remember as you use this technique that you'll have to read food labels as carefully as a detective reads through the files of each suspect. Corn, for example, appears in a huge number of processed convenience foods. And in order for the elimination diet to work, you need to completely abstain from *all* the suspect foods in all their various forms for the first two weeks.

But what if you discover that you're allergic to a food you love? The good news it that you may not have to eliminate your favorite foods forever. In one Italian study, most allergic adults who followed a strict elimination diet for one or two years were then able to eat the culprit foods without having any allergic reactions. They had essentially starved out their food allergies—a happy result that Dr. Yoder says can sometimes occur in as little as one or two months. Allergic chocolate lovers, take heart!

Another encouraging fact is that allergies appear to be related to hormone levels, which fluctuate as we age, says Dr. Yoder. As women begin menopause, for example, and their hormonal levels change, they sometimes develop food allergies. But by the time they reach their sixties, the same women may find that their allergies have subsided.

In other words, the food you're allergic to may be like the friend you had a falling out with and carefully avoided for years. Given time and patience, you may someday enjoy a renewed rapport!

emetics   Poison control experts say there are few things people *won't* put in their mouths. That helps explain the estimated 4.8 million poisonings—caused by everything from drugs and plants to cosmetics and household cleaners—that occur in the United States every year. When poisoning occurs, remedies that induce vomiting—emetics—can be lifesavers. They make sure that what goes down also comes up. Sweet-tasting and inexpensive, syrup of ipecac is "the drug of choice when you have to induce vomiting in an overdose or emergency situation," says Karen J. Tietze, Pharm.D., associate professor of clinical pharmacy at the Philadelphia College of Pharmacy and Science.

Syrup of ipecac contains substances, derived from the dried roots of Brazilian and Central American plants, that work on the stomach and brain to stimulate vomiting. Sold over the counter, syrup of ipecac goes to work in 15 to 20 minutes. If vomiting doesn't occur, a second dose usually does the trick.

Even though syrup of ipecac belongs in every first-aid kit, people should *always* call a doctor or poison center before using it, warns Joseph A. Barone, Pharm.D., chairman of pharmacy practice at Rutgers University and pharmacy clinician at Robert Wood Johnson University Hospital in Piscataway, New Jersey.

"If you've ingested a drug that causes central nervous system depression, for example, that's an indication *against* ipecac," Dr. Barone says. "People also swallow acids and alkalies, like drain openers. There's a rule of thumb: If it burns going down, it's going to burn coming up. You want to avoid that dual burn by *not* inducing vomiting."

Another reason to consult an expert, Dr. Barone says, is that syrup of ipecac, by itself, isn't always effective. Ipecac-induced vomiting will evacuate 35 to 40 percent of the stomach's contents—not always enough for someone who has taken a really dangerous overdose. In the emergency room, doctors may initiate treatment with syrup of ipecac, then follow it with activated charcoal or gastric lavage (stomach pumping).

WHAT *NOT* TO DO

Forget the folk remedies, Dr. Barone warns. Emetics such as mustard or raw eggs—or putting your finger down your throat—don't always work. They also waste valuable time. Warm saltwater may induce vomiting,

but it can "increase blood levels of sodium that, in kids, can cause convulsion," Dr. Barone says.

Properly used, syrup of ipecac is extremely safe, doctors say. However, its frequent use by people with binge-and-purge eating disorders may be extremely dangerous, and some experts believe syrup of ipecac should be sold only by prescription. Others think that it should continue to remain available in pharmacies, supermarkets, and convenience stores.

"Poisonings occur at odd hours of the day, on vacations and holidays," Dr. Tietze says. "The product has to be available immediately." *See also* **charcoal, activated**

emollients. *See* **moisturizers**

endoscopy (en-DOS-kuh-pee) What would you think if your surgeon turned out the lights before operating? Wait, don't leave. With endoscopy, doctors often work in the dark. After all, ceiling lights just won't reach inside your knee joint or light up your lower intestine—both places where endoscopy shines.

Endoscopy refers to any procedure in which your doctor peers through a hollow tube at your insides. There are many types of endoscopy: arthroscopy, for instance, looks at your joints; laryngoscopy peeks at your larynx; colonoscopy snakes through your large intestine.

Some endoscopes are like telescopes: The doctor presses his eye to an eyepiece and a lens system does the rest. Other scopes contain tiny cameras, which transmit clear color images to viewing screens.

Naturally, the cameras are a bit smaller than the family camcorder. Doctors like endoscopy precisely because the apparatus is *very* small. For instance, the hollow, flexible tube the doctor slips inside your injured joints—or inside your abdomen, nose, or throat—may be as small as 2 millimeters in diameter. (To put things in perspective, a pencil's diameter is about 5 millimeters.)

LESS DISCOMFORT, FASTER RECOVERY

Endoscopes let doctors work inside your body without making the large, painful incisions used in conventional surgery. In fact, endoscopy is often used both to diagnose a problem and to treat it—at the same time. A gastroenterologist, for instance, might use an endoscope for a routine bowel cancer screening. If a precancerous polyp is found, it may be removed right away by inserting an electrocautery (a cutting device) right inside the tube. That's good, because rapid intervention is often the best defense against cancer.

Endoscopy really isn't all that new. Many of us have been examined with proctoscopes, and surgeons long have used a type of endoscopy—sometimes called "belly-button surgery"—to remove renegade endometrial tissue. However, modern endoscopy started in the early 1970s when flexible fiberoptics and microtechnology allowed endoscopes to fit into increasingly smaller places.

Many medical specialties use endo-

scopy, says William Ruderman, M.D., chairman of the Department of Gastroenterology at the Cleveland Clinic in Florida. Sinus disorders, for example, may be evaluated and treated with nasal endoscopy. Upper endoscopy is used to seek out (and sometimes cauterize) bleeding ulcers. Endoscopy even goes after gallstones.

Endoscopy often is preferred because people recover a lot faster than with conventional surgery, Dr. Ruderman says. The incision in open abdominal surgery, for example, takes weeks or months to heal. The punctures used for endoscopy, which are small enough to be sealed with an adhesive strip, heal much faster.

Endoscopy appears to work as well as other surgeries, Dr. Ruderman says. After all, it's doing the same job—just going in through smaller incisions or taking advantage of the body's natural openings.

Endoscopy's access advantages can make a big difference, he says. "I had a patient with two large polyps in the colon. She was high risk, with cardiac disease and a previous stroke. The only way in the past [to remove the polyps] would have been to operate on her, and she might have died during surgery." Instead, Dr. Ruderman removed the polyps colonoscopically—that is, with a lower endoscope requiring no incision.

"If you have surgery for a polyp, recovery involves seven to ten days in the hospital and serious pain," he says. "To do it by a colonoscopy, it typically takes 2 or 3 hours, and you're ready to go home that night."

Doctors often use endoscopy to treat endometriosis, which by some estimates may affect half of the nation's premenopausal women. The endoscope—here called a laparoscope—is inserted through the navel to look for uterine tissue growing outside the uterus. If renegade tissue is found, it's removed with an electrocautery or laser. Women recover a lot faster than with open abdominal surgery, often going home within a day.

PICTURE PERFECT

Doctors agree endoscopy produces extra-sharp images of our insides. Indeed, in certain cases endoscopy has already replaced x-rays as the diagnostic tool of choice.

"X-rays are sort of shadows of what's going on inside, but when you go in endoscopically, you're actually looking at the anatomy," says one internist. "We can see things in the body that in some cases we've never seen that clearly before."

As technology improves, doctors will continue to find new uses for endoscopy, Dr. Ruderman says. Neurosurgeons already have used endoscopy to destroy brain tumors, and laser endoscopy has vaporized arterial plaque. Some doctors are even discussing the possibility of endoscopic heart surgery. *See also* **arthroscopy; proctosigmoidoscopy**

epinephrine (ep-i-NEF-rin) There are some families you don't want to mess with. You never mess with folks wearing trenchcoats and diamond pinkie rings. And if an allergy has made you dangerously hypersensitive to life's insect encounters, you never, *never* mess with the Hymenoptera family—the bees, wasps, hornets, and fire ants responsible for many of the approximately 40 insect sting fatalities that occur in the United States every year.

Of course, there's not much you can do about bad human neighbors, but you *can* beat the bees. Epinephrine, injected soon after a bite or sting, tremendously boosts your chances for survival. In fact, epinephrine generally is considered the first-line defense for *all* life-threatening allergic reactions, says Fang L. Lin, M.D., an allergy specialist at the San Diego Naval Hospital in California.

Some people suffer these potentially fatal allergic reactions—or anaphylaxis—from bee and wasp attacks. Others react to foods—peanuts and shrimp are two common culprits. Some people even are intensely allergic to a butterfly's touch!

Regardless of the cause, anaphylaxis is an *emergency.* An anaphylactic reaction may shut your airways, lower your blood pressure, and, in some cases, end in cardiovascular collapse. Epinephrine turns it all around. It quickly expands the airways, so you can breathe again. It stimulates the heart and raises blood pressure. It saves lives.

ADRENALINE ON CALL

Even if you're lucky enough not to have serious allergies, you've still felt the jolt of epinephrine. Only it was produced by your body, and you may have referred to it as your "adrenaline flowing." Actually, epinephrine and adrenaline are one and the same: the stuff your body churns out when you're excited—when you have to speak in public, or when the policeman waves you to the side of the road.

In large amounts, synthetic epinephrine is so powerful that doctors may use it as a heart stimulant when the heart stops beating, Dr. Lin says. Epinephrine helps relieve severe asthma attacks. It also constricts blood vessels, which helps stop nosebleeds and other bleeding, and prolongs the action of some local anesthetics.

As you might expect from such a powerful drug, epinephrine isn't without risks. Acute high blood pressure sometimes occurs, as do heartbeat irregularities called ventricular arrhythmias, which are potentially fatal in some patients. That's why epinephrine is only used for emergencies.

For some people, of course, a bee sting definitely is an emergency. According to one medical journal, "Anaphylaxis is the most dreaded consequence of insect sting hypersensitivity." People who know they're sensitive often carry doctor-prescribed emergency epinephrine kits, says Peter Hauck, director of scientific affairs at Center Laboratories, a company that makes the kits.

Epinephrine self-injectors are charged and spring-loaded at the factory. If you're stung by a wasp, for example, "You place the tip of the injector against your thigh and press, and that will activate the unit," Hauck says. A needle goes in about ½ inch

and "it will automatically inject ³⁄₁₀ milliliter of epinephrine," says Hauck.

Speed is essential, Dr. Lin says. Once injected, epinephrine goes to work in minutes. There's no mistaking its effect, Hauck says. "If you've ever been in a situation where your body produced its own adrenaline, you certainly know the feeling."

Epsom salts   Using Epsom salts will get you into hot water, but some experts think you'll love every minute of it.

Epsom salts is an old home remedy that isn't anything like the salt in your shaker. This remedy is actually magnesium sulfate in a crystal form that's had all its impurities removed, says Richard Hansen, M.D., medical director of the Poland Spring Health Institute in Poland Spring, Maine.

The stuff is mined out of the ground and then chemically processed, says Dr. Hansen. Its rather enigmatic-sounding name isn't much of a mystery after all—Epsom salts were first identified in the mineral-rich waters of Epsom, England, back in the days of Shakespeare.

SOOTHES SORE FEET

Although Epsom salts soaks aren't as popular as they once were, they remain an effective remedy for tired, aching feet and sore hands, says Dr. Hansen. Some of his patients say it helps soften up their corns—although he cautions that it may just be the hot water alone that accomplishes that feet accompli.

Another benefit of bathing in Epsom salts is that it makes strained, bruised, and sore muscles feel better, Dr. Hansen says. It also takes some of the soreness out of stiff joints—"although we don't claim that it heals rheumatoid arthritis," he adds.

How does Epsom salts work? It has the concentrated power to draw toxins or sweat from the pores, says Dr. Hansen. All that salt also takes the swelling out of your feet and leaves them feeling swell again.

The amount of Epsom salts to use depends on whether you're soaking in a basin or tub, says Dr. Hansen. A basin might require you to sprinkle ½ cup into warm or mildly hot water, while a bathtub might require 2 cups or more, he says.

Epsom salts also has other uses. It's used in the relaxation devices called flotation tanks to add buoyancy and keep people from sinking below the surface of the water. Ages ago, people used to take a teaspoonful dissolved in water whenever they needed a laxative, but a high-fiber diet and gentler laxatives have replaced it.

Epsom salts is sold by the box in grocery stores and drugstores. It is a very inexpensive product, says Dr. Hansen, so you won't have to worry about getting soaked until you actually run the hot water. *See also* **flotation tanks**

ergot (ER-got) Like many things in life, ergot is a paradox. Years ago this poisonous black or dark purple fungus that grows on wet grain was a big headache for farmers. It invaded the rye fields of Russia and other European countries, causing convulsions and gangrene in cattle and humans who ate the grain.

But now drugs derived from it are hailed as a *remedy* for headaches. Ergot derivatives also may alleviate memory loss and enhance concentration in some elderly people.

One of these drugs, ergotamine, is used to relieve and prevent vascular headaches, including migraines and cluster headaches. It constricts blood vessels and reverses the dilation (widening) associated with migraines. When taken at the onset of a headache, it can work within 30 minutes and provide relief for up to 48 hours. The drug may be combined with caffeine to enhance its absorption.

TOUGH HEADACHE CHALLENGE

Ergonovine is another ergot-derived drug that has the ability to constrict blood vessels. It's used to end uterine bleeding following childbirth. It is also being investigated as a migraine treatment.

Ergonovine may be particularly effective against migraines caused by menstruation, says R. Michael Gallagher, D.O., of the University of Medicine and Dentistry of New Jersey School of Osteopathic Medicine in Stratford.

"There are women who, when their hormones act up during menstruation, defy all of the guidelines that we normally use to treat migraine patients," he says. "In those instances, we have to go to extraordinary means such as ergonovine to help them out."

In a study of 40 women who had suffered menstrual migraines for at least two years, Dr. Gallagher found that half of those treated with ergonovine had fewer and less severe headaches at the end of the six-month trial.

However, both ergonovine and ergotamine have some nasty side effects. Both can cause nausea and vomiting and may be dangerous for patients who have high blood pressure, poor circulation, or a history of or high risk for stroke or heart disease.

Another promising ergot derivative, dihydroergotamine mesylate, also known as DHE, is a powerful weapon against migraines but has fewer side effects than ergotamine, says Stephen Silberstein, M.D., co-director of the Comprehensive Headache Center at Germantown Hospital in Philadelphia.

At the center, Dr. Silberstein and his associates conducted a study of 300 patients with chronic headaches. They determined that 91 percent of those treated with injections of DHE became headache free, usually within 48 hours.

Unfortunately, DHE is currently available only as an injection. Doctors anticipate that it will be available in a nasal spray soon, however.

Another drug, ergoloid mesylates, is a mixture of three substances produced by the ergot fungus. Unlike other ergot derivatives, it relaxes blood vessels and increases circulation to the brain. It's primarily used to alleviate memory loss and impaired concentration in the elderly.

estrogen replacement therapy   You wake up in a cold sweat at 3:00 A.M., your face and arms smarting as though they've been rubbed with a red-hot coal. Your hair is matted to your scalp, and your soaked nightgown is sticking to your skin. You wish you could hurl yourself into a snowbank.

Welcome to "hot flash hell," a tormenting sensation of intense heat that happens to some women when their periods stop and their ovaries no longer produce the hormone estrogen. When your body goes through estrogen withdrawal, your blood vessels react and your skin flushes with heat.

But lack of this precious hormone can also cause other problems: vaginal dryness that makes intercourse painful or impossible; changes in the urinary system that can cause embarrassing leakage; bones that become so brittle that bumping your hip could cause a fracture. And without estrogen's help, you may be at a higher risk for heart disease or stroke.

Fortunately, you can relieve the midlife miseries that may occur when your estrogen supply dwindles. Estrogen replacement therapy (ERT) puts back the hormone lost to natural menopause (or surgical menopause if you've had your ovaries removed). ERT given in continuous doses may benefit the cardiovascular system and bones.

The hormone is usually prescribed in pill form, but it is available in creams, vaginal suppositories, or patches that adhere to the body and release estrogen through the skin. The form you use depends upon your symptoms.

SAFER THAN EVER

ERT was once quite controversial because it increased a woman's risk of cancer. When it was first prescribed in the 1960s, estrogen was administered in large doses and was later linked to an increased risk of cancer of the endometrium (the lining of the uterus). Today, ERT is given in much lower doses, and when the uterus is present, it is prescribed along with another female hormone, progesterone (typically a progestin, a synthetic form) which counters estrogen's negative effects in the uterus.

Should all menopausal women go on ERT? Definitely not, according to the experts. "ERT is not for everyone," says Wulf Utian, M.D., Ph.D., director of obstetrics and gynecology at University Hospitals of Cleveland and author of *Managing Your Menopause.* "Some women do not need ERT and others cannot take it. To determine whether you should take ERT, you and your doctor need to carefully weigh the pluses and the minuses based on your own personal profile of potential health risks and benefits."

HOW ERT HELPS

In general, there are certain compelling reasons for taking ERT.

Severe hot flashes. If you're getting up several times a night to wring out your bedclothes, ERT may end your misery. "You don't have to suffer for the year or two it usually takes hot flashes to pass," says Valery Miller, M.D., associate research professor in medicine at George Washington University in Washington, D.C. "ERT helps reset your internal thermostat and regulate your blood vessels to reduce flushing. As a result, you'll sleep better, think better, and feel less irritable."

Vaginal deterioration. Estrogen withdrawal can cause the vaginal walls to shrink and dry, resulting in maddening itching and painful intercourse. An estrogen-containing vaginal cream applied twice weekly may help where lubricants fail. "A few weeks of estrogen cream may be all that is needed to restore vaginal tissues to a more youthful state—thicker, moister, and more flexible," says Lila E. Nachtigall, M.D., associate professor of obstetrics and gynecology at New York University School of Medicine and author of *Estrogen: The Facts Can Change Your Life.* As a bonus, estrogen cream may also halt recurring vaginal infections.

Weak bladder. Because a lack of estrogen weakens tissues supporting the bladder, over a third of all postmenopausal women may experience stress incontinence (bladder dribbling) when they cough, sneeze, or laugh. By improving the health of vaginal tissues and lending more support to the urinary tract, ERT can often relieve urinary incontinence.

Bone loss. Estrogen controls the absorption of calcium in the bones.

"When you no longer make much estrogen, your bones quickly start losing more bone bulk than they gain," says Dr. Nachtigall. So by the time you reach 85, the chances are one in three that you will have had a serious bone fracture—a fracture that could be fatal.

Doctors have been recommending since 1984 that women at high risk for bone-thinning osteoporosis take ERT. That was the year that a special panel of the National Institutes of Health concluded that ERT was the best way to retard or halt bone loss and fractures in postmenopausal women. While weight-bearing exercise and calcium supplements can also help keep bones strong, they said, estrogen is a better bone protector.

In a pioneering study conducted by Dr. Nachtigall, a group of age-matched women were given either estrogen (with progesterone) or an inactive substitute. Those who were given ERT within three years of menopause actually *increased* their bone mass. Among the women who started taking ERT three or more years after their last period and had already lost bone, "the condition was stopped in its tracks with no additional loss," says Dr. Nachtigall. Women who received the estrogen substitute continued to lose bone mass.

More recent studies have underscored ERT's benefits to the bones, no matter at what point after menopause the therapy is begun. In one, ERT reduced hip and wrist fractures by half. "It's never too late for ERT to protect bone," says Dr. Miller.

"There is no question that if you are at risk for osteoporosis, you should take ERT," adds Dr. Utian. You are at risk if you've had a surgical or natural menopause before age 50, if you smoke, abuse alcohol, are thin, or have a family history of osteoporosis.

Heart disease. A major, multicenter study conducted by the Lipid Research Clinics Program of the National Institutes of Health followed more than 2,000 women, some who used ERT and some who didn't, for an average of 8½ years. The result: ERT users had a 70 percent reduction in risk of death from cardiovascular disease than nonusers.

"We're not exactly sure how estrogen protects the heart," says Dr. Miller, who is the medical director at the Lipid Research Clinic in Washington, D.C. "It appears to affect the waxy plaque that can build up in arteries and plug them, leading to heart attacks." This plaque is deposited in arteries by LDLs (low-density lipoproteins) and carted off by HDLs (high-density lipoproteins). Estrogen raises HDLs and lowers LDLs.

EVALUATING THE RISKS

If you're starting ERT and you still have your uterus, doctors recommend that you take estrogen's sidekick hormone, progestin, at the same time. Why? Estrogen's main job is to build up endometrial tissue, while progestin's job is to make sure that this buildup is not the sort of *uncontrolled* growth that becomes cancer. The excess tissue is shed in menstrual flow.

Concerns have also been raised about a possible estrogen/breast cancer link. "According to the bulk of the evidence, estrogen taken solo in low doses does not increase the risk of breast cancer," says David Page, M.D., professor of pathology at Vanderbilt Medical Center in Nashville.

But one study did show a very modest increased risk of breast cancer for current ERT users. "Estrogen probably does not cause cancer directly, but perhaps it may encourage tumor cells to spring up in women who have the beginnings of a tumor that otherwise would not have grown," says Meir Stampfer, M.D., associate professor of epidemiology at Harvard School of Public Health. Dr. Stampfer stresses that the risk was small.

Adding a progestin may not protect your breasts in any way and may, in fact, overstimulate breast tissue. In a Swedish study, researchers found that the breast cancer risk was highest in a group of women who took estrogen *with* progestin for long periods. There is also some new evidence that progestins may undo estrogen's positive effects on blood fats.

In light of these concerns, it's more important than ever to weigh all the factors before taking estrogen (either with or without progestin), says Dr. Stampfer. "There is no recommendation that applies to all women."

Until long-term studies give us more information, most doctors agree with Dr. Stamfer: "The benefits of taking estrogen replacement therapy (with or without progesterone) outweigh the risks for women who have severe hot flashes or vaginal atrophy or who may be at high risk for bone loss or heart disease."

POINTS TO CONSIDER

If you eat a low-fat diet, maintain your ideal weight, exercise regularly, and reduce stress, you may be able to reduce your risk of heart disease without ERT, reminds Dr. Miller. "But why not improve your risk in all ways?"

If you have an intact uterus but don't wish to take a progestin along with the estrogen, your physician may recommend that a sampling (biopsy) of your endometrial tissue be done periodically to check for abnormalities.

Before taking any hormones, have a blood pressure check, a pelvic exam, and a Pap smear, says Dr. Utian. You should also have a mammogram both before starting ERT and every year thereafter. To play it safe, have semiannual breast exams by a physician (in addition to monthly breast self-exams).

Always report any irregular vaginal bleeding to your doctor.

If you have a history of breast cancer or estrogen-dependent cancer (meaning estrogen makes it grow), uncontrolled high blood pressure, thrombosis or thromboembolic disease, abnormal uterine bleeding, gallbadder disease, fibroids, or endometriosis, ERT may not be right for you. In any case, find a doctor who is knowledgable about ERT and is willing to discuss all your options.

eucalyptus (yew-cuh-LIP-tuss) Bet you've never seen a koala bear with a cough.

That could be a standing joke among herbalists, based on the fact that these cuddly marsupials spend most of their day in eucalyptus trees, munching on the long, scythe-shaped leaves. Oil from eucalyptus leaves (called eucalyptol, or cineole) has proven anticough properties and is officially recognized by the Food and Drug Administration for that purpose.

Eucalyptol is added to cough and cold medicines as an expectorant (a substance that loosens phlegm in the chest, making it easier to cough up). And the oil adds a crisp, cool smell and flavor. It's the primary ingredient in Hall's Mentho-Lyptus and is used in small amounts in Noxzema Medicated Skin Cream, Vicks Vapo-Rub, and Listerine mouthwash.

Herbalists have traditionally recommended eucalyptus oil as an antiseptic to be applied on the skin, as a gargle for sore throats, and as an inhalant for bronchitis and nasal congestion. Some health spas put eucalyptus leaves or oil in their steam rooms to impart a refreshing, nose-opening scent.

Like many other essential oils, eucalyptus may indeed have antiseptic properties, says James A. Duke, Ph.D., a botanist and toxicology specialist with the U.S. Department of Agriculture in Beltsville, Maryland. A few studies suggest eucalyptol kills influenza A virus, which causes a serious form of flu. And it kills some bacteria, meaning it may help prevent bacterial bronchitis, a common complication of colds and flu.

Used in liniments or ointments for aches or minor skin problems, eucalyptus oil will make your skin redden, so it feels warm. That same effect may reduce swelling by helping to increase blood flow to the affected area, and it may also reduce the sensation of pain. (Because of its irritating effect, eucalyptus oil should never be applied to cuts or broken skin.)

If you are planning to use eucalyptus oil on your body, massage therapists say it's best to dilute two drops in 1 ounce of bland vegetable oil such as almond or jojoba oil. That way, you may avoid a possible allergic skin reaction to the eucalyptus.

To use as an inhalant, simply put a few drops of the eucalyptus oil, or a few leaves, in a pot of steaming water and inhale, says Dr. Duke, adding the caveat that some individuals may be allergic to eucalyptus. Or add a few drops to warm bathwater. But never swallow the oil, Dr. Duke warns. Less than 1 teaspoon of pure eucalyptus oil has been reported fatal.

evening primrose oil The primrose plant provides more than spires of small yellow flowers. Evening primrose oil is a rich, natural source of gamma-linolenic acid, or GLA, which the body requires for a range of functions.

One of the ways the body uses GLA is to convert it into short-lived hormones called prostaglandins. The prostaglandins serve the body in a number of ways: They regulate the chemicals that send messages between brain cells, help control blood sugar, aid in the clotting of blood, keep arteries and veins strong and firm, play a role in regulating your digestion, and maintain your body's balance of salt and water. Different prostaglandins act in very different ways.

Because prostaglandins serve so many important functions in the body, some researchers theorize that changes in the metabolism of prostaglandins may be responsible for certain health problems. If so, perhaps a good source of GLA might help heal those problems. That's the basis for studies examining the effects of evening primrose oil supplements on atopic eczema, bronchial asthma, cyclical breast pain and cysts, rheumatoid arthritis, and cardiovascular disease.

Yet only the rheumatoid arthritis research shows much promise, and even these studies don't all agree.

"GLA is known to increase production of a series of prostaglandins that have inflammatory lowering effects, so it is not unreasonable to expect that it might be helpful in the treatment of arthritis," writes University of California, San Diego, faculty member Sheldon Saul Hendler, M.D., Ph.D., in *The Doctors' Vitamin and Mineral Encyclopedia.*

FEWER SYMPTOMS

In one study, 90 percent of rheumatoid arthritis sufferers who took 540 milligrams of GLA per day reported significant improvement at the end of a year-long treatment period. They required fewer nonsteroidal anti-inflammatory drugs than patients in a second group who received a nontherapeutic placebo. Only 30 percent of the people in the latter group reported a decrease in symptoms.

However, a 12-week Finnish study of 18 rheumatoid arthritis patients showed that 20 milligrams of evening primrose oil a day also raised levels of body acids that might trigger symptoms of the disease. The authors concluded that this finding makes evening primrose oil a questionable treatment for this condition.

Evening primrose oil may offer limited help for women suffering from cyclical breast pain. A Welsh study showed that evening primrose oil reduced breast pain compared with a placebo. But in a follow-up study of 200 women, evening primrose oil was unable to reduce the recurrence of breast cysts, which are common in many women with cyclical breast pain.

Experts say evening primrose oil merits further study. Right now, however, the claims are unproven. Chances are, your diet provides you with all the essential fatty acids that you need.

exercise therapy   Once upon a time, most people who exercised did so because they wanted to compete in a sport. These days, however, more and more people exercise just for the health of it.

"Exercise therapy is any regular and continuous physical activity performed to improve health," says Edward

A. Palank, M.D., director of the New Hampshire Heart Institute in Manchester. "It is used both to prevent and to treat illness."

A VERSATILE REMEDY

Let's take a look at some of the conditions exercise can help.

Minding the weight. There's no doubt that exercising is the best therapy for burning calories, says Dr. Palank. "Exercise expends energy and uses up calories to lower body mass and lower weight," he says.

If you're over your ideal weight, exercise is the ideal way to banish obesity, says Dr. Palank.

Kiboshing cholesterol. While it is important to eat a low-fat diet, to really put cholesterol down for the count, people need to exercise, says Dr. Palank. "Exercise does something special that really nothing else can do," he says. "It raises your good cholesterol."

Cholesterol, as you probably have heard, is divided into good and bad varieties. The good cholesterol in your bloodstream—termed HDL (high-density lipoprotein)—does a fine job of housecleaning in your arteries. The bad cholesterol—LDL (low-density lipoprotein)—helps clog arteries.

To reduce your chances of some-day developing coronary heart disease, therefore, you'll want to improve the ratio of HDL—the cholesterol that wears a white hat—to total cholesterol, says Dr. Palank.

Even mild forms of exercise such as walking or playing golf (sans cart!)

help raise HDL slightly, says Dr. Palank. And marathon runners or others who enjoy regular aerobic activities such as jogging, bicycling, riding a stationary bike, or swimming reap even greater benefits—plus, they can significantly lower their total cholesterol, he says.

To lower your cholesterol to your heart's content, you need 30 minutes of moderately vigorous exercise three or four times weekly, says Dr. Palank. "You should try to get your heart rate above 70 percent of what's normal for your age and sustain it," he explains. (Always check with your doctor before beginning any new exercise program.)

Going off the fritz. "When someone who is injured or out of shape exercises to bring tissues back to normal, the process is called rehabilitation," says Robert P. Nirschl, M.D., medical director of the Virginia Sportsmedicine Institute in Arlington. The goal is winning good health—not beating or performing better than someone else, he says.

If rehabilitation of disabled muscles or joints is your intent and you decide to give exercising a shot, it is imperative that you see a doctor who can help you learn your limitations and work around them.

Countering diabetes. Sometimes exercise can help restore the whole body to good health—especially when a program of good nutrition is also started, says Michael Walczak, M.D., a physician from Sherman Oaks, California, and past president of the International College of Applied Nutrition.

People with diabetes, for example, frequently are helped by exercising, he notes.

"In borderline diabetes, improving the diet and adding exercise could bring them back to normal so that they could stay off medication," says Dr. Walczak. "In cases of severe diabetes, exercise might help prevent some of the side effects of the disease by improving circulation and lowering blood sugar levels enough that they could decrease the amount of insulin they take," he adds.

Exercise may also benefit people with high blood pressure, says Dr. Walczak. "In borderline cases, exercise could eliminate the need for medications," he says.

Fighting stress. Exercise is an excellent way to work off stress, says Dr. Nirschl. "Aerobic activities—those things like jogging that increase the pulse rate—blow off the adrenaline in our bodies," he says. The adrenal glands normally secrete excess adrenaline in stressful situations.

Beating depression. Regular exercise can help give depressed people a lift by triggering the release of mood-elevating natural chemicals called endorphins and by shifting their general outlook. One of the best mental benefits of exercise is that "it allows you to focus on something other than your depression," says D.W. Edington, Ph.D., director of the University of Michigan Fitness Research Center in Ann Arbor. Exercise also tends to raise one's self-esteem. "It gives you a sense

of accomplishment and a feeling that you're healing from within," Dr. Edington says.

You don't have to try out for an Olympic berth to give your body a boost with exercise, says Dr. Walczak. "I don't recommend strenuous aerobics for older people, but I do recommend walking, bicycling, or swimming as a very basic, minimum activity that's easy to do," he says.

Walking, in particular, is something that many people can do. "It doesn't require any equipment," he says. "Simply go out and walk as fast as you can." Dr. Walczak prefers that people walk daily, but he says that three days weekly is the bare minimum.

Start off walking just 10 minutes a day the first week and add a minute per day each week until you're able to walk for 30 minutes daily, he suggests. "As you get in condition, you'll start feeling better as your circulation improves."

If you have access to a pool or a bicycle, you might want to alternate these activities with walking, says Dr. Walczak. "Exercise doesn't always have to be the same thing," he says. "People can swim one day, or bicycle, or walk."

Weight training. In addition to conditioning the body, people would do well to strengthen it, says Dr. Walczak. He recommends simple isometric (resistance) exercises with light weights—either in addition to walking or in place of it.

Besides building muscle tone, lifting light weights helps reduce stiffness in many people—including those who have arthritis, says Dr. Walczak. "The less you use your muscles, the stiffer you get," he warns. In addition, some people with diabetes find that their blood sugar stabilizes and their insulin works better when they follow a weight-lifting program, he adds.

Another benefit of isometric training is that it helps maintain the strength of your bones, says Dr. Palank. If you are concerned about developing osteoporosis, therefore, you may want to bone up on this uncomplicated exercise, he says.

Water workouts. Exercise in the water—also known as aquacize—is a nonpainful, comfortable way to work out that is particularly good for people with bad knees or a weight problem, says Dr. Edington. "The buoyancy of the water gives them a way to exercise without pounding the joints," he says.

Professional football teams such as the San Francisco 49ers have used

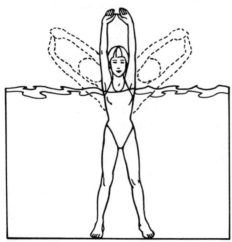

Water exercise

aquacize to give injured players workouts they otherwise might have skipped.

One popular exercise that you might do with your doctor's permission is to go for a slow jog in the water, says Dr. Edington. "If you've ever been to the beach and tried running in water up to your thighs, you know that's really hard work," he says.

In tight quarters, such as the pool at your local Y, you can get the same benefit by buying and using a special tether that anchors you to one spot, says Dr. Edington.

Oriental originals. There are a variety of Asian techniques that are valuable both for the exercise they provide and for the philosophies they teach, says Dr. Edington. The exercises can vary greatly in the demands they place upon you, he says.

One approach that provides a great deal of benefit with a minimum of exertion is t'ai chi, an ancient Chinese activity involving meditative movements that many modern people use as a form of exercise.

"T'ai chi is very good for many people," says Dr. Edington. Noting that many of the gentle, flowing movements mimic the movements of animals, he says, "It gives people a full range of motion."

More grueling oriental martial arts such as Tae Kwon Do, aikido, and karate are popular with conditioned athletes, says Dr. Edington. "These get to be very, very strenuous," he says. "But there is motivation for people to keep coming back to the activity because they move from one belt to another as they reach higher levels of achievement."

How do you choose an exercise therapy that's right for you? There are two conditions that should be met, says Dr. Edington. First of all, "find an exercise you enjoy. If you count it as a job it just won't last very long." Second, if you have any history of illness—or just to play safe—follow a doctor's advice on whether you need to limit your exercise activities. If you have special physical problems, your doctor can send you to a physical therapist, who will work with you to design a long-term exercise program. Even if you're handicapped, there is probably some sort of exercise program that you can do, says Robert S. Brown, M.D., Ph.D., clinical professor of behavioral medicine and psychiatry at the University of Virginia in Charlottesville. "Any exercise is better than no exercise," he says.

WISE WORKOUTS

Warming up before a workout is a wise precaution that can help prevent injury. In the not-so-good old days, however, people tried to warm up by stretching—a practice that may have hobbled as many runners as it helped, says Dr. Nirschl. "Stretching is not a warm-up," he says. "A warm-up is an activity that increases your body heat to make your tissues more pliable."

The goal of any warm-up is simple—to achieve a light sweat, says Dr. Nirschl. "Stretching doesn't do that."

If you don't warm up by stretching, how do you do it? Two ways—passively and actively, he says.

A passive warm-up requires a source of heat to get you jump-started. Some people go into a sauna or soak in a hot bath or whirlpool bath, says Dr. Nirschl. Others with a troubled lower back or other ailments may opt for a heating pad.

An active warm-up is preferable to a passive one—although a passive warm-up beats having no warm-up at all, says Dr. Nirschl. The purpose of an active warm-up is to get your muscles working and generating heat on their own, he says.

One way to actively warm up is to simply do the activity you had planned to do—walking or bike riding, for example—but at a much slower speed for a few minutes until your temperature gauge tells you it's all right to go full throttle at what you're doing, says Dr. Nirschl. Other ways to warm up include slowly riding a stationary bike, jogging in place, or doing jumping jacks and calisthenics—"something basic that gets you stirred up on a gradual basis," he says.

Even after you've fully warmed up, it pays to know your body's limits and respect them. Attempting to do too much too soon only invites injury, says Dr. Edington.

"Keep the exercise at a moderate level so that you don't end up feeling soreness or fatigue," he advises. If you're very sore—or worse, in pain—you've likely gone overboard with your program, he says.

Whether you're lifting weights, jogging, or doing any other type of exercise, know your body's warning signs. "If you get dizziness or chest pain, stop immediately and get a doctor's evaluation," says Dr. Walczak.

Exercise is certainly worth doing, but it's not worth overdoing. *See also* **stretching**

eyedrops These liquid medications can be used to cure and prevent eye problems, as well as to relieve eye discomfort, lubricate dry eyes, and—as TV commercial watchers all know—"get the red out."

There are many kinds of eyedrops, says Eric Donnenfeld, M.D., a corneal specialist and ophthalmologist in Rockville Center, New York. But they can be divided into two broad categories: prescription and nonprescription.

GLAUCOMA CONTROL

Among the most important prescription medications are drops used by glaucoma patients to lower excessive pressure inside the eye. By controlling intraocular pressure, antiglaucoma drops can help prevent progression of the disease, which, if unchecked, can lead to blindness.

No drops can restore destroyed vision, unfortunately, says Dr. Donnenfeld. "Once you have glaucoma, any vision that you've lost is gone permanently—the drugs only prevent worsening of the condition," he says.

Other prescription drops contain antibiotic medications that either fight infection or keep infections from forming in the event of an eye injury such as a scratched cornea. The most common reasons antibiotic drops are prescribed are for conjunctivitis ("pinkeye") and corneal ulcers, Dr. Donnenfeld says.

Another common class of prescription drugs is used mainly by ophthalmologists and optometrists. These are dilating drops used for retinal examinations. By causing the pupil to open wider, they enable the doctor to look at the back of the eye.

Finally, some prescription drops help hay fever and other allergy sufferers and also get the redness out of sore or tired eyes. These drugs are more effective in controlling allergy symptoms than are their over-the-counter counterparts, says Dr. Donnenfeld, who has conducted comparison studies of these medicines.

WETTER IS BETTER

Over-the-counter eyedrops are subdivided into two categories—lubricating drops and decongestant drops, says Dr. Donnenfeld.

The lubricating drops are better known as artificial tears. "These are used by people with dry eyes to supplement natural tears," Dr. Donnenfeld says, noting that about 30 percent of all women over 50 have this problem. A different variety of artificial tears is used as wetting drops to assist contact lens wearers whose eyes tend to feel dry.

The decongestant drops are used either to soothe "red eyes" or to help people with watery eyes caused by allergies. These medications usually are only effective for the short term, says Dr. Donnenfeld. Long-term use can lead to dependency—the condition becomes worse unless people continually use the drops, he says.

GETTING AN EYEFUL

A word of caution: People frequently are prescribed more than one type of eyedrop medication, says Dr. Donnenfeld. Those with glaucoma, for example, may be assigned three different prescriptions. If that's the case with you, always allow at least 5 minutes between insertion of drops, recommends Dr. Donnenfeld. "If you put in a second drop right away, it will wash out the other drop and your medication won't be as effective," he warns.

Also, eyedrop users should be aware of certain warning signs that indicate they need to see a doctor, says Dr. Donnenfeld. These include red eyes accompanied by any discharge, pain in the eyes, decreased sharpness of vision, and sensitivity to light.

You should be very careful with drops, never sharing medications and making sure that the contents don't become contaminated with bacteria, says Dr. Donnenfeld. Also, "no bottle should be used past its expiration date or if the drops become discolored," he says.

Putting eyedrops into your eye is not quite as difficult as making sure bombs dropped from a warplane hit the target, but nonetheless, many people feel intimidated by the process of getting an eyeful. There are many incorrect ways to put in drops, but there is one correct way you should know, says Dr. Donnenfeld.

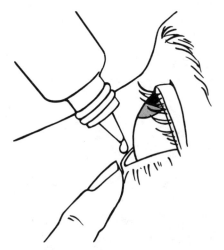

Inserting eyedrops

"Pull the lower lid down with one hand while the other hand holds on to the dropper," he says. "Look up at the ceiling, then look at the dropper while you drop the drop into the space created between your eye and lower lid."

What if your aim was off and you fear that you might have partly missed with the first drop? Then go ahead and put a second drop in—although chances are the first drop is going to prove effective anyway, says Dr. Donnenfeld.

"There's no harm in putting a second drop in if you're not sure," he says. "The volume of tears that are held in your eye is much smaller than a drop, so most of each drop doesn't stay in the eye regardless—only about one-third of a drop does." *See also* **tears, artificial**

eye exercises. *See* **vision therapy**

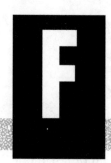

fasting For the desperately overweight, going without food for an extended period—fasting—is a unique type of lose-lose situation. You're almost guaranteed to lose weight. You're almost guaranteed to harm yourself.

A total fast that you supervise yourself is never called for medically, says Patrick O'Neil, Ph.D., director of the Weight Management Center of the Medical University of South Carolina in Charleston. "I can't think of a reason on earth why it would be good for the body," he says.

Others share this opinion.

"It's a really bad method of dieting. Besides losing out in the vitamin and mineral area, there are a lot of biochemical processes going on in the body when you fast which are just not healthy," says Heidi Dufner, a registered dietitian with the University of Vermont extension system in Burlington.

A WASTE OF MUSCLE

"If you go on a total fast and you're not a certain percentage above your weight, then you increase your risk of burning up your own muscle tissue because you don't have enough fat stores," explains Eileen Stellefson, a registered dietitian and associate director of the Weight Management Center. She reminds patients at the Charleston center that the heart, too, is a muscle. "So you're not just losing a little muscle in your legs and arms. Wasting of vital organs can occur," she says.

And if you reason that just a short fast won't hurt anything, think again. "When the body goes on a total fast, it loses the most amount of muscle tissue and protein in the first three days," Stellefson says. "It's very dangerous."

Yet you *will* lose weight on the total fast.

"People say, 'I can fast and lose 4 or 5 pounds in two days.' And I'm sure they can; they are just urinating it away," Dr. O'Neil says.

"When you quit consuming calories through food and drink, your body has to turn to its own internal stores of energy to operate. The first ones it turns to are its glycogen stores," Dr. O'Neil says. Each of us carries about a pound of this fuel source, he explains. While using up the glycogen, we eliminate about 4 to 5 pounds of water. This is the water weight you lose.

Your body may eventually reach a state known as ketosis, Dr. O'Neil says. When this occurs, your system produces ketone bodies, which serve as fuel for certain brain cells. You may notice a fruity odor to your breath, and perhaps loss of appetite and a feeling of euphoria, yet doctors aren't sure if ketosis produces these appetite or mood changes, Dr. O'Neil says. When you begin to eat again, you shift out of ketosis.

Still, this can be a dangerous time. "There are certain by-products of this process that may enter the blood at too high a rate during fasting," Dufner says. "It's dangerous to have this happen. You don't want to experience ketosis."

Although experts advise against fasting, if you do decide to try it, you should be aware of these warning signs, and if you experience them, start eating or see your doctor: dizziness, headache, muscle cramps, diarrhea, or constipation.

You may end a day-long fast by eating just about anything you want. If you've fasted for several days, though, to avoid stomach discomfort, take it easy and start with liquids or juices, avoiding fibrous or rich foods.

A Safer Way

There is a safer way to help obese people lose weight under medical supervision: the supplemented or modified fast. "Unlike a total fast, we supplement with some calories, good-quality protein, and vitamins and minerals that the body needs to survive," Dr. O'Neil says.

At the Weight Management Center, modified fasters drink five specially formulated shakes daily, Dr. O'Neil says, providing them with up to 800 important calories and necessary protein, electrolytes, vitamins, and minerals. These are not the liquid diets of the past or the powders you buy at the grocery store.

The modified fast is recommended only for people who fit the following categories, Dr. O'Neil says: (1) at least 30 percent or 50 pounds overweight and (2) healthy enough to pass a screening assuring there are no underlying problems that would make the fast unsafe.

People who are less than 50 pounds overweight should not use modified fasts because they lose too much muscle and can endanger their health, Dr. O'Neil stresses.

Does the modified fast work?

"The fast is 100 percent successful in getting the weight off for those who comply with it," Stellefson says.

The problem arises when the last lump of shake has been sucked from a straw. "There has to be a maintenance component in order for people to keep the weight off," Stellefson says.

Dr. O'Neil offers these suggestions for finding a safe and effective modified fast program.

• Make sure that the program is hospital based, with a team composed of a physician, registered dietitian, behavioral specialist such as a licensed psychologist or clinical social worker, and an exercise specialist.

• There should be a time limit for the fast, usually 12 to 16 weeks, for health reasons.

• Check for medical screening, testing, and monitoring, including a weekly check by a physician.

• There should be a behavior modification program to help make postfast lifestyle changes.

• Check for nutrition and exercise instruction.

Costs vary, ranging from $2,000 to $4,000 for a total program, and may include all medical tests, consultations, and supplements. *See also* **weight loss**

Feldenkrais Method It might seem far-fetched to suggest that a series of lessons designed to teach small, very subtle changes in everyday body movements can bring improvement to those suffering from a condition as serious as cerebral palsy or help those who've had a stroke. Yet, says Mark Reese, Ph.D., a practitioner of the technique in San Diego County, California, these are areas where the Feldenkrais Method really shines as a healing tool.

"These people often come to us after their therapists tell them they can't get any more improvement," says Dr. Reese, a coauthor of *Relaxercise.* "But we find continual improvement. In Feldenkrais, we emphasize the plasticity of the nervous system. I think anyone at any age, and in any condition,

has the ability to forge new neuro-muscular pathways that allow freer movement."

People suffering from injuries, as well as chronic aches and pains, also turn to Feldenkrais for help. Lessons are dispensed in two forms: group classes and private hands-on table work. Both approaches are gentle and very practical in their orientation, says Larry Goldfarb, a practitioner in Champaign, Illinois, who teaches clinical applications of Feldenkrais to physical and occupational therapists.

NEW WAYS TO MOVE

"Generally, you can expect to learn a new way of doing something by the end of each lesson, whether it's getting in and out of a chair or throwing a baseball," he says. "Each lesson shows you a unique movement. You may not know where you're headed initially, but that's part of the surprise. In Feldenkrais, you're discovering something new about how your body is designed to move."

"Feldenkrais works with the unconscious," he says. "It is not something you have to practice or always be thinking about. People love doing it."

The method was devised by the late Moshe Feldenkrais, an Israeli physicist and judo expert who drew upon both his areas of expertise in an effort to discover how the body was designed to move. He developed hundreds of movement lessons, based on his analysis of patterns in judo, yoga, and other fields—including animal evolution and child development. But there are no

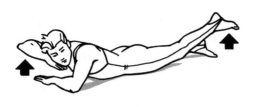

A Feldenkrais exercise

formal studies completed yet to prove that the method can do what its practitioners claim.

Goldfarb says he considers the Feldenkrais Method a good support therapy for people with neuromuscular disorders.

"Most of the people I work with haven't been helped with more traditional methods," he says. "I have one client who was what they call a 'wildcaner' [a reflection of his lack of muscle control after a head injury]. After working with him off and on for a period of two years, he's able to go mountain climbing now."

PAIN REDUCED

Another area where the method can bring "spectacular results," according to Dr. Reese, is chronic joint and muscle pain. "If people commit themselves to a sufficient number of sessions, they are able to get lasting improvement," he says. (He recommends 12 to 24 private lessons, over a 4- to 12-week period, depending on the severity of the condition.)

"We had a psychologist who suffered for 20 years from chronic pain in her back, neck, and jaw. She had shingles—that's what caused the problem to begin with. Within three months of intensive work with us, she's become almost pain free," Dr. Reese says. "For the first time, she has tools she can use that help her eliminate the muscle tightness and pain."

Dr. Reese says people with knee and shoulder injuries might also stand to benefit from Feldenkrais's unique approach. "More traditional therapies focus on the injury itself, by trying to strengthen or stretch the muscles in the affected area. Feldenkrais looks at the person's movements as a whole, to see ways in which other parts of the body may be contributing to the problem." In the same way, says Goldfarb, the method can be used to prevent certain occupational injuries, by teaching people the correct way to move *before* they hurt themselves.

To help locate a practitioner, contact the Feldenkrais Guild, P.O. Box 13285, Overland Park, KS 66212–3285.

fennel   If you should ever dine out at an Indian restaurant, don't count on getting the standard after-dinner mints. More likely, once you've eaten your fill of fiery lamb vindaloo or highly spiced vegetable curry, your waiter will approach with a small, complimentary bowl of fragrant, greenish brown fennel seeds.

Why fennel seeds? "If you eat fennel as part of your meals, you won't have a gas problem," claims Rajul Gupta, owner of Albuquerque's India Kitchen restaurant. "It creates a lot of saliva in your mouth, and that helps you digest your food," she says.

Fennel and other highly flavored foods do indeed increase your saliva output and they also reduce flatulence, says pharmacist David Spoerke, director of the Denver-based POISINDEX Information System, a toxicology computer network. Fennel contains large amounts of anethole, a volatile oil with an antispasmodic effect on the intestinal smooth muscles, Spoerke says, and that inhibits gases from building up.

In the past, fennel was used to soothe tired eyes, boost the production of breast milk, and stimulate menstruation. Traditionally, fennel oil has been regarded as an antibacterial agent.

STICK WITH SEEDS

Unless you're allergic to fennel seeds—which actually are small, dried fruits—they appear to be entirely safe. Fennel extracts, however, may be too concentrated for at-home use, so stick with the whole seeds.

To assist your digestion, munch a tablespoon of fennel seeds after supper, Gupta suggests. Or brew a cup of fennel tea. Simply bruise 1 to 2 tablespoons of seeds and steep them for 10 minutes in a cup of hot water. It tastes like licorice! *See also* **anise**

feverfew   Interest in feverfew is heating up—again. In ancient times, folk wisdom alleged that this herb was good for bringing down fevers (hence its name) as well as treating headaches, menstrual irregularities, and stomachaches. During the 17th century, Europeans relied on feverfew to treat the intermittent fevers caused by malaria. (They even planted feverfew around their homes as an "air purifier" in an effort to ward off the disease, which they mistakenly believed to be caused by putrid air.) But after the discovery of quinine as a malaria treatment, fervor for feverfew cooled down.

FEWER MIGRAINES

Today this member of the daisy family—often confused with another family member, chamomile—is enjoying somewhat of a comeback, this time in connection with migraines. In a 1988 study, University Hospital researchers in Nottingham, England, gave each of 30 people susceptible to migraines one capsule of feverfew per day. Thirty other sufferers took blank capsules. No one knew which group was taking the feverfew. After four months, the two groups switched capsules for another four months. The result: While taking feverfew, the migraine victims had 24 percent fewer headaches than they did while taking the placebos. And the migraines they did get brought less pain and vomiting.

Migraines are now recognized as being a combined neurological and vascular disorder involving fluctuating levels of serotonin—a chemical that causes blood vessels to contract, says Dennis Awang, Ph.D., noted feverfew expert and head of the Natural Products division of Canada's federal

Health Protection Branch. Laboratory studies have identified ingredients in feverfew called sesquiterpene lactones, and one in particular called pathenolide, which appear to inhibit the release of serotonin.

"We're certainly not knowledgable enough to set a precise level for parthenolide needed," Dr. Awang says. And analysis of commercial sources of feverfew in North America revealed that their parthenolide content was much lower than that of the British feverfew used in the Nottingham study, he adds.

Other research suggests that sesquiterpene lactones may prevent the body's production of prostaglandins, thought to be involved in arthritis pain.

HELP IN SMALL DOSES

If you do try feverfew for migraine control, be aware that the herb suppresses these headaches but doesn't cure them. When the therapy stops, migraines typically return, so sufferers might end up taking the herb for years. As for dosage, herb expert Varro E. Tyler, Ph.D., from Purdue University, says, "If you take feverfew by eating the leaves, it should be in very small doses—from 50 to 60 milligrams each day, which is three or four of the little feverfew leaves." Because the herb has a bitter taste, you might want to mix it into other foods to hide the flavor.

So far, no one has reported serious toxic effects in people taking feverfew. But Dr. Tyler cautions that some commercial feverfew products currently available do not contain as much of the herb as they claim. And

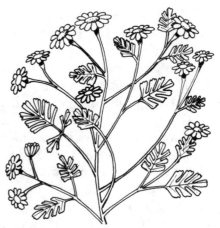

Feverfew

in some people, feverfew causes swollen lips, dulled taste buds, and sore mouth and tongue. Finally, pregnant women shouldn't take chances with feverfew, experts say, until they know more about how it works.

One note: Do not confuse feverfew with the plant known as Santa Maria feverfew, which grows along the Gulf Coast and in other subtropical climates. This plant may be responsible for allergies previously blamed on ragweed. Researchers say that many people who experience watery eyes, runny noses, and itchy throats may be reacting to Santa Maria feverfew rather than the ragweed that grows in the same areas. If you think you might be affected, see your allergist.

fiber   Food trends come and go, but fiber is forever. Every other day, it seems, doctors find new ways to use this food factor as a remedy for . . . well, for almost everything.

When high cholesterol threatened, fiber rushed to the rescue. When constipation, diverticulitis, hemorrhoids, and other lower digestive tract afflictions made life miserable, fiber brought relief. Fiber came through for diabetics . . . for heavy people trying to lose weight . . . for slender people trying to stay thin. High-fiber magic? You bet.

There's a catch. Fiber works, but only if we eat enough of it. And most of us don't. A survey of 11,658 adults revealed they consumed an average of 11.1 grams of fiber a day—a long way from the National Cancer Institute's recommendation of 20 to 35 grams (about 1 ounce) of fiber daily.

It's easy to have a high-fiber day. A serving of broccoli, for example, holds 2.4 grams of fiber—about one-tenth of your daily requirement. Do you like whole wheat spaghetti with mushroom sauce? One serving delivers up to 4.2 grams of fiber. An apple holds 2.8 grams, and a double handful of dried apricots packs 4 grams. If you eat a large oat bran muffin and a plate of baked beans, you get 11.4 grams.

That's the wonderful thing about fruits, vegetables, and grains. You don't have to eat a truckload to get your fiber fill.

What is fiber, really? It's the parts of a plant you don't digest. It's as simple as that. Of course, there are many different forms of fiber—including cellulose, pectin, and gums—all of which have parts in our high-fiber play. However, the various fibers are generally grouped in two broad categories: soluble and insoluble.

Soluble fiber—oat bran is a rich source, as are beans, apples, and carrots—dissolves in water and is absorbed into your bloodstream. Insoluble fiber, abundantly present in wheat bran, rice bran, and lentils, remains relatively unchanged on its intestinal journey. But these aren't the only differences, so let's take a closer look.

Cholesterol Cut

Soluble fibers have received a lot of attention for their cholesterol-lowering abilities. For instance, volunteers in a study conducted by the Department of Medicine at the University of California at Irvine ate two oat bran muffins a day for 28 days. They lowered their total cholesterol 5.3 percent. If that doesn't sound like much, remember that for every 1 percent you lower your cholesterol, you reduce your risk for heart disease by 2 percent.

Score one for soluble fiber.

Doctors agree obesity is a killer. They also agree foods rich in fiber trim the fat. For one thing, most high-fiber foods contain very little, if any, fat. And by rapidly inducing satiety (a feeling of fullness), they leave less room for hamburgers, shakes, and fries.

Non-insulin-dependent diabetics can also benefit from high-fiber diets. Because dietary fiber increases the time it takes to digest and absorb foods, tissues get a steady supply of glucose, and that reduces uncomfortable swings in blood sugar.

Insoluble fibers also deserve a tip of our high-fiber hats. They soak up water in the lower intestine, so stools become larger and softer. Bowel movements become easier and more regular. If you eat the recommended level of enough fiber, you'll rarely be constipated. If you do get hemorrhoids, a fiber-rich diet can make your stools less painful to pass.

Even though dietary fiber is a must for a smoothly functioning digestive tract, newcomers to high-fiber diets should proceed carefully, says Barbara Harland, Ph.D., a nutritionist at Howard University in Washington, D.C. Dietary fibers absorb a lot of water, so you should increase your fluid intake. In addition, your innards are used to your old ways of eating. If you eat too much fiber before they have a chance to adjust, "you just won't feel good. There will be a lot of bloating, gas, and flatulence," Dr. Harland says.

Take about a month to work up to your goal of a total of 20 to 35 grams of fiber a day, she says. And enjoy it. Eating more fiber isn't supposed to be hard work—just good sense. *See also* **bran**

fish   Most Americans eat one fish meal a week. If that describes you, be advised that many doctors would like to see you eating fish two to three times more often.

Why? One reason is that fish is a very lean alternative to red meat: 3 ounces of cooked Atlantic salmon (one of the fattiest fish) has less than one-third the total fat of 3 ounces of broiled rib-eye steak. Other fish, especially white fish like flounder, haddock, and cod, have almost negligible amounts of fat.

But what really clinches fish as a superfood is that whatever little fat you do find in fish—quite unlike the fat of land animals—may actually be *good* for you! A number of studies show that the omega-3 fatty acids found in fish fat may protect against heart disease and other ailments like rheumatoid arthritis and psoriasis.

FISH FOR THE BEST

If fish fat is good for you, does that mean you should go out of your way to pick fish high in fat, like sardines or herring? Not necessarily. "Research shows that even a small amount of fish fat can provide substantial protection for your heart," says Virginia F. Stout, Ph.D., a researcher at the Utilization Research Division of the Northwest Fisheries Center of the National Marine Fisheries Service.

Since all fish contain some omega-3's, it's hard to go wrong with whatever fish you eat, and you should enjoy a variety, says Dr. Stout. Aside from the fat factor, a variety of fish will also supply your body with important nutrients like magnesium, potassium, iron, and zinc.

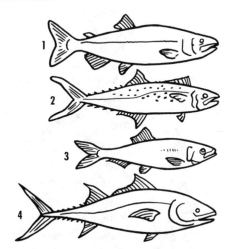

Fish rich in omega-3 oils: (1) salmon, (2) mackerel, (3) herring, (4) tuna

But what about *shellfish?* Aren't they just swimming in cholesterol, a leading contributor to heart disease? Well, there are two kinds of shellfish—mollusks and crustaceans. Mollusks (clams, oysters, scallops) aren't as high in cholesterol as was once thought. And crustaceans (shrimp, lobster), while high in cholesterol, are low in saturated fat, the main villain in heart disease. The American Heart Association says that one serving of lobster or shrimp a week is perfectly all right for people on a prudent (low-fat, low-cholesterol) diet.

Is any kind of fish *not* all right? The only one that deserves a red flag is squid, or *calamari,* as it's known in most Italian restaurants. "The cholesterol content of squid is comparable to that of egg yolk," says Irena B. King, Ph.D., a research scientist with the University of Washington School of Medicine. "Squid should be eaten only occasionally and preferably not fried," she says. *See also* **fish oil**

fish oil   Down, down in the ocean deep, where temperatures can hover near freezing, our fair-finned friends swim about oblivious to the intense cold. How? Partly, because of their body oil. Unlike the body fat of land animals, which is solid and turns even harder when chilled, fish oil stays liquid even when cold. This difference may be significant if you're concerned about the health of your heart.

Fish oil contains substances known as omega-3 fatty acids. These not only keep fish oil liquid, they also make it a healing factor of the first order. Eskimos, who eat sled-loads of fish, seem to have a remarkable power to ward off heart disease. That's why so many doctors are saying that by getting more fish oil in *your* diet, *you* may be able to do the same.

A cold look at the Eskimos is what first brought fish oil into the public eye. That was 20 years ago. Since then, numerous studies have lent only more reason to consider fish oil as a firm friend of a firm heart. One such study, from the British medical journal *Lancet,* looked at more than 2,000 men who had already suffered heart attacks and concluded that those who went on to get the most fish oil significantly boosted their chances of warding off the Grim Reaper.

The men in the study were separated into three groups. One group was advised to cut down on total fat while increasing the ratio of polyunsaturated to saturated fat in their diet. Group two was told to eat more fiber. Group three was advised to eat more fish. Although all three suggestions were good ones, the best—the very best—turned out to be the last. After two years, 29 percent more of the frequent fish eaters were around to celebrate the good news.

WHY IT WORKS

Scientists are grappling to better understand how fish oil works its magic. One theory is that it interferes with the stickiness of the blood, making it less likely to form artery-blocking clots. Fish oil may also make red blood cells more flexible, so they can dart around sharp curves in arteries without creating logjams. Fish oil also seems to somehow evict heart-threatening triglycerides and cholesterol from the bloodstream.

Researchers at the University of Washington have provided new clues as to how fish oil may offer even greater health benefits. In a study published in the *American Journal of Clinical Nutrition,* the cholesterol-lowering powers of two distinct kinds of omega-3 fatty acids—docosahexaenoic acids, or DHA, and eicosapentaenoic acids, or EPA—were put to the test. One group of people received supplemental pollack oil that was rich in EPA, while the rest got tuna or salmon-blend oil, rich in DHA. The DHA group had the best luck. Their overall cholesterol levels were reduced by 23 to 31 percent.

Until now, omega-3 fatty acids were not well understood, but this is changing, says Irena B. King, Ph.D., research scientist in the School of Medicine at the University of Washington and one of the authors of the study. In the future, she says, additional research may help us better understand the healing power of fish oil and how we can best make use of it (perhaps by separating the DHA and EPA).

WHERE TO GET IT

For now, doctors agree that the very best way to get fish oil is by eating fish, just as the people in igloos do. It's difficult to pick a fish that's higher in DHA than EPA, because the level of these substances in a particular species varies depending on where the fish is in its spawning cycle. Some fish, however, are higher in *all* omega-3's.

What kinds of fish? You guessed it—those fish from the nippiest ocean waters, like mackerel and bluefish. But all fish have some oil, and studies show that you really don't need much to reap the maximum benefits for your heart. Dr. King recommends three fish meals a week, with perhaps one of the three being a particularly oily fish and the other two, "simply what you like." The important thing, she says, "is to enjoy it."

What about fish-oil supplements? Doctors advise caution. In such concentration, fish oil can interfere *too much* with the ability of blood to clot and, in some people, may even cause excessive bleeding. Eating fish rather than taking supplements is the preferred route to a healthier heart.

Dr. King, who is also with the Cancer Prevention Research Laboratory at the Fred Hutchinson Cancer Research Center in Seattle, says her next study will track the effects of fish oil on breast cancer. There's good reason for such a study—"breast cancer, like heart disease, is extremely low among Eskimos," she says.

And who knows what other health benefits from fish oil may emerge in the future? Preliminary research has indicated that this natural remedy may also help those with rheumatoid arthritis, psoriasis, Raynaud's disease, and asthma. *See also* **fish**

flotation tanks Why would anyone want to float in a dark tank for an hour? People who drift in the silent void of a flotation tank do it to beat stress, combat high blood pressure, ease headache pain, kick bad habits, and boost concentration.

When you float in a tank, you are essentially drifting in warm, buoyant liquid inside a light-free, soundproof chamber. Today's tanks barely resemble the earlier coffinlike structures known as "sensory deprivation" or "isolation" tanks, once tucked away in research labs. The updated tanks can be found in pain clinics, stress-management centers, and athletic camps, as well as commercial float centers.

And the new models are user-friendly. One state-of-the-art tank is shiny, red, and looks like a Porsche without windows or wheels. Certainly not designed for sensory deprivation, it's equipped with a Jacuzzi and switches to control dim lights, an intercom, and even a video screen.

The primary purpose of a flotation tank, however, is to tune *out* distractive stimuli. In your own private sea, you see only blackness. You hear nothing but your own breathing. The water is heated to skin temperature, so you barely feel it on your skin. Your body seems to melt. Eight hundred pounds of dissolved Epsom salts keeps you bobbing weightlessly. As one floater put it, "It's as if you are suspended somewhere between the earth and moon."

Floating, free of light, sound, and touch, you are now able to tune in to profound relaxation that, scientists have found, triggers the same positive physical and mental effects that occur during meditation.

And even more significantly, this deep relaxation seems to linger long after the float is over, according to Thomas Fine, assistant professor of mental health at the Medical College of Ohio.

When researchers there tested people who had floated for 1 hour, they found that the subjects' heart rates and breathing had slowed down and their blood pressures dropped. This favorable drop in blood pressure may be due to the additonal finding that floaters had lower levels of cortisol and other stress hormones that influence high blood pressure. Moreover, these stress hormone levels remained lower for several days. This suggests that after a float, you may increase your tolerance to stress. Floating, it appears, changes your blood pressure to a lower "set point," according to Fine.

NATURAL PAINKILLER

If you are suffering chronic back pain, headaches, or some other painful condition, floating can be a part of your pain management program, according to Gib Koula, program coordinator of Stress Lab Services at St. Elizabeth's Hospital, Appelton, Wisconsin. Researchers have found that when flotation is used as a primary method of relaxation training, chronic pain conditions improved. For one thing, pain is eased because buoyancy reduces pressure on the body and thus brings blessed relief. Even more significant is the fact that floating triggers the production of endorphins, your body's natural painkillers.

Gratefully, this special painkilling

effect continues after you step out of the tank. Roderick Borrie, Ph.D., director of the Sensorium Clinic, East Seatauket, Long Island, found that when people who suffered from rheumatoid arthritis floated twice a week, they were able to remain pain free for up to five days.

The big advantage of using a flotation tank for pain management is that it serves as a natural form of feedback. Without outside stimulation you can zero in on your breathing, heart rate, and muscle tension. "This feedback helps you learn how to deeply relax and alter bodily functions at will for the times you need pain relief when you are not floating," says Koula.

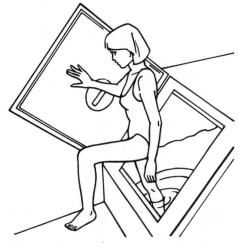

Flotation tank

TANKS FOR THE MEMORY

Some people are floating before they make a speech, have a tennis match, or take exams. Sound farfetched? It's not. Preliminary studies show that flotation can help improve concentration, boost memory, and enhance learning, according to Dr. Borrie.

When you float, your brain waves switch to a lower frequency and you enter a trance state much like the early stages of sleep or meditation. Experts such as Fine theorize that in this state your mind is more receptive to suggestions and visualizations. When you are starved for stimulation, you go into "stimulus hunger." Your mind gobbles up whatever images or information you feed it—whether from your own imagination or from a tape played through the tank's intercom.

Suppose you would like to make a successful speech. It's possible to imagine a perfect state of performance while floating and then be able to duplicate it in your active life.

If you would like to kick the smoking habit, stop overeating, or overcome your fear of heights, you might try the "floating couch" therapy. While floating, you become more open to positive behavioral suggestions communicated by the therapist through the intercom. For this reason, therapists have found that floating works better than hypnosis for helping patients break bad habits, says Lloyd Glauberman, Ph.D., a Manhattan clinical psychologist.

If you wish to break a habit or control pain, hypertension, or some other problem, see a specialist who uses a flotation tank for stress management. "Flotation is more effective when used as part of a relaxation training program," says Dr. Borrie.

If you would like to float away from everyday stress and tension, you can rent a float tank on an hourly basis at commercial centers or health clubs. It may take a few sessions before you are able to fully relax in this pitch black, silent environment. To locate a float tank for recreational or therapeutic purposes, contact the Flotation Tank Association, P.O. Box 1396, Grass Valley, CA 95945.

fluids "Drink plenty of fluids, take two aspirin, and call me in the morning." Is there a doctor *anywhere* who has never said that? We all know that aspirin is helpful for aches and fever when you're under the weather. But what is it about *fluids?*

The fluids doctors recommend when you're out of sorts are not always intended to cure your illness. Chicken soup, whatever Grandma says, is no antibiotic. But extra fluids are critical to replace all the extra water your body is using while trying to heal itself. You can easily lose 1 quart or more a day through vomiting, running to the bathroom with diarrhea, or sweating under your covers, says Hinda Greene, D.O., staff internist with the Cleveland Clinic in Fort Lauderdale, Florida.

Experts recommend that you drink extra fluids any time anything is causing you to sweat—including exercise, hot weather, or (for women) "hot flashes" associated with menopause. If you spend long periods of time in air-conditioned, heated, or other dry environments (airplanes are infamously dry), bottoms up. Extra fluids are also commonly recommended for a number of ailments, most notably kidney stones (to help pass the stones) and urinary tract infections.

FILLING YOUR QUOTA

Under normal conditions, your need for fluids (beyond those contained in your food) will range from 6 to 8 cups a day, says Kathleen M. Zelman, a registered dietitian, spokeswoman for the American Dietetic Association, and dietetic internship director at Ochsner Medical Institutions in New Orleans. Fill those cups with water, milk, juice, soup, lemonade, or just about any other fluid. But don't depend on alcoholic and caffeinated beverages. Alcohol, although a fluid, actually dries the body out. And beverages containing caffeine tend to pass through you too quickly, says Zelman.

How much additional liquid do you need when you're sick? If you have a mild fever, you should try to drink roughly 1 quart or more above the normal requirement, says Dr. Greene. If you're having trouble keeping things down, she recommends that you take your fluids in frequent small amounts—for example, a tablespoon every few minutes. "This may help you avoid stomach contractions that can make you throw up," she says.

When you're feeling ill, clear fluids, like apple juice or broth, are usually the best. These are most easily tolerated by an upset tummy. Of course, water is the clearest of all liquids, and most experts recommend you drink lots of water. But when you're sick, and your appetite hasn't been so hot, you might be better off sipping something containing a few calories and extra nutrients, says Zelman. (Water has neither.)

Is Grandma's chicken soup a good option? Yes, perhaps—but let it cool a bit before digging in. With an upset stomach, you're better off avoiding anything too hot or too cold, says Dr. Greene. *See also* **chicken soup; electrolytes; water**

fluoride In the phobia hall of fame, even the fear of being audited or the terror of getting stuck in an elevator pales next to the sheer dread of the dentist's drill. The mere thought of a shrieking, spinning tool boring deep into a cavity is enough to make even Stephen King shudder.

Today's kids are lucky. Many of them may never know such "drill dread" at all. Thanks to the use of fluoride, nearly half of the 5- to 17-year-olds in the United States don't have a single cavity in their teeth, studies show.

But the need for protection is lifelong. To keep avoiding the drill and a mouth full of fillings, root canals, and dentures, experts say you must continue bathing your teeth with fluoride even as an adult.

Fortunately, you don't have to look far for this natural element. Fluoride is an essential mineral found in soil and water in various concentrations. Added to oral treatment products in small amounts, and to drinking water in even smaller amounts, it fortifies your teeth against decay in a number of ways,

depending on whether you swallow it or a dentist swabs it on.

If you swallow a sufficient amount of fluoride starting as a baby when your smile is all gums, the mineral is absorbed into your bloodstream, deposited in developing teeth, and incorporated in their crystalline structure. Years later, when your permanent teeth come in, they are harder, denser, and more resistant to decay.

Once your permanent teeth are in, there's no longer a need to ingest fluoride into your system.

But bathing your teeth regularly with fluoride is important for people of all ages. "Topically, fluoride works by making the surface enamel on your teeth less likely to dissolve in acid," explains John Bogert, D.D.S., executive director of the American Academy of Pediatric Dentistry. Acid is produced from bacteria growing in the sticky plaque that builds up on tooth surfaces. "When you apply fluoride topically, the enamel absorbs it and forms calcium fluoride, which acts like a protective shield against acid," says Dr. Bogert. At the same time, fluoride helps remineralize (build up) the enamel surface against acid onslaught.

There's more. Fluoride also interferes with the decay-causing bacteria that produce acid.

This means that applying fluoride faithfully keeps bacteria at bay, remineralizes your teeth, and even reverses the early decay process. "Fluoride can arrest the microscopic holes that form in the enamel," says Gary M. Whitford, D.M.D., regents professor of oral biology at the School of Dentistry of the Medical College of Georgia in Atlanta.

NOT JUST IN TOOTHPASTE

For most of us, it's not practical to continually visit the dentist for a professional application of a super-strong fluoride solution. So more than half of all U.S. communities have added fluoride to the drinking water supply in extremely low amounts. This addition adjusts the fluoride level up to the optimal level (one part per million) recommended by the American Dental Association (ADA).

For kids living in nonfluoridated areas, pediatric dentists routinely prescribe fluoride drops or tablets to be taken daily from the time the child is in diapers until close to driving age.

The ADA also recommends that children as well as adults brush with a fluoridated toothpaste twice daily—no matter how much fluoride is in the water.

Compared to drinking water, toothpastes are concentrated fluoride sources, says Dr. Bogert.

If you are cavity-prone, your dentist may recommend that you use one of the newer, super-strength fluoridated gel toothpastes or add a fluoride mouth rinse product to your cavity-control routine.

A fluoride rinse may be particularly important if you take antidepressants or other medications that dry out your mouth, or if you have a reduced saliva production for other reasons. Saliva is your body's built-in defense against decay-causing bacteria.

It washes them away. "When you are older or take certain medications, saliva production may come to a standstill," says Phillip Trask, D.D.S., associate clinical professor at the University of California, Los Angeles, Dental School. "In that case, swishing with a fluoride rinse at bedtime may be advised."

Likewise, a fluoride rinse may help if your gums have started to recede. Receding gums expose a part of the tooth that has never been treated with topical fluoride. The rinse could help reduce cavities around these vulnerable roots, says Dr. Trask.

Because fluoride in excess amounts is toxic, topical fluoride rinses and gels are intended for you to swish and spit out. "They are not to be swallowed or used as mouthwashes or breath fresheners," says Dr. Bogert.

So don't let children under 12 use them without supervision. Ingesting high concentrations of fluoride could cause permanent teeth to come in with fluorosis, chalky white patches in the enamel, says Dr. Whitford.

BUILDS BONE, BUT...

Fluoride has also been prescribed as a treatment to strengthen bones as well as teeth. Because of the mineral's ability to stimulate new bone growth, doctors considered it a promising treatment for the bone-thinning disorder known as osteoporosis.

But a four-year study conducted by the Mayo Clinic has cast doubt on this approach. One group of women with osteoporosis was given 75 milligrams of sodium fluoride a day. (This is more than 30 times the amount provided daily by fluoridated water.) A second group was given a nonactive substitute. Both groups were also given 1,500 milligrams a day of calcium, which helps the body utilize fluoride.

The researchers found that while bone mass in the spine increased by more than a third in the fluoride-treated women, the overall rate of fractures did not decrease significantly. In fact, the number of hip and wrist fractures was *higher* in the treatment group.

"The sodium fluoride did stimulate the bone-forming cells, but the bone formed was laid down in a less organized pattern and was less elastic and more brittle than normal bone," says the study's coauthor, Steven Hodgson, M.D., associate professor of medicine and endocrinology at the Mayo Medical School in Rochester, Minnesota. "Using fluoride treatment for osteoporosis is like constructing a faulty bridge. If it's thrown together with weak materials, it won't hold up."

The bottom line: Sodium fluoride gets a definite thumbs-up for preventing tooth decay and a possible thumbs-down for preventing osteoporosis. "Sodium fluoride in the dosage used is not an effective or safe treatment for osteoporosis," says Dr. Hodgson.

folate. *See* **nutritional therapy**

foot odor remedies If taking off your shoes gets the same reaction as lifting the lid off a garbage pail, foot odor products may be your foot-pollution solution.

A quick, convenient way to elim-inate offensive foot fumes is to spritz on a foot deodorant spray. Most of these products contain antibacterial agents that can kill odor-causing bacteria on contact.

Deodorant products are more effective if you attack the underlying cause of foot fumes, says Richard L. Dobson, M.D., a professor of dermatology at the Medical University of South Carolina. Foot odor usually occurs because your feet get overheated, sweat pours from the sweat glands just under the skin, and then bacteria acts upon the sweaty secretions. Therefore, Dr. Dobson says, the best way to stop the stench is to reduce perspiration and get rid of bacteria buildup.

Just as you probably wouldn't apply an underarm deodorant before washing, you should apply a foot deodorant to clean feet. Use an ordinary antibacterial soap, or a special foot soap containing antibacterial agents such as borax and iodine. Be sure to dry each and every toe, too. Between washings, keep bacteria in check with your foot deodorant spray or by sprinkling powder containing the antibacterial tricosan into a fresh pair of socks. Don't forget to powder the insides of your shoes, too.

Avoid foot powders containing boric acid. This antibacterial ingredient is extremely toxic and may be absorbed into your skin if you have a cut.

Not all acids are bad for your feet, though. In fact, the higher the level of acidity on your skin, the more you can reduce bacteria. That's why some experts recommend soaking your feet in ½ cup of vinegar (vinegar is very acidic) mixed with 1 quart of water. This easy-to-make solution makes the surface of your feet more acidic and less hospitable to odor-causing bacteria. Try soaking for 15 minutes at a time, twice a week.

If your feet reek like Limburger or Camembert cheese, you may need more than drugstore remedies. A pungent, cheesy odor could mean that your feet are harboring certain bacteria similar to those used in making those cheeses. If so, you may benefit from a prescription for an antibiotic liquid containing clindamycin. A dermatological researcher at the University of Miami School of Medicine has found that with regular use, this liquid can keep the bacteria under control and eliminate odor.

No-Sweat Tactics

Another important way to fight foot odor is to keep your feet dry. Some doctors recommend using an underarm antiperspirant product containing aluminum salts on your feet. But underarm antiperspirants may not be effective. "The skin on your feet is thicker than the skin under your arms and may not absorb the aluminum chloride in commercial products," says Jerome Z. Litt, M.D., assistant clinical professor of dermatology at Case Western Reserve University School of Medicine in Cleveland, Ohio. This explains why there are so few foot antiperspirants available.

Dr. Litt says the best home remedy for reducing excess foot perspiration is to soak your feet in a drying solution such as tea. Place two tea bags in a pint of boiling water for 15 minutes. Pour the brew into a tub filled with 2 quarts of cool water and soak your feet for 20 to 30 minutes. Do this daily for a week to ten days, and after that use only as needed. The tannin in tea literally tans the hide on your feet, blocking the pores and choking off the sweat. If odor lingers, try the same approach using *four* tea bags.

In between soaks, let your feet "breathe" as much as possible. Avoid rubber-soled or plastic shoes, or any other airtight footwear material that seals in moisture. Wear sandals around the house. Slip into light-colored or white, all-natural fiber socks. Dust your feet, socks, and shoes with absorbent powders that contain cornstarch or talc. You might also find that wearing shoe inserts containing activated charcoal will help absorb moisture and odor, Dr. Dobson says. Be sure to change these inserts often.

Keeping your feet clean and dry can eliminate most foot odor problems. If the bad smell persists, your doctor can prescribe Drysol, a strong solution of aluminum chloride and alcohol that obstructs the pores. Dr. Dobson says it works for 95 percent of people with persistent foot perspiration and odor.

foxglove. *See* **digitalis**

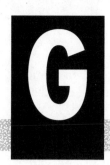

gamma globulin   There are three good things you can say about the majority of infectious diseases: They usually occur *once* during a person's lifetime. They help make your immune system stronger. And they leave something in your blood that can prevent *other* people from getting sick. Here's how.

When a disease bacteria enters the body, your immune system begins producing antibodies—made by attack cells that recognize and fight that particular bug. Those same antibodies, taken from blood donors like yourself and made into gamma globulin, then can protect other people before *they* catch the disease.

Also called immune globulin, gamma globulin actually contains many kinds of antibodies, says Stephen L. Cochi, M.D., a pediatric epidemiologist with the federal Centers for Disease Control in Atlanta. That means one shot can protect people from diseases such as measles and hepatitis A.

Another type of globulin, called the hyperimmune globulin, works the same way. But it's more selective, usually containing large amounts of antibodies for only one disease—rabies,

for example—instead of many different kinds.

"The immune globulins generally are used to prevent the disease before the exposure actually occurs, although in some cases they're given very soon after the exposure to abort the illness," Dr. Cochi says.

Although both are typically given by injection, it's important to differentiate between immune globulins and vaccines, Dr. Cochi says. Vaccines usually are made from weakened or killed forms of the disease-causing virus or bacteria. Those vaccines made from weakened forms of a disease-causing virus or bacteria are not strong enough to make you sick, but they do stimulate your body's production of antibodies, which can later protect you from disease. Immune globulins, on the other hand, are borrowed antibodies; when they leave your bloodstream, you're once again susceptible to the disease.

QUICK PROTECTION

They have the advantage, however, of being fast acting. People who receive immune globulins don't have

243

to wait several weeks for their immune system to crank out antibodies—they're fully armed, as it were, right away. That's why vacationers on tight deadlines often receive immune globulins before they depart for distant climes, Dr. Cochi says.

"The risk of hepatitis is probably the most common reason for using immune globulins," he says. "For example, if a food outbreak [of hepatitis] has been identified, people who have eaten at the implicated restaurant may be given immune globulins."

There are many types of immune globulins. People exposed to rabies, for example, might receive a rabies immune globulin (RIG). (They would be given a rabies vaccine, too.) The varicella zoster immune globulin (VZIG) protects against herpes zoster, and tetanus immune globulin (TIG) may be given after some puncture wounds.

While some vaccines and immune globulins are given at the same time (to protect against tetanus, for example), the immune globulins usually are used alone, Dr. Cochi says.

"In order for a vaccine to take, the weakened virus has to multiply many times and get into your bloodstream before your immune system will produce antibodies against it," he explains. "If you gave immune globulin at the same time, it would attack the virus and prevent it from multiplying."

gargling If you've ever soaked in a Jacuzzi, you know how soothing the swirling bubbles can be to sore muscles.

Gargling is like a Jacuzzi for your sore throat—at least for the raw, upper portion you see in the mirror and that hurts like the dickens when you swallow. The gurgling liquid bathes the back of your mouth and helps gently scrub away mucus, phlegm, and debris, which can irritate inflamed throat tissues. Discomfort and pain float away.

If they held a contest for the gentlest gargling liquid, the antiseptic mouthwashes would lose. When you swish with these tingly tasting products, you feel a coolness as if you've just inhaled an ice cube. That's because the phenol, menthol, and other antiseptic ingredients irritate nerve endings so they tingle when exposed to the air. Unfortunately, these ingredients may also irritate throat tissues. "They can make a sore throat worse," warns John Henderson, M.D., assistant clinical professor of ear, nose, and throat surgery at the University of California School of Medicine in San Diego.

Moreover, just because these mouthwashes smell mediciny doesn't mean they can cure your sore throat or shorten your cold. Antiseptic mouthwashes wipe out only the harmless bacteria that normally reside in your mouth. It's a temporary victory, anyway. Soon after you spit the stuff out, new bacteria move in.

And mouthwashes are no match for cold viruses. These menacing microbes invade deeply into cells—well out of the range of mouthwashes. What all this means is that "chemical gargles may kill millions of germs, but your cold lingers on," says Neil

Schachter, M.D., associate director of pulmonary medicine at Mount Sinai Medical Center in New York City.

If you really want to help your sore throat, go for a gentle gargle with *real* medicinal power: saltwater. That's right. Ordinary table salt mixed with warm water in a weak solution is the throat tonic doctors recommend most. Why? "Saltwater mimics the body's natural saline content, so it doesn't irritate nerve endings," says Dr. Henderson. What's more, salt reduces swelling in infected cells by sucking them dry of germs and fluids. And the warm water acts like a magnet, drawing healing white blood cells to the infected area.

Another benefit: Saltwater doesn't dull your taste buds as the harsh antiseptic gargles can. Just be sure you don't swallow any of the solution if you're on a sodium-restricted diet.

GARGLING GUIDELINES

Make your saltwater gargle by mixing 1 teaspoon of salt in 1 pint of warm water.

To assume the proper gargling position, imagine you are auditioning for the Metropolitan Opera. Sip a small amount of saltwater, gently drop your head back, and blow air bubbles. Now, in your best Pavarotti vibrato, hum the musical scale.

"Making noise helps direct the soothing saltwater more deeply into your mouth," says Dr. Henderson.

But if you have laryngitis, nix the noise. "The vibration can actually harm inflamed vocal cords," says Robert J. Feder, M.D., former chief of otolaryn-

gology at Cedars-Sinai Medical Center in Los Angeles.

If you have laryngitis or are hoarse or have a cough, it means that the sore spot is further down—too far for gargling to help.

"Gargling may not reach down into the larynx where the irritated or inflamed tissue is," says Dr. Feder. He found this out by taking x-rays of 15 volunteers after they gargled with a harmless radio-opaque substance. In all cases, the fluid made it only to the back of the tongue, not deep into the throat.

When you gargle, your tongue rises and acts as a barricade, blocking the fluid from reaching down past the soft palate at the back of your mouth.

Still, a saltwater gargle can make swallowing more bearable when you have a sore throat. If your throat hurts for more than two days, however, stop gargling and see your doctor. *See also* **sore throat remedies**

garlic Eating this culinary cousin of the lily won't sweeten your kisses, but it just might give you a hardier heart. Garlic's potential to treat—and prevent—a number of cardiovascular diseases has been suggested in a spate of studies. There have been many claims made for this ancient folk remedy, but this one, scientists say, has the most support.

If you've ever minced a clove of garlic or crushed one, then you know some of its active ingredients by smell. Garlic contains over 200 different compounds. The important ones, medicinally, include the same sulfur compounds that release garlic's pungent odor when the clove is cut or bruised. (Cloves are the individual segments in a "head" or bulb of garlic.)

One of these compounds, allicin, has been shown in the lab to kill bacteria even in concentrations as low as 1 part per 125,000. Allicin has also been shown to reduce the tendency of blood platelets to clump together and form clots that could potentially cause heart attacks.

HEART HELPER?

Garlic seems to have a special talent for keeping the arteries clear and improving blood circulation. Preventing platelets from clumping is just one of the ways in which it does this, says Robert I-San Lin, Ph.D., the Irvine, California, clinical researcher who organized the first world congress on garlic health effects. Garlic also enhances fibrinolytic activity — the blood's mechanism for breaking up potentially dangerous clots.

But the most consistently demonstrated property of garlic in humans is its ability to reduce artery-clogging cholesterol. Five out of six studies on people found this effect. The drawback is that volunteers had to consume the equivalent of 7 to 28 breath-fouling cloves a day. (Some of the studies used garlic extracts.) In another study of ten people with high cholesterol, garlic powder — in a daily dose equivalent to 64 cloves of garlic — brought their blood fat levels 10 percent lower than a low-fat diet alone. Levels of trigly-

cerides, which can contribute to artery clogging, also dropped.

There's also indirect evidence for garlic's protective benefits: Several population studies show that the more garlic consumed, the lower the incidence of coronary heart disease among that population.

Garlic's promise as a heart helper is nothing new to the Chinese. For centuries, herbalists there have used garlic aged in wine or vinegar to treat people suffering from the chest pain attacks of angina, Dr. Lin says. And a close relative of garlic is one of five standard herbs Chinese physicians still prescribe for people with circulatory disorders, he adds.

AN AID TO DIGESTION

Garlic may aid other body systems, too. Purdue University herb specialist Varro E. Tyler, Ph.D., says that eating garlic can improve digestion by aiding peristalsis, the rhythmic squeezing and releasing process that moves food through the intestines. There are even hints of a possible link between garlic-laced meals and lower rates of stomach and colorectal cancer. Dr. Lin says the Chinese have long used garlic as an herbal treatment for tumors.

The bulbous herb is also a mild antibiotic. In the lab, it's been shown to conquer the types of bacteria that cause typhoid fever, yeast infections, and intestinal ailments like diarrhea. Ancient warriors used to tote garlic so they'd have it on hand if they were wounded, says Judith Dausch, a registered dietitian and coauthor of a National Cancer Institute review of the healing properties of garlic.

Eating garlic for this purpose is safer than rubbing it on the skin, however. Its irritant effects were amply demonstrated by three young Israeli soldiers who, intent on getting a medical discharge, rubbed raw garlic on healthy skin until they developed debilitating sores, says Eric Block, Ph.D., chairman of the chemistry department at the State University of New York at Albany and a world expert on the constituents of garlic.

Given the evidence, should you make garlic a regular part of your diet? While there is no conclusive proof that garlic will cure anything, tossing a few minced cloves in with salads, marinades, or pasta can't hurt and just may help, experts say.

Just don't go overboard. Eating more raw garlic than your tummy can handle can easily upset it. And eating garlic paste by the jar could actually burn the lining of the stomach and esophagus and even cause anemia, Dr. Block warns.

Cooked or dried garlic is kinder to your insides but may not be as potent. Most experts believe that both processes destroy many of garlic's healing agents. But commercially available powdered garlic extract apparently gets around this problem. "Aged garlic extract contains potent cholesterol inhibitors," says Asaf Qureshi, Ph.D., president of Advanced Medical Research in Madison, Wisconsin.

Other garlic supplements, in tablet and capsule form, are also available.

Most of these products can spare you from that garlicky smell.

"I still think the fresh plant is the best, the safest, and the most time-tested," Dr. Block says. "It's undergone 3,000 years of use and there have been minimal reports of serious problems. The other products are relatively new on the scene."

gentian violet (JEN-shun) Not long ago, when a woman had a vaginal infection, the cure was nearly as bad as the condition. Doctors used to swab a gentian violet solution in the vagina to treat vaginitis. This substance with the genteel name is a powerful microbe killer that works agains fungi, parasites, and bacteria living in moist environments of the body.

Gentian violet doesn't do its work invisibly, however. Whatever it touches — you, your clothes, your furniture — is left with a deep purple stain. "If I were rating the messiest liquids on a scale of one to four," says one doctor, "gentian violet would rate a five!"

Gentian violet gets its colorful name not from a plant but from triphenylmethane, a coal tar derivative that provides the basis for a number of purplish red staining products. Also known as crystal violet and methylrosaniline chloride, gentian violet is used as a staining dye for viewing microscopic slides, for typewriter ribbons, and in hair dyes.

Therapeutically, a number of newer, less messy antifungal and antibacterial products have replaced gentian violet as the first line of defense against most infections.

According to one Australian report, there is the possibility that gentian violet may disappear from pharmacies altogether if studies confirm the suspicion that this purple liquid could be cancer causing. Earlier studies on gentian violet seem to indicate that it could cause cellular changes in lab animals.

CANDIDIASIS TREATMENT

Occasionally, gentian violet is still used to treat very resistant cases of mucocutaneous candidiasis, an itchy, yeastlike fungal infection that affects the mucous membranes of the mouth, intestine, and vagina. "Gentian violet is old-fashioned, but it is a bit faster and more effective for treating resistant candidiasis than nystatin or some of the newer antibacterial or antifungal drugs," says John Lawsen, M.D., professor of obstetrics and gynecology and genetics at George Washington University.

If you have recurring vaginal candidiasis, your doctor may suggest that you insert a gentian violet tampon for 3 to 4 hours once or twice daily for 12 days.

To boost your fight against the fungi, your doctor may also prescribe an antiyeast cream or tablets along with gentian violet. "We find that using gentian violet along with an imidazole antifungal product is very effective for knocking out candidiasis," says Giles Monif, M.D., professor of obstetrics and gynecology at Crayton University Medical School in Omaha, Nebraska.

You may also be asked to make some dietary changes—such as avoiding yeast-based foods like breads, wine, and cheese and limiting sugar—to help restore the microbial balance in your body.

Gestalt therapy As psychological therapies go, Gestalt is among the most free-wheeling and dramatic. As a client in Gestalt therapy, you might be asked to shout your lungs out, bash your fists into pillows, or jump back and forth between chairs pretending to be two different people.

When Richard lost his teenage daughter to suicide, he grieved. He gained weight. He overslept. He grew depressed. After two years, he turned to Gestalt. The next thing the 40-year-old professional knew, he was play-acting the role of Mr. Spock, the pointy-eared alien from "Star Trek." As Spock, he would zoom back in time to meet again with his lost child.

A CLEARER PICTURE

The goal of such theatrics is not to win an Oscar but to help the client to better know himself and to more accurately perceive the world around him, says Robert Barcus, Ph.D., clinical associate professor at Wright State University School of Professional Psychology and a Gestalt psychologist in private practice in Yellow Springs, Ohio. The word *Gestalt,* which comes from the German word for "form," means "meaningful whole."

Gestalt therapists say that if your perceptions of yourself and your world are clouded, you may experience psychological thunderstorms. "We see a lot of people who are depressed, anxious, or feeling overcontrolled and restricted," says Dr. Barcus. Other Gestalt therapists claim success working with people suffering from phobias, obsessions, panic attacks, alcohol and drug problems, or even more serious psychological problems, such as various forms of psychoses (in which a person loses contact with reality).

In Richard's case, his funk came partly from feelings of self-blame over his daughter's death. He also felt furious at her for taking her own life. In one session toward the end of a year's therapy, during an imaginary conversation with his daughter, "his face softened, and he came to a resolution," says Dr. Barcus. Richard was finally getting in touch with his feelings and was beginning to express them. His depression started to lift.

Why the Spock role? In Gestalt, "we often use what's 'in the air,'" says Dr. Barcus. "I knew he was a fan of 'Star Trek,' and the Spock role became a convenient vehicle." Richard was afraid to confront his feelings, but by taking on the role of someone else, "it encouraged him to move toward his feelings by creating the safety of emotional distance," says Dr. Barcus.

AN ACTIVE THERAPY

Action and creativity are hallmarks of Gestalt, says psychologist Elizabeth C. Stirling, Ph.D., director of the Washington (D.C.) Gestalt Center. "I don't sit behind a couch and do needlework while other people talk," she says. When a client gets angry, for instance, Dr. Stirling may give them one of many cushions she keeps in her office and tell the client to pummel away.

Gestalt may be done one-on-one, in groups, or in workshops, where a therapist works with one person as others watch. Workshops were a favorite of Gestalt pioneer Frederick S. "Fritz" Perls. His California workshops during the 1960s gained fame not only for their vitality but also for their often confrontational approach. More often, however — contrary to popular misconception — "Gestalt is *not* a confrontational scream-in-your-face therapy," emphasizes Dr. Barcus.

Gestalt is also not a scientifically proven therapy. Some modern psychotherapies, like cognitive and behavioral therapy, have scientific studies to indicate their effectiveness at battling problems such as depression and phobias. But Gestalt, like its older cousin, psychoanalysis, has little of the kind. "The research isn't there," says Dr. Barcus. But he contends that thousands of improved lives (like Richard's) attest to Gestalt's therapeutic gift.

Most Gestalt therapists hold Ph.D.'s; some have master's degrees in social work or other fields. The length of therapy varies from several months to years.

The way to find a therapist, says Dr. Stirling, is to drop a note to an established training center, such as the Gestalt Institute of Cleveland (1588 Hazel Drive, Cleveland, OH 44106) or the New York Institute for Gestalt Therapy (P.O. Box 20742, New York, NY 10025).

ginger Modern studies have proven what ancient fishermen riding the waves of stomach queasiness on stormy seas discovered long ago: Powdered gingerroot may calm a churning stomach and quell dizziness.

Nausea associated with motion sickness arises when your brain expects one thing (the stability of solid ground), but your eyes and ears tell your brain something else (that there is movement all around you). The feedback response from your brain to your stomach triggers motion sickness.

Ginger seems to interrupt the response from the nausea center in the brain. In fact, this pungent spice from the Far East and Jamaica quells queasiness even better than the leading antinausea drug, according to a study conducted by Daniel Mowrey, Ph.D., director of the American Phytotherapy Research Laboratory in Salt Lake City.

"I first became interested in ginger's antinausea effects when I discovered that the encapsulated version of the herb kept me from losing my lunch during a bout with the flu," says Dr. Mowrey. "I decided to conduct a study on ginger and motion sickness and see how it stacked up compared to dimenhydrinate, the ingredient found in the over-the-counter antinausea drug Dramamine."

CALMED SEAT-SICKNESS

Dr. Mowrey, then at Brigham Young University in Provo, teamed up with a colleague from Mount Union College in Alliance, Ohio. They asked 36 students to swallow either 940 milligrams of powdered gingerroot, 100 milligrams of Dramamine, or two capsules of a neutral herb. Then the students took turns sitting blindfolded in a tilted and revolving chair. The ginger group was able to endure 5.6 minutes in the torture seat compared to 3.6 minutes for the Dramamine group and 1.5 minutes for the herb group (three of whom vomited).

And ginger seems to have another advantage. Because it appears to work directly on the gastrointestinal tract rather than the central nervous sytem, it doesn't cause side effects like drowsiness and blurred vision, Dr. Mowrey says.

In other studies, Dr. Mowrey found that gingerroot reduced or eliminated morning sickness in more than 75 percent of the women who took it. "The women found that when they took a few capsules at the slightest hint of nausea, the queasiness went away," he says.

If you're scheduled for surgery, you might want to check with your doctor about taking some ginger capsules to offset the nausea commonly felt after anesthesia. Researchers in London found that postsurgical patients who took gingerroot capsules had less nausea and vomiting than patients who were given an inactive capsule.

Ginger's thousand-year-old reputation as a digestive aid for gas and heartburn seems to have some scientific merit as well.

One of ginger's ingredients, zingibain, stimulates the flow of saliva and increases the concentration of digestive enzymes in the saliva, explains Dr. Mowrey. Ginger also helps stimulate blood circulation in the gastrointestinal tract.

Researchers have also started to check out ginger's reputation in India as an anti-arthritis spice. They speculate that ginger consumption may reduce the amounts of prostaglandins, substances that play a part in joint inflammation.

"All in all, ginger has some very interesting pharmacologically active substances with very few downsides," says Sheldon Saul Hendler, M.D., assistant clinical professor of medicine at the University of California in San Diego.

TAKING THE GINGER ROUTE

You might have been told as a child to drink ginger ale to settle your upset tummy. For very mild stomach upset, this may work. But generally, ginger ale and gingersnaps don't contain enough of the spice to do you much good.

You are better off taking capsules purchased from a health food store, says Dr. Mowrey. The prescription for motion sickness: Take two to four capsules 15 minutes before your trip. Repeat every 4 hours or as needed.

It takes about 10 minutes for the ginger to wind its way through your system. As the effect wears off, you may have to take more. When you get a ginger aftertaste in your mouth, though, you know you have taken enough, Dr. Mowrey says. Just don't overdo it. Too much could make your upset stomach worse, and large overdoses have the potential to disturb your heart rate and nervous system. Preg-

nant women are advised to talk to their doctor before taking ginger capsules. *See also* **antiemetics; motion sickness remedies**

gingko.   *See* **Chinese herbs**

ginseng   Russian cosmonauts have taken it to counteract the rigors of orbiting the earth. Some American runners take it to zoom ahead in races. And the Chinese take it to keep themselves young, virile, and disease free.

We're talking about the root of the ginseng plant. According to the ancient doctrine of signatures, healing herbs supposedly resemble the body part they cure. So ginseng's human-like shape makes it a whole-body tonic. And because some specimens of this "man plant" have a third, shorter root, ginseng has been especially prized as an aphrodisiac.

Despite its suggestive shape, there's no evidence that ginseng enhances sexual performance, experts say. And even ginseng's reputed power as an energizing and revitalizing agent is open to scientific debate. Nonetheless, there are an estimated five to six million ginseng users in the U.S. alone. Avid ginseng diggers have made American ginseng an endangered species.

Most of the ginseng research has been conducted overseas—primarily in Russia, Japan, and Britain. As far as physical stamina and energy go, researchers have reported that ginseng increased race times in soldiers, boosted work speed and accuracy in radio operators, and reduced fatigue among night-shift personnel.

"The ginseng studies are intriguing, but most of them lacked controls [they were not tested against nonactive substitutes] and few have been convincingly confirmed," says Sheldon Saul Hendler, M.D., Ph.D., assistant clinical professor of medicine at the University of California at San Diego and author of *The Doctors' Vitamin and Mineral Encyclopedia*.

MIXED RESULTS

What's more, says Dr. Hendler, many of the studies contradict each other. For example, some ginseng research showed reductions in blood pressure, while others suggest the herb can dangerously elevate pressure.

Part of the confusion may stem from the fact that saponins, some of ginseng's active compounds, which exist in the root in large numbers, may not be the same in every sample. These saponins have been called "adaptogens" because experiments show that these compounds adapt or increase resistance against certain physical, chemical, or biological stresses. Solid studies on ginseng are tricky to do because saponins may occur in any combination in the plant, and their strength is affected by geographic location, growing conditions, and time of harvest. Furthermore, these saponins' effects on the body are believed to differ, depending on where the plant comes from. The Chinese believe that their own ginseng has a stimulating effect, while American ginseng supposedly has a calming, antistress effect.

"The most that can be said for any of the ginseng herbs themselves is

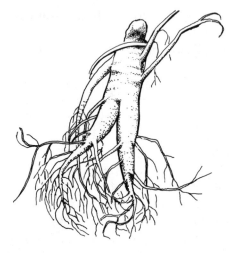

Ginseng root

that they yield mixed results," says Dr. Hendler. But when *extracts* of the herbs were used, study results have been more consistent.

Of particular interest is work showing that ginseng extract may stimulate the immune system. One animal study conducted by the Systemic Toxicology Branch at the National Institute of Environmental Health Sciences in North Carolina showed that Asian ginseng extract stimulated natural killer cell activity and provided some degree of protection against infection.

Because the Food and Drug Administration does not consider ginseng to be a drug, there is no quality control over the products sold. One study showed that more than half of the ginseng products analyzed were worthless and a fourth contained no ginseng at all.

Some preliminary studies seem to indicate that long-term use of 3 grams a day of ginseng may result in insomnia, nervousness, and elevated blood pressure. But other subjects have shown an opposite reaction—the ginseng acted like a tranquilizer and lowered blood pressure. Other studies have shown that ginseng, including topical applications, can cause vaginal bleeding in postmenopausal women.

Generally, Siberian ginseng, called eleuthero, seems to have fewer side effects, less estrogen-like activity, and somewhat more predictable actions than Asian or American ginseng, notes Dr. Hendler.

But until more studies have been completed, many experts advise against prolonged, regular use of ginseng. Pregnant or nursing women, children, and people with high blood pressure should not use ginseng at all.

glandulars   Back in the days of ancient Rome, glandular therapy for "rejuvenation" was the rage. The prescription: Ingest the ground-up testicular gland of a donkey.

As unappetizing as that sounds, the practice of ingesting concentrates of various glands from livestock animals is making a comeback. Some of the glandular products available today include pituitary, thyroid, adrenal, prostate, ovary, and yes, even testicles. The glands are freeze-dried, pulverized, put into tablets, and sold in health food stores.

As in the old days, people take glandulars in the hopes of rejuvenating their body and overcoming everything from impotence to anemia. Supposedly, ingesting glandular material from a cow, pig, or sheep will give

you a dose of hormone and revive your own sluggish gland.

Several decades ago, doctors used pulverized thyroid gland from slaughtered animals to treat what was then called an "underactive thyroid." Your thyroid gland, located beneath your Adam's apple on your neck, helps regulate a number of body processes, including energy metabolism. It was once believed that if you had low energy or were overweight, a bit of animal thryoid gland could spark your own sluggish thyroid into action.

Today, synthetic equivalents of your own thryoxine hormone (the hormone produced in the thyroid) are the prescribed treatment for clinically diagnosed thyroid problems. A recent survey showed, however, that many older people still take animal-derived thyroid gland to combat fatigue, speed up weight loss, and even to counteract hair loss.

Moreover, many not-so-old people are also using glandulars. One formula touted as the "steroid alternative" for body builders contains pituitary and testicular glandulars. Supposedly, growth hormone from the pituitary glandular would help bulk up muscle while testosterone from the testicular glandular would increase strength. But do they?

PROOF IS LACKING

Despite their renewed popularity, there is no convincing evidence to prove glandulars work. Nor is there any biochemical reason to even suspect that they would be useful, experts point out.

"The theories are half-baked," says

Luke Bucci, Ph.D., biochemist and clinical nutritionist in private practice in Houston. "The idea is that the DNA patterns in these glands will help program your own organs to function better. But DNA is broken down during digestion and inactivated."

On the other hand, ingesting too much animal hormone could be harmful, according to Marie Gelato, M.D., Ph.D., associate professor of endocrinology in the Department of Medicine at the State University of New York at Stony Brook. If you took too much thyroid hormone, for example, it could actually turn off your own thyroid production.

There is also the danger that the concentrates may contain antibiotics, pesticides, and many other toxins to which livestock are exposed, warns Sheldon Saul Hendler, M.D., Ph.D., assistant clinical professor of medicine at the University of California in San Diego. His advice? "Avoid glandulars."

And if you've been taking animal thyroid because it was once prescribed for you years ago, ask your doctor if synthetic thyroid might be a better choice.

gold   Just the promise of it lured explorers to the New World. Just a speck of it sparked a mad scramble to California. And now just a bit of it may relieve arthritis pain, battle skin ailments, and yes, even help some people blink their eyes.

The healing potential of gold can be traced back to ancient doctors who used it to treat itching of the palms. In 1890, physicians began using inject-able gold particles to treat tuberculosis and other infectious diseases. Forty years later, doctors turned to gold injections to combat rheumatoid arthritis.

Today, doctors continue to find other uses for the precious metal.

Some plastic surgeons, for example, are implanting gold weights in the eyelids of patients who have lost their ability to blink, says Monte Keen, M.D., director of facial, plastic, and reconstructive surgery at Columbia Presbyterian Medical Center in New York City.

The patients can open their eyes but can't close them because of nerve damage. Without the ability to blink, the eyes dry out and become susceptible to infections, Dr. Keen says.

The gold implants, which weigh less than $\frac{1}{28}$ ounce, allow patients to use gravity to mimic blinking. Gold makes a perfect implant because it is pliable and it won't affect surrounding tissue or enter the bloodstream.

Some dermatologists use gold pills to treat pemphigus, a rare disease that causes blisters on the face, chest, groin, and neck.

ARTHRITIS FIGHTER

Even more significantly, however, the metal continues to be a primary weapon in the fight against rheumatoid arthritis. "Studies clearly show that gold has a major impact on the disease in about one-third of patients when it is used properly in those who can tolerate it," says Sanford Roth, M.D., medical director of the Arthritis Center in Phoenix.

Unfortunately, the patient's tolerance is a key problem because when used as a drug, gold has many nasty side effects, including skin rashes, kidney damage, jaundice, diarrhea, and suppressed blood cell production in the bone marrow.

In fact, because of the severity of the side effects, fewer than one in four arthritis patients who begin taking gold pills or receiving injections are still on the medication five years later, says Ronenn Roubenoff, M.D., a rheumatologist at Tufts University in Boston.

Gold also has other drawbacks. A slow-acting drug, it can take up to six months for a patient to notice that it's working. Even when it does work, many patients develop a resistance to the drug that limits its effectiveness.

THE GOLD STANDARD

So why do doctors still use it? Researchers believe that gold is able to do something that many other arthritis medications can't: It signals the body to stop destroying joint tissue and bone. Many doctors believe that rheumatoid arthritis is caused by out-of-control immune cells. These cells, called phagocytes, start attacking healthy joint tissue as if it were an enemy. Gold apparently tells the phagocytes to stop attacking those joints.

Some doctors treat arthritis with gold pills, but most consider gold shots more effective. And as you might guess, they're not cheap. Injectable gold, along with the doctor's fee to administer it, costs about twice as much as oral gold and four times as much as penicillamine, another slow-acting drug often used instead of gold.

But gold's days as a preferred treatment for arthritis may be numbered. Another arthritis drug, Methotrexate, is gaining popularity because it works faster than gold and is less likely to produce severe side effects, Dr. Roth says. In addition, a few physicians are beginning to question the role of gold as an effective arthritis treatment.

In a five-year study of the long-term effects of treating rheumatoid arthritis patients with injectable gold, researchers at the University of California, San Francisco, concluded that the 162 patients who received gold shots had no better mobility and about the same number of painful joints as patients who didn't receive the treatment.

"Gold therapy has shown itself to be frequently toxic and usually ineffective as a treatment of [rheumatoid arthritis]. . . . It may be a drug whose time has gone," according to Wallace Epstein, M.D., of the Rosalind Russell Arthritis Center at the University of California, San Francisco.

goldenseal   Years ago, Cherokee Indians would not go on the warpath without two things: a supply of arrows and a supply of goldenseal juice for treating arrow wounds.

Modern herbalists still insist that goldenseal is a good remedy for treating everyday cuts and scrapes and to stave off infectious germs that target any part of your body. In fact, they consider this brilliant yellow plant (also called hydrastis, after its Latin name, *Hydrastis canadensis*) to be one of nature's best antiseptics.

Over the years, goldenseal has been

used to treat everything from pinkeye (conjunctivitis) to infected pinkies.

"A nice feature about goldenseal is that it can be used in a variety of forms to treat a number of ailments, especially mucous membrane infections," says Cathy Rogers, a naturopathic physician (one who treats without drugs or surgery) in Seattle.

Rogers uses goldenseal tea to treat urinary tract infections and gastrointestinal problems, and goldenseal cream to treat impetigo, a skin infection caused by staphylococcus bacteria. She even uses a goldenseal powder for diaper rash.

EVIDENCE IS SPARSE

There is only a smattering of scientific evidence to support some of goldenseal's popular uses. Its active ingredients berberine and hydrastine are alkaloids that are astringents with mild antiseptic properties, say scientists.

"Used externally, goldenseal could have mild antiseptic and hemostatic [stops bleeding] properties that would make it a local treatment for rashes, cuts, and minor skin ailments," says Ara Der Marderosian, Ph.D., professor of pharmacognosy and medicinal chemistry at the Philadelphia College of Pharmacy and Science.

Furthermore, some studies show that berberine sulfate (a derivative of berberine) may assist in fighting internal infections.

Researchers at the Veterans Administration Medical Center and the University of Tennessee in Memphis found that, in the test tube, berberine sulfate blocked the adherence of streptococcus bacteria (the culprit in strep throat) to cells taken from the mouth. They also found that berberine blocked adhesion of *E. coli*, the bacteria that cause gastrointestinal infections.

But perhaps even more intriguing is the evidence that the berberine extract showed antitumor activity in the test tube.

It's important to keep in mind, however, that these studies used concentrated extracts, not the actual herb. "There is no documentation that goldenseal itself has any of these activities," says Sheldon Saul Hendler, M.D., Ph.D., assistant clinical professor of medicine at the University of California, San Diego. What's more, the potency of the active ingredients may vary from one sample of the herb to another. "Even if it were shown that goldenseal containing high amounts of berberine did display some antitumor activity, this is no guarantee that the goldenseal that you obtain at your local distributor would have similar activity," says Dr. Hendler.

Based on the scant evidence, some experts say that goldenseal's medicinal power is just a colorful part of native American legend. What's more, goldenseal's alkaloids can be hazardous to your health at concentrations powerful enough to tackle infectious germs, they say. Even some herbalists agree that goldenseal is overused and that cautions are often not emphasized enough.

Other experts warn that, unless you really water them down, goldenseal remedies could damage mucous membranes instead of healing them. What's more, taking too much goldenseal internally could cause nausea and vomiting and decrease your white blood cell count.

Goldenseal tea, however, is fairly mild-mannered in moderate amounts, says Dr. Der Marderosian. Serious infections need a doctor's attention, however.

gotu kola　(GAH-too KO-lah) On the other side of the world, in the land of exotic spices, silks, and monsoons, vast herds of elephants once roamed freely through an unspoiled, tropical landscape. According to Far Eastern legend, these massive beasts owed their long life span and remarkable memory to the gotu kola herb, their prime food source.

Today, in the United States, many people have begun to ingest gotu kola (also called Indian pennywort) with the hope of boosting their memory power, strengthening their body, and extending their longevity.

In other parts of the world, this practice is not new. The Chinese have regarded gotu kola as an anti-aging herb and brain food for centuries. In fact, in China, gotu kola is considered a revitalizing tonic rivaled only by another major "fountain of youth" herb—ginseng.

"Gotu kola has traditionally been used to treat worn-out bodies," says Ara Der Marderosian, Ph.D., professor of pharmacognosy and medicinal chemistry at the Philadelphia College of Pharmacy and Science. But is there any scientific basis for such a use? Per-haps the herb's reputation for revitalization stems from saponin glycosides, believed to be gotu kola's active ingredients, Dr. Der Marderosian says.

In India, gotu kola (known botanically as *Centella asiatica*) is so highly regarded that it is called brahmi, a sacred herb of the highest order.

"Gotu kola ghee [gotu kola mixed with clarified butter] is a popular Ayurvedic [Indian medicine] pick-me-up," according to Vasant Lad, an Ayurvedic doctor of herbal remedies who practices in Alburquerque, New Mexico.

APPLIED TO SKIN

Applied to the skin, gotu kola can make wrinkles fade away, Lad contends. That's quite a strong claim to make about a bunch of tropical leaves. Yet, around the world, gotu kola has been touted for its skin-healing powers. It has reportedly been used to treat blisters, psoriasis, and even leprosy.

In one study, 17 of 22 patients had their chronic skin uclers healed when treated with an extract of gotu kola. "Further research along these lines is warranted," says Sheldon Saul Hendler, M.D., Ph.D., assistant clinical professor of medicine at the University of California, San Diego, and author of *The Doctors' Vitamin and Mineral Encyclopedia*.

There really isn't any research to substantiate gotu kola's reputed anti-aging or energizing effect, however. Perhaps the herb's notoriety as an energizer stems from confusion over its name, he says. Gotu kola is often mixed up with kola nut, a completely different herb that contains caffeine, a well-known stimulant.

"Whatever else it may be, gotu kola is certainly not a stimulant," adds Varro Tyler, Ph.D., professor of pharmacognosy at Purdue University. "In relatively large doses, gotu kola has definite sedative effects in small animals."

gravity inversion Even a monkey could understand the logic of this technique: Hang upside down and you might help reverse stress on the spine created by standing right-side up. An estimated one million Americans were going head over heels over gravity inversion during the mid-1980s, most in search of relief from low back pain. But the popularity of the technique seems to have fallen off since then, perhaps in part because of warnings of possible stroke or eye injury from blood pooling in the chest and head. Few actual problems have been reported, however. "Done properly, it's relatively safe for most people and effective for the short-term relief of a lot of back pain conditions, but it simply no longer enjoys its fad status," says Robert Goldman, D.O., Ph.D., of the National Academy of Sports Medicine in Chicago.

Inversion therapy uses the force of gravity to stretch the muscles and ligaments of the spine. Advocates of the technique say this helps to reduce pain by relaxing tight muscles, which allows space between the spinal vertebrae to increase and relieves pressure on compressed structures. They claim the therapy's ability to decompress the spine is like getting the benefits of weeks of bed rest in just a few hours.

"There's no question that the procedure can cause vertebrae to separate to a considerable degree and that pain caused by pressure on spinal nerves can be relieved," says physical therapist and certified athletic trainer Larry Nosse at Marquette University in Milwaukee. "The effects do appear to be only temporary, however, which means the technique has to be practiced regularly to be of maximum benefit. I recommend that patients use the therapy three times daily, starting with sessions lasting only 30 seconds or so but working up to periods lasting 2 to 4 minutes each."

HANGING HARDWARE

Also to be considered is *how* to hang. Inversion therapy can be approached by hanging upside down directly—via the use of boots that hook over a bar, by lying on a tilting table that oscillates between horizontal and vertical positions, or by lying over a triangular stand that allows the upper half of the body to hang, supported by the thighs.

"All things considered, I recommend the stand," says Nosse. "Compared with hanging by your feet, you get even more force directed specifically at stretching the lower part of the spine, and there's less strain on the joints of the ankles, hips, and knees."

The triangular stand—and also the oscillating table—are thought to reduce the potentially harmful effects on the cardiovascular system and the eyes created by hanging upside down by the feet. "Some research has shown that blood pooling may occur, which can elevate blood pressure, increase pulse rate, and raise the pressure of fluid within the eyes," says Nosse. "But these effects appear to be reduced when only the upper half of the body is inverted, or when inversion is intermittent, as with the oscillating table."

Even so, anyone with a heart condition, high blood pressure, sinus infection, or problems with the inner ear should avoid gravity inversion, Nosse says. Other conditions that should put the procedure off-limits are glaucoma, detached retina, conjunctivitis, lung disorders, a tendency toward fainting or dizzy spells, osteoporosis, hiatal hernia, extreme obesity, or recent surgery. "I'd suggest people check with their doctor before giving inversion therapy a try," Nosse says. "And I'd even recommend having blood pressure and heart rate checked the first time the procedure is done. Sometimes

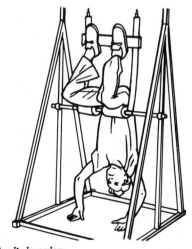

Gravity inversion

the experience itself can cause an exaggerated cardiovascular response even in healthy people."

If you're up to it, however, and low back pain has been a problem for you, inversion therapy—past its popularity prime or not—might be worth a try. In one study, 133 of 155 patients suffering from severe back pain were able to return to work following an average of just eight sessions of inversion therapy lasting 5 minutes each. Other research designed to measure the separation between vertebrae with the use of x-rays found that the procedure does, in fact, produce significant changes. "If separation of the lumbar vertebrae indeed plays a role in the symptomatic relief of low back pain . . . then gravity-facilitated traction may be an effective modality in the treatment of these conditions," concluded researchers in a *Journal of Orthopaedic and Sports Physical Therapy* report.

As a final note of caution, however, Nosse adds that you should let your pain be your guide. "If inversion seems to aggravate your condition, by no means should you pursue it. This isn't to say brief periods of discomfort won't be experienced at the very beginning of an inversion session, as the spine begins its stretching process, but if pain persists longer than 5 seconds or so, you should stop, because you could be doing more harm than good."

group therapy If you believe two is company but three is a crowd, skip this entry. Group therapy harnesses the powerful medicine of human interaction—usually between six to ten people—to help overcome personality problems or deal with crises.

Experts today rank group therapy superior to individual therapy for certain emotional problems, such as those stemming from mastectomy, death of a spouse, drug or alcohol abuse, or having survived the horrors of combat. It has also proved beneficial to those suffering from generalized anxiety, panic attacks, or obsessive-compulsive behavior.

WELCOME TO THE CIRCLE

Most often, a group will meet for 2 to 3 hours per week, under the guidance of a professional therapist, often two. Typically, members of the group, along with the therapists, arrange their chairs in a circle.

What actually happens during a session depends on the therapist's training and personal philosophy. Some counselors are "directive." That means they lead the discussion into helpful areas. They also tell you if they notice habitual, unproductive ways of dealing with people and feelings. Other therapists are more passive. They let the group discussion follow its own path and intervene only rarely.

With the therapist's help, group members learn to trust each other. They may find comfort in hearing others describe similar problems and find useful advice from others who've *been there*. They get to try out new ways of behaving, like assertiveness, in safe surroundings. And positive group pressure can sometimes help a member kick an addictive habit. "If you can get someone into a group of people who have similar problems, a whole lot of therapy can be short-cut," says Warren P. Edwards, Ph.D., a clinical psychologist with Crossing Point, a treatment center for chemical dependency and stress at Fort Madison Community Hospital in Fort Madison, Iowa.

A bonus of group therapy is economy. Depending on your therapist and the number of members in the group, it can cost a fraction of what you'd pay for individual therapy.

Group therapy is used in areas you might find surprising. In one study, 12 weeks of group therapy helped ten people with stubborn eczema stop scratching, allowing their reddened and scaling skin to clear. (Symptoms of eczema are often linked to emotional stress.)

DON'T BE SHY

Although it may seem odd, group therapy can also help overcome shyness. "If severe shyness involves discomfort around people, a group makes all the more sense," says Steve Hampl, Ph.D., director of group treatment programs at the Cleveland Center for Cognitive Therapy and director of the Center for Healthy Lifestyles, a private psychological service in Akron, Ohio. Shy people "don't know how to start or maintain a conversation. Individual therapy is helpful to a point, but group therapy is an opportunity to practice and to check out how people respond to them," says Dr. Hampl.

Overall, says Dr. Hampl, of the people who join his groups, at least 75 percent make very significant progress toward their goals after just eight to ten sessions. Nancy, for instance, often trembled around strangers. The 42-year-old health professional started group therapy. "We helped her to focus on the disturbed and negative thoughts she was having in social situations," says Dr. Hampl. In therapy, Nancy would comment, "These people don't like me." But in fact, she was *very* likeable—and the group was able to tell her so. "Group therapy allows people to share thoughts, ask questions, and speak freely—much more than in normal social settings," says Dr. Hampl.

Agoraphobia, a fear of public places, is also amenable to group therapy. Dr. Hampl starts these groups in his office, eventually moving them into public settings, like airports and shopping malls. An otherwise wrenching situation is eased by the company and comfort of the group.

Note, however, that group therapy is *not* the best option for serious mental illnesses, such as schizophrenia. The very disturbed generally need the more focused attention of one-on-one therapy.

To find an appropriate group in your area, call the social services department at your local hospital or your local government mental-health agency, or ask your family doctor. You can also get more information by contacting the American Group Psychotherapy Association, 25 East 21st Street, 6th Floor, New York, NY 10010.

growth factors Remember the first time you learned about regeneration in biology class? You made the amazing discovery that a starfish could grow back a whole new appendage.

Your body has its own built-in repair kit called growth factors, dozens of natural proteins that are released from injured cells. While these growth factors can't exactly grow back a new limb, they can regulate the growth and healing processes of cells and help rebuild new tissues. When you scrape your knee, for instance, a scab forms, the skin growth factors kick in, and new skin cells are made. In a few weeks, you have a smooth-skinned, healed knee.

But suppose your natural growth factors can't make it to the site of the wound because you have poor circulation due to diabetes. Your sore may then remain unhealed, only to fester with infection.

Fortunately, scientists have been able to isolate and reproduce several dozen growth factors that stimulate new cells to grow—in your skin, bone, and blood—when your natural growth factors can't do the job.

These man-made growth factors have several healing applications. In some experimental tests, for instance, patients are receiving a mix of skin growth factors that are all applied to a wound at once, each with a different job to do.

This healing team may work in much the same way as several housebuilders constructing a house. One growth factor puts a roof of skin over the wound, while another factor lays the supporting framework of collagen (connecting tissue). This is the scaffolding upon which new skin forms. Still another factor puts in blood vessels, the plumbing system.

David R. Knighton, M.D., head of the Wound Healing Clinic at the University of Minnesota in Minneapolis, has developed a process in which he takes a sample of a patient's blood, pulls out the growth factors, and embeds them in gauze bandages that are laid directly on the open wound.

Dr. Knighton's studies have shown that growth factor bandages can knit wounds that previously did not knit. In one study, 16 people with nonhealing leg ulcers were treated with a combination of growth factors soaked into bandages. Sixteen other patients got normal bandages. Within eight weeks, 81 percent of the wounds covered with growth factors were healed, compared to just 15 percent in the other group. When the untreated group switched to growth factors, 100 percent of their wounds healed in seven weeks.

Other researchers are exploring the use of skin growth factors for treating severely burned patients. It's now possible to grow skin in a lab dish using growth factors from the patient's body and then graft the lab-grown skin onto the patient's wound. In another study, skin growth factors helped speed cellular growth at skin-graft donor sites in burn victims and shortened healing by a day and a half.

Some doctors hope that if growth factors can regenerate tissues and blood vessels in the skin, perhaps one day we may be able to regenerate other organs such as the heart or brain. Applying growth factors to cardiac tissue following a heart attack, for example, might help the organ repair itself.

IMMUNE ENHANCEMENT

Using growth factors to regenerate new organs may be several years off. But growth factors that stimulate blood production and the immune system are already being used outside the laboratory setting.

Red blood cell growth factors are being used to replenish red blood cells in patients who have low blood counts because of disease. And white blood cell growth factors are now being used to help prevent infections that plague cancer patients during chemotherapy and radiation.

"The real devastating side effect of chemo and radiation is not hair loss," explains David T. Scadden, M.D., assistant professor in medicine at Harvard Medical School in Boston. "It's having your bone marrow wiped out along with the tumor cells." Bone marrow is the birthplace of infection-fighting white blood cells. When the chemotherapy destroys bone marrow, cancer patients must get transplants.

Preliminary studies at Duke University Medical Center showed that giving test-tube-grown growth factors along with bone marrow transplants speeded up the creation of defender cells by the replaced bone marrow. This means that patients can start fighting off infection sooner.

"Blood cell growth factors are as dramatic a discovery as antibiotics for treating disease," says Dr. Scadden. "The white cell stimulators can help keep cancer patients out of the hospital with infections and enable them to tolerate stronger doses of tumor-killing drugs."

Likewise, growth factors may someday improve survival of some auto-immune deficiency syndrome (AIDS) patients and others who have immune deficiency diseases, says Dr. Scadden.

growth hormone Genetic engineers have come up with a way to synthesize a version of growth hormone, the pro-tein substance that is naturally secreted in your pituitary gland. This is the hormone that stimulates bone growth and allows you to reach your genetic growth potential. Growth hormone also plays a major role in fat break-down and muscle buildup.

Currently, the only approved use for growth hormone is to treat chil-dren who have short stature because of a malfunctioning pituitary gland that does not make adequate amounts of growth hormone. If these kids receive the hormone early in life, they can achieve normal height.

What can growth hormone do for adults? Some studies indicate that it may make your body harder and leaner looking.

In a study conducted at St. Tho-mas' Hospital in London, growth hor-mone was given to 24 adults who had growth hormone deficiency as a result of having their tumorous pituitary gland removed. After six months of treatment, their muscle mass—which had been abnormally low—increased, while fat tissue decreased by about 20 percent.

Even more intriguing is a Uni-versity of Arizona study involving a group of healthy men and women who were highly conditioned from years of exercise training. Each person was injected with growth hormone for six weeks. At the end of that time, the athletes showed a 12 percent decrease in body fat and an 8 percent increase in lean body mass (muscles).

Dreams of having bulging mus-cles like Arnold Schwarzenegger's have led to growth hormone abuse among body builders.

In the drive to look bigger and stronger, these muscle men and women are injecting contraband growth hor-mone into their bloodstreams. Aside from being dangerous and illegal, the injections may be just plain useless for improving strength, experts say.

"Growth hormone may give you bigger-looking, rippling muscles, but there's no solid proof that it will increase strength or power," says Peter Lemon, Ph.D., professor of exercise physiol-ogy at Kent State University in Ohio. In fact, there is some evidence that the hormone actually makes muscles weaker.

And using growth hormone to lose weight could backfire. "What researchers have shown is that growth hormone breaks down fat in obese people," explains Marie Gelato, M.D., Ph.D., associate professor of endocri-nology at the State University of New York Medical School at Stony Brook. "But this fat breakdown did not result in increased weight loss." In response to added growth hormone, your system could start down-regulating, theoretically slowing your metabolism so that you potentially could *gain* weight, says Dr. Gelato.

AN AGE REVERSER?

At the Veterans Affairs Medical Center in Milwaukee, 12 healthy men, aged 61 to 72, who had low growth hormone levels were given growth hormone three times a week for six months. After that, the men had a 14 percent decrease in body fat and a 9 percent increase in lean body mass. They also had nearly a 2 percent increase in the bone density of their spine.

According to the authors of this clinical study, the measured changes "amounted to a reversal of the effects of 10 to 20 years of aging on lean body mass and fatty tissue mass."

"This study shows that growth hormone may have potential for helping the frail elderly—those who have lost muscle mass and who may be wheelchair bound," says Axel G. Feller, M.D., associate professor of medicine and head of geriatrics research at the North Chicago Veterans Affairs Medical Center, a coauthor of the study. "For those people, even a minor increase in muscle strength could determine better functioning.

"Follow-up studies will look at what growth hormone can do for an aging liver, spleen, and kidneys. But we're a long, long way from recommending growth hormone for all elderly," cautions Dr. Feller. "The substance is no fountain of youth."

guided imagery. *See* **imagery**

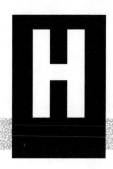

hair dryer You may think we're full
of hot air if we claim that hair dryers
do much more than just dry your hair.
Sure, they can turn a soaking scalp
into some terrific tresses in just a matter of minutes. But you're not using
your head if you think their handi-
work is so limited.

In fact, even the most basic model
hair dryer is capable of lots more.

BOTTOM-LINE RELIEF

Diaper rash is not a pretty sight.
Junior's bottom becomes redder than
Rudolph's nose and his skin is . . . well,
not exactly as smooth as a baby's bottom. Sure, keeping the diaper area clean
promotes healing, but place a towel or
one of those alcohol-soaked diaper
wipes on that ever-so-tender tush and
WHA-A-A-A-A-H-H!

Enter your handy hair dryer. After
bathing the half-pint, "dry his skin
with a hair dryer on the low setting
instead of using a towel," says Rodney
Basler, M.D., assistant professor of internal medicine at the University of
Nebraska Medical Center and a practicing dermatologist in Lincoln. "You
have to keep the skin dry, and since the
skin is so sensitive, a blow dryer is a
good way to do it." However, we stress
it again: Use the *low* setting to avoid
burning the tender skin.

A hair dryer can be put to good
use in other ways, too, according to
Dr. Basler. As full-figured gals know,
large breasts can create special problems.
"It's dampness and perspiration that
cause many skin problems, and there's
no question that the skin under heavy
breasts, or any heavy skin fold, can
become damp and spongy—perfect
breeding grounds for a fungal infection," says Dr. Basler. "Many people
compensate by using a hair dryer to
keep those areas free of dampness."

Women can do it by lifting a breast
with one hand and using a hair dryer
with the other. "It's great prevention
because fungus won't penetrate dry
skin—only damp skin. It's the dampness that breaks down the skin's natural barrier," Dr. Basler says.

Men aren't free from such skin
irritations. The groin area is a damp-
and-perspiring area ripe for fungus—
in this case, jock itch. And while

we're on locker room talk, hair dryers can also help prevent athlete's foot. Again, the dry-prevents-infection theory applies.

What about the notion that a hair dryer makes a good chill chaser? "A hair dryer can warm your skin when you're cold, but a hot bath is definitely quicker," says Dr. Basler. Of course, there are times when a bath is out of the question: When you've left the windows in your parked car open, for example, while it was raining. But you didn't realize that fact until you sat down. Just something to keep in mind the next time you have a wet seat and a public bathroom nearby has one of those hand dryers.

USE WITH CAUTION

But let's not forget the main purpose of a hair dryer: to dry hair. And like everything else, there's a right and wrong way: "Lower settings are definitely easier on your hair," says Dr. Basler, an expert on hair care. "Avoid high settings because they dry out your hair and can cause split ends."

Those with psoriasis or sunburn may want to avoid hair dryers altogether. "A hair dryer may aggravate psoriasis more than not using it. I would suggest that if you use one, put it on the coolest temperature and at the lowest speed. If you're still bothered [by psoriasis] or it makes you itch more—which it very well might—then don't use it at all," he says. "As far as sunburn goes, a hair dryer *does* dry skin by contributing to the dehydrating effect—and that makes the sunburn hurt more.

So if your hair is thinning and you have sunburn on your scalp, don't use your hair dryer."

And one more thing: Dr. Basler knows from personal experience just how important it is to heed the warning on most hair dryers. "Last year, my kids' 18-year-old babysitter electrocuted herself while drying her hair in the bathtub. So please pay attention to those warnings and do *not* use a hair dryer while in the bathtub or anywhere around water."

hearing aids Hearing aids can help many hearing-impaired people regain the ability to clearly understand speech—even in a boisterous crowd. These "substitute ears" also help the wearer hear a doorbell . . . crickets chirping on a summer night . . . and countless other everyday sounds that make life sweet.

Like a miniature public address system, a hearing aid has three parts: a tiny microphone to pick up sound, a battery-powered volume amplifier, and a miniature speaker to deliver amplified sound directly into your ear.

Even though hearing aids can reopen a world of sound, less than one-fourth of the people who need them use them, experts say. Many people feel that a hearing aid broadcasts to the world that they are old and handicapped.

Fortunately, the hearing aid stigma is fading, thanks in part to our 40th president. "When President Reagan began wearing a hearing aid, sales of the devices soared 25 percent," says Maurice Miller, Ph.D., chief audiologist at Lenox Hill Hospital in New York City and professor of audiology at New York University.

ALL BUT INVISIBLE

If you didn't notice President Reagan's hearing aid, it's because he was wearing one of the miniature, barely visible models. Today, over 80 percent of all hearing aid devices are in-the-ear types, making more conspicuous models, like the eyeglass type with microphone, amplifier, and receiver built into the temple, seem as outdated as bell-bottom trousers.

If you have mild to moderate hearing loss, for example, you might be fitted with a small device that consists of a microphone, amplifier, and receiver in a crescent-shaped unit. It nestles in the opening of your ear canal and is no bigger than a quarter.

Or you might get the smaller, in-the-canal hearing aid like President Reagan wore. Dime-size, it fits entirely into the ear canal and is barely noticeable.

The drawback to this tiny model is that the miniature adjustment knobs can be a challenge for anyone with arthritic fingers or other dexterity problems. The unit can also be difficult to insert and the minuscule batteries hard to change. In-the-canal models also cost a few hundred dollars more than in-the-ear models.

In contrast, a behind-the-ear hearing aid is a bit larger, but it is less expensive. This device has two parts: an earmold shaped to fit inside the bowl of your ear and the hearing aid iteself, which fits behind your ear. A behind-the-ear aid has controls that are easier to manipulate and a bigger battery, making it more powerful for a wide range of hearing loss, from mild to severe.

A behind-the-ear model is also capable of housing more of the new electronic circuitry available to help you get clearer, crisper sound.

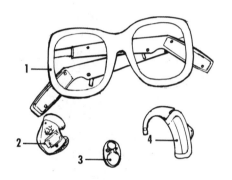

Hearing aids: (1) eyeglass, (2) in-the-ear, (3) in-the-canal, (4) behind-the-ear

"Special circuits enable you to fine-tune the pitch and tone of sounds like you would a stereo," explains William McFarland, Ph.D., head of audiology at the House Ear Clinic in Los Angeles. You can tune in a little less bass here or a little more treble there, and the amplification is customized to match your particular hearing loss. A behind-the-ear model gives you several tuning adjustments, compared with only one or two in the smaller models.

Another plus: Behind-the-ear loaner aids may be available while yours is being repaired—a convenience not available with the smaller hearing aids. On the downside, the behind-the-ear aids may interfere with wearing eyeglasses.

CONVERSATION PIECE

Aside from being smaller and offering improved sound quality, the newest hearing aids also overcome a major problem of traditional hearing aids: They can screen out background clatter, making speech easier to understand.

"Most hearing-impaired people can hear low-frequency (low-pitched) sounds such as footsteps but have poorer hearing in the higher frequencies where the consonant sounds of speech such as b, t, c, and d occur," explains John House, M.D., president of the House Ear Clinic. "The low-frequency sounds drown out speech, distorting it."

Imagine attending a cocktail party wearing a hearing aid that doesn't discriminate between high- and low-frequency sounds. All sounds (unwanted and wanted) that come near the microphone are amplified. You feel like you're standing at the Tower of Babel. Trying to carry on a conversation is impossible.

The newer computer-chip-driven hearing aids let you program out background din and zero in on speech using a pocket-size remote control device.

So-called "smart" hearing aids have also hit the market. These high-tech wonders use computerized digital programming to automatically alter amplification of sounds as you move from a noisy meeting room to a quiet car to talking on the telephone.

But for all the dazzling technology, there are some drawbacks: The digitals are bigger and more conspicuous and cost a few thousand dollars—about three times as much as behind-the-ear models.

Experts say you shouldn't wait for the digital devices to become widely available. "The smaller aids currently on the market are better than ever and can give you good-quality hearing," says Dr. House.

If you have severe hearing loss, though, you may need a more powerful body hearing aid. With this model, a long wire connects the earpiece to a powerful amplifier carried in your clothing.

If your cochlea (inner ear) is damaged to the point where you are deaf and not able to benefit from a hearing aid at all, your doctor may recommend a cochlear implant. A tiny audio receiver is implanted in the bone behind the ear. Sounds are picked up with a microphone and transmitted through the skin into the implanted receiver. A wire connects the receiver to the cochlea, where it delivers electrical impulses to the auditory nerve. The impulses are then carried on to the brain.

Cochlear implants do not restore normal hearing but can help the wearer identify voices, listen to music, use the telephone, read lips better, and hear some sounds and pitches.

AUDITORY ADVICE

If the word "What?" frequently crops up in your dialogue with others, see your doctor for a hearing check. Depending on the results, you may be advised to visit an audiologist—a professional trained to fit hearing aids.

You can expect to pay anywhere from about $500 to a few thousand dollars for an aid, depending on the features and style you select.

Don't be surprised if your audiologist suggests two aids. Most hearing loss is caused by aging and occurs in both ears, says Dr. House. A binaural (two-aid) fitting enables you to determine where particular sounds are coming from, gives you better depth perception, and will help you pick out conversation in a noisy room. "It's like seeing with one eye compared to two. Two just make it better," he says.

Break in your hearing aid gradually, suggests Dr. McFarland. Your own voice will sound louder. Sounds of birds chirping and cars whooshing by may seem uncomfortable at first. So give yourself time to get used to all this. Start by wearing your hearing aid in a relatively quiet environment for a few hours. Then, as you become better at filtering out unwanted sounds, venture into noisier territory such as the grocery store or a family gathering.

Be sure to follow instructions for the care and maintenance of your hearing aid. Earwax can clog some. Batteries will need to be replaced every three weeks or so. Remember, too, that the average life of a hearing aid is three to five years.

heat therapy If you suffer from painful muscle spasms, stiff joints, or a localized infection, turning on the heat may bring you the relief you've been seeking.

Long before aspirin or antibiotics, heat was used to a treat a variety of aches and pains and to fight infections.

Today, people still undergo heat therapy at old-fashioned spalike hospitals as well as state-of-the-art rehabilitation centers and sports medicine clinics, where they're draped with hot compresses, pressed with hot packs, and bombarded with ultrasonic heat waves. In fact, at these facilities there is no escaping the heat. Why? "Heat appears to enhance healing of many conditions, although there are few studies around to prove it," says William Mitchell, M.D., staff physician for the Brookline Sports Medicine Clinic in Brookline, Massachusetts.

RELAXES AND REVIVES

Although the exact mechanism behind this ancient healing method remains a mystery, it's believed that applying surface heat cooks up relief two ways: It relaxes muscles and brings a rush of healing blood to damaged tissues.

When you use a hot water bottle to ease a painful muscle spasm, for example, the heat does not actually penetrate deeply enough to relax your muscles directly. That's because the insulating layer of fat lying just under your skin protects your muscles from heat just as a pot holder protects a countertop. So heat takes a roundabout route to rescue a muscle in distress, says Glen Halvorson, M.D., medical director of Sport Training and Rehabilitation of Tempe/Tucson, Arizona. What happens, he says, is that heat stimulates nerves lying within the top inch of your skin and muscle. That impulse travels to your brain, which signals "relax" to all muscles near the heat source.

A warmed-up muscle can also help thaw out joint stiffness, helping arthritis sufferers move more freely. "Heat increases the flexibility of muscles and soft connective tissue around joints, and it also relieves nerve sensitivity," says John Arbruzzo, M.D., director of the Division of Rheumatology at Thomas Jefferson Hospital in Philadelphia. All this makes for a more mobile joint.

By dilating (widening) the blood vessels, heat draws a greater volume of blood to inflamed or infected tissues, studies show. Researchers at the University of California at San Francisco put wet towels—sealed in plastic and as hot as tolerable—on the upper arms of hospital patients. Then, using probes under the skin, they found that as temperature increased, so did the release of oxygen from the bloodstream into surrounding tissues.

Oxygen is very important for wound healing, according to the study's coauthor, John Rabkin, M.D., fellow in transplantation surgery at the University of California, San Francisco. Phagocytes, the white blood cells that gobble up bacteria in wounds, need plenty of oxygen to do their work. Collagen, the protein that helps mend wounds, also requires oxygen. "Our results reconfirm the value of the age-old remedy of heat for healing superficial infections, bruises, and open wounds," says Dr. Rabkin.

An Immune Booster?

Traditionally, folk healers have attempted to fight colds and flu by heating the body into a sweat-producing fever. The doctors at health resorts who still recommend this remedy say that the application of moist heat to raise body temperature temporarily boosts the white blood cells. They also point to the fact that cancer treatment centers such as the one at the Stanford University School of Medicine in Palo Alto, California, use deep-penetrating ultrasonic heat waves along with radiation to bombard tumors into remission.

"There are few scientific studies that demonstrate a direct reduction of wound infection though direct application of heat," notes Dr. Rabkin. But the doctors who prescribe heat therapy for common ailments insist that warmth works wonders. "Heat stirs up the immune system and may activate the body's natural antibodies," says Milton Crane, M.D., director of medical research at Weimar Institute in Weimar, California. "At our center we've found that a hot bath or hot compress may short-circuit colds, flu, and other viral infections."

Dry vs. Wet

Heat therapy can be delivered two ways—as dry heat or wet heat. Dry heat agents such as hot water bottles and heating pads are believed to penetrate less deeply than wet heat but may be better tolerated, enabling you to use a higher temperature. The good old-fashioned hot water bottle, for example, can work quite well to ease menstrual cramps or a stomachache, reports pain consultant Margo McCaffery, R.N. A hot water bottle placed on the stomach for 10 minutes can help relax the smooth muscle of the stomach wall and reduce gastric acidity, she says.

An electric heating pad gives the advantage of continuous heat. You can choose an all-purpose heating pad, a sinus heating pad that covers the upper face, or an arthritis muff that delivers heat to both hands at once.

On the minus side, a heating pad could burn if you leave it on too long. Be sure to look for a pad with several heat settings and a timer. Set it to mild heat and shut it off after a half hour. Do not fall asleep using your heating pad. Another warning: Don't use mentholated, methyl salicylate arthritis and muscle ache creams like Ben-Gay with a heating pad. Heat makes the skin absorb so much of the cream it can become toxic and cause bad blistering.

For a safer, nonelectric alternative to heating pads, moist hot packs called hydrocollators are available. They consist of a canvas case filled with clay and usually a silicate that you heat in boiling water and wrap in several towels. The amount of heat depends on the thickness of toweling used. After 5 minutes, though, check your skin. A blotchy, uneven redness could be a sign of overheating, indicating that you need to wrap your hot pack with more towels.

Here's another convenient method of applying moist heat to ease muscle strain or arthritis pain: Place a wet hand towel in the microwave for a few minutes. (The temperature is safe if you can pick up the hot towel with your bare hand.) Lay the hot towel on the area you want to treat and cover it

with moisture-retaining plastic wrap, then a dry towel to hold in the heat. Uncover and substitute a fresh, moist towel about every 5 minutes. Use this moist compress treatment three times a day, limiting each session to 20 minutes. Never leave a hot pack on longer than 30 minutes, advises Dr. Mitchell. And to be on the safe side, never use a heat pack of any kind under your body. Your body could trap the heat, causing blistering and burning on your skin.

ALL STEAMED UP

For many who turn to natural healing remedies, moist heat means steam. People have been wrapping all or part of their bodies in fomentations—woolen blankets surrounding steamy, moist compresses—for centuries. For one thing, fomentations induce sweating, which is said to purify the body. Because steamy towels also seal in heat, they can be a useful way to ease sore, tight muscles such as in the calf of the leg, notes Dr. Mitchell.

Fomentations are still used occasionally to fight colds and flu. A common remedy for sore throat: Steam a small towel (in a rack over water just as you would steam vegetables), enfold it in a wool or cotton cloth, and wrap it around your neck. Cover the wrapping with plastic. According to healing lore, if you wear this fomentation all night, your sore throat should be gone by morning.

Wet, hot compresses are still another way to apply moist heat. An unsightly boil on the neck, for example, might be cleared up rather easily with a compress, says Rodney Basler, M.D., assistant professor of internal medicine at the University of Nebraska Medical Center. Simply place a warm wet cloth over the infected area for a half hour, three to four times a day. The heat will generate additional blood flow to deliver your body's own infection-fighting cells to the site. Also, the enhanced circulation will carry off destroyed bacteria and the poison they release. It may take a week for the boil to come to a head and break, Dr. Basler says. He recommends continuing the compress treatments for three days after the boil opens, to thoroughly drain it of bacteria.

DON'T GET BURNED

If your shoulders feel tight from driving in bumper-to-bumper traffic or your joints are stiff and creaky, you could try cranking up the heat on your sore area. But for acute problems, such as a flare-up of acute rheumatoid arthritis or a sprained ankle, you are better off using ice to help reduce the swelling for the first 24 to 72 hours, says Dr. Mitchell. Heat applied any sooner can cause excessive inflammation and swelling that may interfere with healing.

Also, do not use heat therapy if you have neuropathy (nerve damage). Because you may be unable to adequately gauge the temperature, you might burn yourself.

Heat application should feel comfortable—not painful. "If mild heat doesn't relieve your sore muscle or joint after applying it 20 minutes three times a day, see your doctor for further advice," says Dr. Mitchell. *See also* **hydrotherapy**

Heimlich maneuver   (HIME-lick) This lifesaving technique is so easy that a four-year-old child can perform it. And it's so effective, it has saved an estimated 25,000 lives in the United States since first being introduced in 1974.

Doctors call it subdiaphragmatic abdominal pressure. But most people know it as the Heimlich maneuver, named for the physician who developed this procedure to relieve foreign-body upper-airway obstruction. That's more doctor talk for choking.

Picture giving someone a hug from behind and you've got an idea of what the Heimlich maneuver looks like. You stand behind the choking person, hug him around the middle, and press in and upward sharply on his upper abdomen. This procedure raises the choker's diaphragm—the dome-shaped muscle just below the chest cavity that assists breathing—and forces air from the lungs. The air flow from the lungs forces out the obstruction.

If you ever have to use this technique, it will probably be in or near a dining area. That's because pieces of food, particularly morsels of meat, are the most common cause of choking, according to Henry Heimlich, M.D., president of the Heimlich Institute in Cincinnati.

In fact, food is so often the culprit in choking that resulting fatalities have been dubbed "cafe coronaries." That term was coined when doctors found that people who suddenly keeled over in restaurants often died from chunks of food blocking the airway, not from heart attacks.

"Whenever food is not properly

chewed, there is a risk for choking," says Dr. Heimlich. At highest risk are people who are talking, laughing, or walking while eating. Gulping your food like there's no tomorrow is also a risk factor. The elderly are prime candidates for choking because they often have difficulty chewing food. Children are also at risk because they often put small toys and other objects in their mouth.

If more people knew the Heimlich maneuver, cafe coronary deaths could practically be wiped out, doctors say. According to one study, accidental choking claims more than 3,000 lives a year. "Most of these fatalities can be avoided if the Heimlich maneuver is performed," the researchers concluded.

BETTER THAN BACK BLOWS

Why not just slap the choking person on the back? Because that action could be fatal. "Back blows are death blows. They have the tendency to move the foreign body in the wrong direction, tighter into the airway," explains Dr. Heimlich.

In contrast, the Heimlich maneuver compresses the lungs and drives air out with enough force to literally pop the obstruction out of the throat and mouth.

The American Red Cross and American Heart Association (AHA), the two organizations that help set emergency lifesaving standards, recommend that only the Heimlich maneuver and not back blows be used for airway obstruction. The exception is infants under one year of age.

As valuable as it is, the Heimlich maneuver is only for individuals over the age of one year, cautions James Seidel, M.D., Ph.D., chairman of the AHA's pediatric resuscitation subcommittee. For children under one year old, ask your pediatrician to demonstrate the proper procedure, says Dr. Seidel, associate professor of pediatrics at the University of California, Los Angeles, School of Medicine.

HOW TO DO IT

The Heimlich maneuver is easy to learn and just as easy to perform. Dr. Heimlich tells of a four-year-old child who was taught the technique by his father. The boy later successfully performed the maneuver on his little sister, who was choking on a piece of meat.

For starters, it's vitally important that you learn to recognize the signs that someone is choking. Collapsing suddenly, for example, may easily be taken as a symptom of a heart attack or stroke.

You should suspect choking if the victim had been eating prior to collapsing. Or if a person is eating and suddenly grasps his throat, it's a pretty good bet that he is choking.

If the victim can breathe, cough, or speak, the airway is not completely obstructed. It's best to leave him alone until he can dislodge the food or other object by throat clearing or coughing.

If the victim cannot cough, speak, or breathe, don't waste time. After the air supply is shut off, there are only about 4 to 6 minutes before irreversible brain damage and death occur.

Yell out to someone to dial 911 or otherwise summon help.

Then stand behind the victim and wrap your arms around his waist. Make a fist with one hand, placing your thumb against the victim's abdomen in the midline, just above the navel and well below the rib cage. Grasp your fist with your other hand and press into the victim's abdomen with a quick, upward thrust. Don't push on the rib cage—you may fracture a bone or injure internal organs. You may have to repeat the maneuver six to ten times before the object is expelled.

If the victim is lying down, turn him face up and straddle his legs. Place the heel of your hand on his abdomen in the midline just above the navel. Push inward and upward with quick thrusts. Repeat until the victim expels the object.

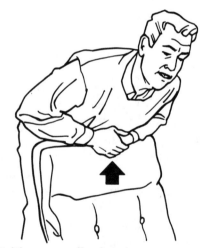

Heimlich maneuver self-performed

You can save yourself with the Heimlich maneuver. If you are choking, try to let people who are nearby know immediately, before you pass out. Grasp your throat with your hand—this is the universal distress signal of choking.

Then, place your fist on your abdomen, slightly above your navel and below your ribs. Grasp your fist with your other hand and press inward and upward several times. If this doesn't work, forcefully press your upper abdomen over any firm surface, such as the back of a chair, side of a table, or porch railing.

homeopathy   (ho-mee-OP-a-thee) Developed as an alternative to bloodletting and other harmful medical procedures practiced more than two centuries ago, homeopathy is a system that attempts to stimulate the body's natural defenses. Its originator, Samuel Hahnemann, was a German doctor who believed that you could treat an ailment by giving a patient an extremely dilute solution of a substance that would *cause* the disease's very same symptoms in healthy people—a concept he called "like cures like." (*Homeo-* means "like," and *-pathy* means "suffering.") Instead of trying to stop a cough with cough suppressants, for example, a homeopath will give as a remedy a dilution of a substance that would normally trigger a cough, "and thus stimulate the ill body to restore itself" (to quote the National Center for Homeopathy, Washington, D.C.).

Homeopaths use a variety of substances, including herb extracts like arnica or potentially lethal substances like snake venom, belladonna, and arsenic. The amounts prescribed are too minute to be toxic, though. In fact, they're so dilute—as little as one part in a million, or less—that, even with sophisticated technology, chemists may find it difficult or impossible to detect any active ingredients, raising the question of whether the remedies have any effect whatsoever, good or bad. Dr. Hahnemann knew that it was unlikely that the solutions he used contained even a single molecule of the original extract. But he believed a "memory" of the original substance remained to stimulate the body's natural defenses and recuperative powers.

A PLACEBO EFFECT?

Homeopathy is still used to treat a wide range of conditions, including colds, flu, hay fever, rheumatoid arthritis, toothaches, headaches, digestive ailments, and sports injuries, among many others. But modern physicians say homeopathy is nothing more than a placebo, a nontherapeutic "imposter" more apt to trigger your belief system than your immune system.

"If you respond well to placebos, homeopathy could work for you," says Varro E. Tyler, Ph.D., an expert in the biological effects of druglike substances at Purdue University. "For example, a cold will go away with or without homeopathic medicine. A cold is a viral infection, and ordinarily there is no remedy for a viral infection."

One homeopathy researcher maintains that there are at least 15 well-designed, carefully controlled scientific studies demonstrating that the technique does have an effect. Critics disagree. Most notably, a study published in the scientific journal *Nature* in 1988 seemed, at first blush, to give credence to homeopathy. But the results were later disproven. Walter W. Stewart, a research physicist in Bethesda, Mary-

land, and one of the investigators who found fault with the study, says, "Any apparent usefulness was due to flaws in the scientific technique. Homeopathy has no accepted scientific basis or support and should not be used for anything that needs medical attention."

Nevertheless, homeopathy is still practiced. In most states, only people with degrees that qualify them to practice medicine in that state can legally prescribe homeopathic remedies. Generally, that includes medical doctors, osteopaths, dentists, naturopaths, and some chiropractors. In most states, however, unlicensed individuals are free to buy homeopathic remedies without a prescription in health food stores, in homeopathic pharmacies, or through the mail—provided they use the substances to treat themselves for minor ailments only.

By law, drugs must be scientifically tested and reviewed by the Food and Drug Administration for safety and effectiveness. But homeopathic medicines are exempt. At the dilutions used, officials have said safety is of little concern—unless you substitute homeopathy for standard treatment of a serious condition that could get worse without medical intervention.

Researcher Stewart says: "Homeopathy is harmless *unless* you need treatment for a medical condition. Then it can be life-threatening. For example, homeopathy may be okay for a headache—unless you have a brain tumor. Then you should see a medical doctor."

Dr. Tyler concurs. "If you have gallbladder pain, there are ways to treat severe pain and avoid emergency surgery. But homeopathy isn't one of them."

The bottom line: Homeopathy shouldn't replace standard medical care.

honey The healing benefits of this sweet, thick liquid made by bees go back to the days of hieroglyphics — somewhere between 2600 and 2200 B.C. The ancient Egyptians used honey to help heal wounds and soothe stomach ailments. Later, generations of Scots used it to treat ulcers and abscesses, and as a gargle to clear phlegm. Russian soldiers in World War I slathered it on battle injuries. And in England, honey mixed with cider vinegar is still a popular folk remedy for rheumatism and arthritis — to the consternation of at least one dentist who says repeated use of the brew can damage the teeth.

Is there scientific evidence to support any one of these uses? Some.

Several clinical studies suggest that honey really can speed healing of open wounds. In a study at a Nigerian teaching hospital, for instance, topical application of unprocessed honey brought "remarkable improvement" to 58 of 59 patients with wounds and ulcers that hadn't responded to more conventional treatment.

The Nigerian study was important for two reasons. It was the first relatively large-scale study to assess the use of honey as a wound healer. It was also the first study to show that honey can separate dead skin tissue from new, healthy tissue — a process doctors call debridement. This allowed the Nigerian surgeons to remove the old tissue with

forceps, without causing pain and without resorting to surgery.

INFECTION CONTROLLED

The surgeons found the honey useful in a number of ways: It maintained the sterility of wounds which were sterile at the outset of the study. And within one week, infected wounds became sterile, too, and their odor disappeared. Swelling also subsided. Weeping ulcers gradually dried out.

Topical treatment with honey, plus skin grafts, spared four diabetic patients in the study from amputations, the surgeons reported. Curiously enough, the honey appeared to have even more potent antibacterial activity in people than in laboratory cultures.

How does honey work? According to doctors who've studied it, honey has several properties that enable it to absorb water from swollen tissue, clean the wound, and protect the wound from further infection.

In the United States, where antibiotics are much more available, there's little call for honey in surgical wards. But Jack Galloway, M.D., a Van Nuys, California, obstetrician/gynecologist, has used it successfully for the occasional Caesarean section or hysterectony incision that's become infected and resisted routine treatment. Improvements in the procedure have greatly cut back on infections, so Dr. Galloway doesn't turn to honey often. But he wouldn't hesitate to use it again, if needed.

Does he consider honey a safe home remedy for minor wounds?

"Sure," says Dr. Galloway. "Just be sure the wound doesn't become infected. If it seems to be getting worse—becoming more and more red—check with your doctor. You may then need to try a standard antibiotic like Neosporin."

horehound Added to candy and syrups, extracts of this herb have been used to quell coughs and tame hoarse throats for generations. Also known as *Marrubium vulgare,* or white horehound, horehound's funny name recalls the plant's hairy leaves and its use by ancient Greeks to treat the bite of mad dogs. While horehound for rabies has gone the way of the chariot, its use as an agent that brings up phlegm (an expectorant) and for silencing coughs endures.

Scientists have isolated a "bitter" called marrubiin from horehound that could account for its phlegm-loosening reputation. But no one has extracted the marrubiin and put it through clinical testing to tell us for sure whether horehound works, says John K. Crellin, M.D., Ph.D., professor of medical history at Memorial University of Newfoundland.

Experts can only guess why horehound might clear chest congestion. For starters, it's believed that marrubiin stimulates the secretions of the bronchial mucosa and makes it easier to cough up excess phlegm. Or it could be that this pungent-tasting aromatic oil helps liquefy mucus, making it easier to move, says Varro E. Tyler, Ph.D., a professor of pharmacognosy at Purdue University.

Horehound's reputation as a cough silencer may be related to its saliva-stimuating ability. Possibly, an increase in saliva helps calm the tickle in your throat that can send you into coughing spasms.

And it's anybody's guess as to why horehound has lasted as a favorite sore throat tonic. "The bitter, tingly taste might very well distract you from the pain sensation," speculates Branton Lachman, Pharm.D., clinical assistant professor of pharmacy at the University of Southern California School of Pharmacy in Los Angeles.

Perhaps you'd like to experiment and discover horehound's secrets for yourself. You may find horehound candy in drugstores or specialty shops ready for the trying.

Finding horehound as an ingredient in cough remedies may be difficult. The Food and Drug Administration is currently sweeping house on all ingredients in over-the-counter products that have never been demonstrated as effective. That means that horehound in commercial syrups and cough drops could soon go the way of hoop skirts.

horticultural therapy. *See* **plant therapy**

humidifiers Heating your home can create the ideal climate—for a cactus, that is. When your furnace is roaring day and night, your household's relative humidity can dip below 15 percent. That's drier than Death Valley! But you need about 40 percent relative humidity for optimum health and comfort, experts say. A dry home means dry, itchy skin and a greater chance of catching colds.

When humidity drops below 40 percent, the mucous film that lines the nose and throat becomes thick and sticky instead of free flowing, says otolaryngologist John Henderson, M.D., assistant clinical professor of ear, nose, and throat surgery at the University of California School of Medicine in San Diego. As a result, bacteria and viruses may get trapped in the stagnant mucus, making you susceptible to sore throats, sinusitis, and other upper airway infections.

Some ear, nose, and throat specialists recommend humidifiers to add moisture to the air and help people avoid these problems. "Humidifying the air can help keep the mucus thin and free flowing so that it can continue to protect you from bacteria and viruses," says Dr. Henderson.

Humidifying the air also keeps precious moisture in your skin. "One of the chief reasons we have dry skin is the low humidity in the air, which allows our own skin water to evaporate," says Joseph Bark, M.D., chairman of dermatology at St. Joseph's Hospital in Lexington, Kentucky. "One solution to dry skin is to increase humidity in the air where you spend most of your time—such as your home."

How to Humidify

For several hundred dollars, you can purchase a humidifier that hooks up to your heating system. "These units are incredibly effective and healthy for the wintertime," says Dr. Bark. You can also add humidity to your whole house with a freestanding humidifier console.

Either way, you'll find there are several different types of humidifiers that operate by different mechanisms.

One type, called evaporative humidifiers, works by driving water through a spongy material. A fan then forces air through the water-moistened material, causing evaporation that adds invisible moisture to the room. An automatic thermostat maintains the desired humidity level, which should be "between 30 and 50 percent for comfort," advises Harriet Burge, Ph.D., an associate research scientist at the University of Michigan Medical Center.

Whether you choose a built-in or freestanding humidifier, pick a model with a flow-through drain rather than a reservoir. A drain is preferable because it doesn't allow water to stand—and standing water can breed mold, bacteria, and other irritants. If you've already selected a model with a reservoir, change the water frequently. "Evaporative humidifiers, including steam and warm-mist models, are not likely to disperse microbes growing in the reservoir, but you should play it safe and make sure the water is changed periodically," says Eva Lehman, a toxicologist with the Consumer Product Safety Commission (CPSC). Likewise, clean and change the filter at regular intervals.

If you don't really require a large, evaporative-type humidifier, you might try running a small cool-mist vaporizer or ultrasonic humidifier in your bedroom while you sleep, suggests Dr.

Bark. Just be prepared to use some elbow grease if you decide to get one of these portable units. The reason? "Our studies indicate that standing water in the cool-mist and ultrasonic tanks can breed microbes which may be spewed out in the water droplets sprayed into the air," says Lehman. There is also some evidence that the ultrasonic machines—which use high-speed vibration to disperse a fine mist—may broadcast irritants that could cause respiratory problems.

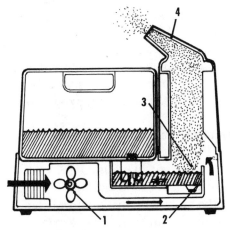

Ultrasonic humidifier: (1) fan, (2) nebulizer, (3) mist chamber, (4) nozzle

With a little effort, however, it's possible to keep your portable humidifier clean and safe. "You must change the water every day," advises Dr. Henderson. "Every third day, scrub the tank with a tablespoon of bleach or hydrogen peroxide mixed in a gallon of water. Rinse thoroughly, and use only demineralized (distilled) water."

Or you could skip all this work and get yourself one of the newer steam humidifiers. "No conclusive data is available yet, but presumably any humidifier that boils water to create a mist is not likely to promote microbial growth," says Lehman. Just be careful: Steam or warm-mist humidifiers can cause scalds and burns if tipped over. Keep these humidifiers well out of reach of small children.

No matter which portable humidifier you use, don't run it nonstop. "Overmoisturizing the air may encourage the growth of mold and dust mites in the house, which could trigger a reaction in allergy-prone people," says Harold Nelson, M.D., senior staff physician in the Department of Medicine at the National Jewish Center for Immunology and Respiratory Medicine in Denver.

A hygrometer (humidity gauge) can help you keep the humidity within optimal limits.

Looking for other ways to help boost the humidity in your house? Boil a kettle of water on the stove. Place large pans of water on radiators. Fill your bathtub with water. Finally, lower your thermostat. "Keeping your indoor temperature lower than 70°F will reduce your need to add moisture," says Dr. Burge. *See also* **vaporizers**

hydrocortisone   You might call hydrocortisone, a steroid produced by your adrenal glands, the granddaddy of the corticosteroids. The natural model for drugs such as cortisone, prednisone, and triamcinolone, hydrocortisone is a powerful anti-inflammatory agent that relieves the swelling caused by asthma, arthritis, and injuries.

Under normal circumstances, your body's own hydrocortisone regulates metabolism. But some people — those with Addison's disease, for example — don't produce enough hydrocortisone to stay regulated. For them, small replacement doses (20 to 30 milligrams a day) make up the difference. Taken in low doses, hydrocortisone doesn't appear to cause many side effects.

Hydrocortisone is quite safe for topical applications, too. Many ointments contain small amounts of hydrocortisone, which help relieve the itchy swelling of skin diseases such as eczema and dermatitis. Topical steroids aren't recommended for long-term use, but they go right to work. Symptoms often disappear in minutes.

Taken in large doses, prednisone (a synthetic relative of hydrocortisone) will suppress your immune system. That helps control diseases such as lupus and rheumatoid arthritis.

HELP FOR ARTHRITIS

Let's say you have a flare-up of rheumatoid arthritis — it hurts to lift your arm, doesn't it? If you've already tried — without success — aspirin, ibuprofen, or other nonsteroidal anti-inflammatory drugs, your doctor might aim a shot of hydrocortisone square into the joint. The swelling is liable to go right down.

Is hydrocortisone starting to sound pretty good? Wait a moment.

Hydrocortisone in some cases packs too powerful a punch. In fact, some doctors bring it out only as a last resort. Here's why.

Hydrocortisone, when taken for a long time, may suppress your body's natural production of some hormones.

That means when you *quit* taking hydrocortisone, all of a sudden you'll have some extra problems.

In large doses, hydrocortisone has been linked with inhibited growth in children. In adults, it may promote osteoporosis by depleting bones of essential minerals. And, because it may suppress your immune system, hydrocortisone puts you at risk for infectious diseases.

On the other hand, hydrocortisone *is* a natural part of your body's chemistry; your adrenal glands, if they're working properly, make some every day. Don't be afraid if your doctor hands you a prescription for hydrocortisone. Used appropriately and with careful monitoring, it can work very well. *See also* **cortisone; prednisone**

hydrogen peroxide In the decorous world of medicine, hydrogen peroxide stands out like a loud tie. Unlike most antiseptics and antibiotics, which do their jobs with maximum efficiency and minimum fuss, hydrogen peroxide goes to work with hisses, bubbles, and pops. With all that excitement, you might assume it is strong medicine indeed.

"It's been advocated for many procedures, but the antibacterial level of hydrogen peroxide is fairly low," says Max Goodson, D.D.S., Ph.D., head of the Department of Pharmacology at Boston's Forsyth Dental Center. "It would be very difficult to make a strong case for its effectiveness."

Hydrogen peroxide reacts with catalase, an enzyme found in most cells, and releases oxygen. The resulting bubbles, responsible for peroxide's brief antibacterial action, quickly bubble to the surface, cleaning the wound by carrying away bits of skin and debris.

Hydrogen peroxide, typically sold as a 3 percent solution, is an excellent disinfectant. Wiped on metal surfaces, it kills germs without leaving a residue. For wounds, however, simple soap and water probably work just as well. As one textbook notes, it is "futile to attempt antisepsis" with hydrogen peroxide.

GUM TREATMENT

Hydrogen peroxide has been used, at home and in the dentist's office, to treat the gum infections that accompany periodontal disease. In a process called the Keyes technique, people pressed a paste—a mixture of baking soda and hydrogen peroxide—into crevices between their teeth and gums. The mix, it was thought, would help eliminate troublesome bacteria.

In a study conducted by researchers at the University of Minnesota School of Dentistry, 171 volunteers with periodontal disease were divided into two groups. People in one group practiced the Keyes technique, while others simply flossed and brushed their teeth. After four years, gum inflammation was decreased in *both* groups. This suggests that thorough oral hygiene, not hydrogen peroxide, was responsible.

Even as a mouth rinse to reduce dental plaque (the sticky invisible film that can lead to gum disease), hydrogen peroxide fails to live up to its reputation, Dr. Goodson says. "It has been difficult to demonstrate convincing evidence that hydrogen peroxide has a significant effect on the retardation of plaque formation or on removal of plaque that has already been formed," he says.

Finally, hydrogen peroxide sometimes is promoted by mail-order quacks, who claim it cures everything from AIDS to Alzheimer's disease. Not only are these claims entirely bogus, doctors say, but the recommended concentrations—35 percent—can be extremely dangerous.

Hydrogen peroxide has other, more legitimate uses. For example, dentists routinely use a 35-percent solution to whiten stained teeth. "The dentist will apply it full-strength to the enamel and irradiate it with ultraviolet light to enhance the bleaching effect," Dr. Goodson says. To protect the rest of the mouth from the concentrated peroxide, however, the tooth first is isolated with a rubber dam, he adds.

Modern medicine chests have little need for hydrogen peroxide, experts say. Oral antibiotics and newer, more efficient antiseptics have supplanted this once-common germicide. On the other hand, hydrogen peroxide has one important advantage: It actually *looks* like it's working.

hydrotherapy Go to the nearest sink or tub. Turn on the tap. Flowing from the faucet is Mother Nature's most versatile wonder drug—a painkiller, sedative, stimulant, muscle relaxant, and possibly even an antibiotic, all swirled into one. Turn the tap to hot and you have the means to help loosen stiff arthritic joints. Turn it to warm if you want to feel soothed and relaxed. Switch from hot to cold and back again to soothe pain. Add a pulsating jet stream and you can massage tired muscles.

For centuries, hydrotherapy—the therapeutic use of water—was relied on to treat everything from paralysis and pneumonia to typhoid fever and tumors. In recent years, though, hydrotherapy has been nearly drowned out by a tide of pharmaceutical painkillers and antibiotics that treat a broad range of diseases. But water therapy continues to make a splash in the treatment of many structural problems and injuries.

"Water is not a miracle tonic. It can't cure diseases. But hydrotherapy does have a very important place in enhancing the healing of certain conditions," says Irene Von Estorff, M.D., assistant professor of rehabilitation medicine at New York Hospital–Cornell University Medical Center in New York City.

INJURIES SOOTHED

At the rehabilitation department in New York Hospital, for example, patients exercise in a therapeutic pool as warm water soothes severe back injuries. Farther up the coast, at the state-of-the-art training camp for the Boston Celtics basketball team, players dunk their limbs in buckets of plain old water. Without water therapy, these athletes might be benched for the season with wracked knees, pulled hamstrings, sprained shoulders, and other problems. "Getting players into a cold or hot bath helps them heal these inju-

ries so that they can get back into the game more quickly," says William Mitchell, M.D., staff physician for the Brookline Sports Medicine Clinic in Brookline, Massachusetts, and a team doctor for the Celtics.

Water therapy also helps arthritis sufferers get back into the game of life. "Water is definitely part of the prescription for easing joint stiffness and improving mobility," says John Arbruzzo, M.D., professor of medicine and director of the Rheumatology Center at Thomas Jefferson Hospital in Philadelphia.

At high-tech trauma and burn management centers, currents of water gently cleanse wounds and soothe exquisitely sensitive nerve endings, with a touch more tender than a nurse's hands. In simpler settings, water is used every day to treat a host of minor discomforts from hives to hemorrhoids.

WHY WATER WORKS

What is it about the earth's most abundant substance that makes it so abundantly healing? For one thing, the buoyancy of a bath lifts away weight and pressure from ailing joints and muscles. Water also provides a form of massage that can soothe a wounded body as well as wounded spirits.

Additional benefits flow from the fact that water is an excellent conductor of heat and cold, according to Richard Hansen, M.D., director of Poland Springs Health Institute, Poland Springs, Maine. Temperature changes can heal your body in a variety of ways, says Dr. Hansen. Warm water causes blood vessels to dilate, then constrict as you cool off. On the other hand, cold water causes vessels to constrict, then dilate as you warm up. This blood vessel workout helps pump more blood through the system. And enhanced circulation can enhance healing. "Stagnant blood flow is like stagnant water—it can breed disease," says Dr. Hansen. "Flowing water, on the other hand, purifies itself. In the same way, hydrotherapy gets the blood flowing and promotes good health."

Just as ice cream comes in more flavors than vanilla and chocolate, hydrotherapy is more than just a hot or cold soak. Here are some of the possibilities.

HOT TUBS

Those giant, family-sized redwood hot tubs have largely been replaced by more sanitary, easier-to-maintain fiberglass tubs. Some scaled-down models even fit nicely in home bathrooms. In rehabilitation centers, a hot tub is usually a huge stainless steel tank.

Whatever form it takes, the hot tub is here to stay. Some claim that 15 minutes sitting in a hot tub is like spending a session with a masseur. A hot soak dilates blood vessels, increases blood flow, and loosens muscles, making kinks disappear, Dr. Hansen says.

For arthritis sufferers, a soak in the hot tub can help joints move more freely. "A hot bath seems to help thin out joint fluid and prevent it from thickening like molasses in January, so it can do its job of lubricating your joints," says Dr. Hansen.

Besides soothing nerves, muscles, and joints, Dr. Hansen thinks that hopping into a hot bath at the first sign of sniffles might help drain away a cold or flu. "A hot bath or shower that increases body temperature to 103°F has been shown to increase the infection-fighting white blood cell count three-fold for 5 hours," says Dr. Hansen. "What's more, most cold and flu viruses don't multiply at temperatures above 101.6°F."

Many doctors remain skeptical that a hot tub could squelch the flu bug or other infectious disease. "We really need to do a lot more research in order to understand the effect of hot water immersion on the body." says Dr. Von Estorff.

Even so, Dr. Hansen, and other physicians at health resorts who routinely prescribe hot baths for a variety of conditions, think the tubs are of value.

"I'm convinced that the best investment you can make for sore muscles and joints and for your health in general is an oversized bath or hot tub so you can really stretch out," says Dr. Hansen.

A hot soak in your standard-sized bathtub can be therapeutic, too, he suggests. Use a water thermometer to make sure that the water temperature goes no higher than 104°F, the limit recommended by most doctors. Turn on a timer, too, since you should not soak for more than 15 minutes, Dr. Hansen says. Also, keep a cold compress on your head to prevent congestion or headache.

Hot tubs are not recommended if you are pregnant or have circulation problems, high blood pressure, heart disease, nerve impairment, or diabetes. Do not take a hot bath right after a strenuous workout—cool down first. And if your muscles or joints are inflamed, treat them with ice for one to three days until the swelling subsides. "Heat is the last thing you want to use on an already hot, swollen joint," reminds Dr. Von Estorff.

After a hot bath, splash your body with lukewarm or cool water. This will help stabilize the blood vessels. "When wide open blood vessels hit the cold air, they could slam shut and create a stress load on your heart," says Warren Howe, M.D., a physician in private practice in Seattle. So cool down slowly.

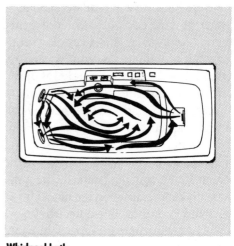

Whirlpool bath

WHIRLPOOLS

If you've ever sat at the seawater's edge and felt the marvelous massaging effect of the currents swirling around you, you have an idea of how soothing a whirlpool can be. "A whirlpool's jets give a boost to a warm bath's positive effects," says Dr. Hansen. Like a thousand tiny fingers, whirlpool bubbles gently knead the muscles and stimulate more blood flow to muscles, joints, and skin.

A home whirlpool unit can be an excellent way to help loosen stiff joints in the feet and ankles, according to Dr. Arbruzzo.

Even if you don't have pain, a whirlpool may be worth buying simply for the positive mental benefits it offers. Researchers at the University of Minnesota found that people re-

ported feeling more relaxed after bathing in bubbles than after bathing in still waters. The researchers concluded that this perception of relaxation could be therapeutic in itself. "For some people, prudent use of whirlpools may serve as a healthy alternative to other recreational activities (such as the use of alcohol and drugs) as a means of reducing tension," commented William Robiner, Ph.D., the study's author, a clinical psychologist with the Health Psychology Clinic and the University of Minnesota.

WARM BATHS

Can't sleep? Turn off the whirlpool and turn down the tap water to about 100°F—just slightly above skin temperature. Soak for half an hour, dry off, and slip immediately into bed. According to a study from Loughborough University in England, people who took a half-hour soak before bedtime fell asleep sooner and experienced deeper sleep than those who did not indulge in this nightly ritual. The researchers theorize that by raising body temperature, a warm bath may cause biochemical changes within the brain that induce deeper sleep.

NEUTRAL BATHS

If you are feeling uptight and jittery, try a bath at about 92°F to 97°F. Called a "neutral bath," this can be a great natural sedative, says Dr. Hansen. Your blood vessels relax, blood pressure goes down, and you actually breathe slower. Your entire nervous system downshifts.

An even cooler bath could leave you surprisingly calm, suggests Hardinger Singh Ghuman, M.D., a psychiatrist at Baltimore's Sheppared and Enoch Pratt Hospital. Cool baths have been used to calm down agitated mental patients for years. "A bath on the cool side makes your blood vessels constrict initially. But when you step out, your vessels dilate and you feel all warm and cozy, profoundly relaxed," says Dr. Ghuman.

But don't try to mimic the members of the Polar Bear club—the hardy bunch who plunge off lakeside docks in midwinter. "To the unaccustomed, a really cold bath or shower could place too much stress on your heart," warns Dr. Von Estorff. To be on the safe side, stick to cool douses, never ice-cold dunks.

CONTRAST BATHS

The alternating hot and cold bath is one of the most widely used forms of hydrotherapy. Using both hot and cold water makes the blood vessels dilate, contract, then dilate again, a pumping action that can greatly boost blood flow and promote healing of a variety of conditions. In fact, if you have joint stiffness or pain in your arms or legs, combined hot and cold baths may double your pain relief, says Margo McCaffery, R.N., pain consultant and coauthor of *Pain: Clinical Manual of Nursing Practice.*

For pain or stiffness in your limbs, first submerge your sore area in a bucket filled with warm water at approximately 104°F for 4 minutes. Then alternate with a dunk in a bucket of cold water at 59°F for 1 minute. Repeat the process five more times. The entire treatment lasts 20 minutes. This contrast bath coupled with exercise during the warm phase of treatment may facilitate earlier range of motion.

You may also be able to ease a migraine by taking a hot shower followed by a cool one. That's the advice of Augustus S. Rose, M.D., from the Veterans Administration Wadsworth Medical Center in Los Angeles. It's speculated that the migraine is interrupted by the temperature contrast, which shrinks swollen blood vessels in the head. Dr. Rose has had success with this technique for 20 years. But anyone with heart trouble, high blood pressure, diabetes, or hardening of the arteries should not try a contrast bath or shower without consulting a doctor first.

FOOTBATHS

Oddly enough, a hot footbath can sometimes relieve a sinus headache or a stuffy nose. According to otolaryngologist Lloyd Rosenvold, M.D., part of that stuffy feeling is caused by sluggish circulation in inflamed mucous membranes. The hot footbath causes blood vessels in the feet to open wider than usual. Blood rushes to fill the enlarging arteries and is drawn away from the head, unblocking the nasal traffic jam.

SITZ BATHS

If you have an infection or inflammation in the pelvic region, a sitz bath—or hip bath—helps you direct soothing water where it's needed the most. Either a cold or warm sitz bath is effective at relieving the swelling and pain following childbirth, studies show. And a warm sitz bath can still be the best treatment for hemorrhoids, according to Dr. Hansen. Simply fill the tub with a few inches of warm water, sit down, and raise your knees. The warm water should help dull the pain and increase blood flow to the area. Ultimately, swollen veins could shrink and you may get relief. *See also* **cold therapy, heat therapy**

hyperbaric oxygen   A few years ago, pop star Michael Jackson was photographed, lying with arms folded across his sequined jacket, inside an 8-foot see-through sealed chamber. Inside this plastic tube, Jackson was breathing hyperbaric (high-pressure) oxygen. Apparently, the singer presumed that flooding his body with oxygen would rejuvenate worn-out cells and bestow eternal youth.

Another clever publicity stunt?

Perhaps. But even noncelebritites have been resorting to hyperbaric oxygen chambers in an effort to treat everything from wrinkles and sagging breasts to senility and cancer.

"Some people believe that aged and diseased tissues are 'oxygen-starved' and that an infusion of oxygen greater than the body normally takes in can help reverse the condition," says Eric P. Kindwall, M.D., associate professor of hyperbaric medicine at the Medical College of Wisconsin in Milwaukee. "But there simply is no evidence to support hyperbaric oxygen [HBO] therapy for use in these cases. People who say that HBO is a cure-all are wrong."

On the other hand, says Dr. Kindwall, those who say that hyperbaric chambers are not good for anything are also wrong.

Since the turn of the century, deep sea divers have used hyperbaric chambers to treat decompression sickness, called the "bends." This condition occurs when divers swim too rapidly to the water's surface, and nitrogen gas bubbles become trapped in the bloodstream instead of dissolving in the lungs and being exhaled. The bubbles cut off circulating oxgyen, producing a dull ache in the limbs, or possibly a total collapse of the blood vessels.

When a diver experiencing the bends enters a hyperbaric oxygen chamber, he receives 100 percent oxygen at greater atmospheric pressure than at sea level—an environment that mimics being underwater. The combined increased pressure and super-high oxygen level shrink the nitrogen bubbles and increase the amount of oxygen dissolved in the bloodstream.

As hyperbaric chamber use (and abuse) grew, the Undersea and Hyperbaric Medical Society (the governing body for legitimate HBO therapy) created a committee to investigate claims regarding other disorders. They recommend 14 therapeutic applications in a hospital setting.

"We found that HBO is a limited but very important tool for surgeons," says Dr. Kindwall, who headed the committee's investigations. That's because HBO is useful for shrinking air bubbles that may occur in the bloodstream during various surgical procedures.

A stint in the chamber could also help spare a badly injured limb from gangrene, a condition in which tissues die from lack of oxygen.

"HBO may help reduce swelling and increase oxygen delivery to the tissues until blood vessels can be surgically repaired," says Pamela Grim, M.D., director of hyperbaric medicine at the University of Chicago.

BURN VICTIMS TREATED

There are some preliminary studies showing that HBO may help heal burns. A few burn centers are already using this method to treat second- and third-degree burns. It was at such a center, in fact, that Michael Jackson was first exposed to a hyperbaric chamber when he was treated for a head burn.

"Hyperbaric oxygen has been hypothesized to play a role in reducing scarring, decreasing swelling, and im-

proving skin graft take after burns," says Dr. Grim.

Burn patients, and other critically ill patients as well, enter a one-person chamber (called a monoplace chamber) that is equipped with an intravenous tube. This allows vital fluids to be administered while the person is being treated with pressurized oxygen.

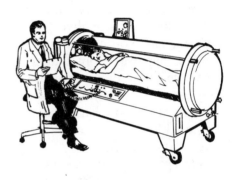

One-person hyperbaric oxygen chamber

More commonly, however, critically ill and injured patients enter a larger, 14-person compressurized chamber. These bigger chambers allow an entire surgical team to continue to care for patients receiving HBO.

Being inside either type of chamber is a little like being inside a pressurized airplane cabin during takeoff. Your ears feel full and your voice sounds funny, rather like Donald Duck's.

But HBO is not to be taken lightly. There are some risks involved, according to Dr. Grim. One hundred percent oxygen under high pressure can cause injury to the ears and sinuses, and in rare cases, to the lungs and central nervous system.

Despite these risks, it's possible that HBO may someday play a role in treating common diseases. But don't hold your breath.

Researchers have begun to take a serious look at HBO to treat myocardial infarction (heart attack), reports Dr. Kindwall. Infarctions occur when a clot stops blood flow. In preliminary studies with dogs, HBO seemed to help maintain blood circulation and keep the heart muscle alive when a clot formed in a coronary artery. "But we are a long way from finding an HBO cure for cardiovascular disease or any other disease," says Dr. Kindwall. "If you hear of hyperbaric chambers being used for this purpose, you can be sure it is not legitimate."

One place you may legitimately come in contact with HBO outside of the hospital may be high in the Rocky Mountains. Trekking up sky-high peaks where the air is thin can give you altitude sickness. Normally the cure is to descend to a lower altitude where there's more oxgyen.

Now you don't have to backtrack. A portable, inflatable sleeping-bag-type hyperbaric device has been invented that essentially "takes the healthier lower altitude up to the patient," according to experts. A foot pump pressurizes the bag, simulating atmospheric pressure of 8,000 feet for example, when you are really up at 14,000 feet. Once inside the bag, your altitude sickness may be alleviated in minutes, says Peter Hackett, M.D., associate professor of medicine at the Center for High-Altitude Health Research in Anchorage, Alaska.

hypnosis   Have you ever driven down a highway, mentally replaying a conversation you've just had, rehearsing your role in a meeting you're about to attend, or visualizing some scene in an audio book you're listening to on the car stereo? And then when you got to your destination, were you so involved in your thoughts that you couldn't remember how you got to where you were going? If so, you may have experienced a hypnotic-like state of mind.

"Hypnosis is a process in which you shift your attention from the activity going on around you and refocus it on the thoughts, feelings, or sensations inside you," explains Gerard V. Sunnen, M.D., associate clinical professor of psychiatry at the New York University Bellevue Hospital Medical Center. There's no hocus-pocus involved. It's a natural state that we all drop in and out of about a hundred times a day. But it's also something you can teach yourself to do "on command."

Why would you want to? Scientists say that you can use hypnosis to control fear and alleviate pain. People who are afraid to do something—speak before a group, drive across a bridge, or meet new people, for example—can sometimes reduce their fear by using hypnosis. Once guided into the hypnotic state, they can be asked to use their imagination to experience the situation that frightens them, in a more successful and less stressful way.

The mind is most open to suggestion when the body is in a very relaxed state, says Dr. Sunnen. So first "we teach someone how to go into a deep state of physical relaxation. Then we ask them to project themselves slowly into a situation they want to handle better, like public speaking, all the while maintaining a profound sense of well-being."

After five or six practice sessions, the relaxation they feel during the mental "rehearsal" will carry over automatically to the real speech.

PAIN CONTROL

As effective as it is in reducing fear, hypnosis may be equally effective in reducing pain. Cancer researchers at the University of Washington, for example, have found that hypnosis allows some people with cancer to dissociate themselves from their pain so that, for all intents and purposes, it is not as disruptive to the quality of life and to the treatment process.

The researchers first enlist a person's attention by asking him to either concentrate on his breathing or focus his eyes on a particular spot. Once the person is concentrating on something other than his pain, the researchers lead him through a relaxation exercise. Once he is fully relaxed, an inspirational mental image or scene is suggested, in which the person should reinvest his attention. The dissociation process is now complete. As far as the patient is concerned, the pain may still exist, but it is now experienced as being separate and disconnected from himself.

Although hypnosis is highly effective in helping people overcome both fear and pain, one area in which it appears to have variable effectiveness is addiction, says Dr. Sunnen. It nevertheless succeeds in helping 30 percent of those who try it to stop smoking and 15 percent of those who try it to lose weight.

For a referral to a qualified hypnotherapist, contact the American Society of Clinical Hypnosis. Check the Yellow Pages of the city nearest you for a branch office listing, or send a self-addressed, stamped envelope to them at 2200 East Devon Avenue, Suite 291, Des Plaines, IL 60018. Generally you can expect to spend at least four to six sessions with a hypnotist before you'll be able to use hypnosis effectively on your own. *See also* **autogenic training; Relaxation Response**

hysterectomy   From the Greek words *hystera,* for "womb," and *ektome,* for "excision," comes the name for this common operation. And we do mean common. Experts say one in three women faces the prospect of having her uterus removed.

The reasons vary.

Two absolutely inarguable reasons to have a hysterectomy are uterine cancer and ovarian cancer. An estimated 13 percent are done for this reason. The other reason for a hysterectomy is bleeding that begins during a Caesarean section or other gynecological operation and can't be stopped any other way.

Hysterectomies used to be the treatment of choice for certain cervical pre-cancerous lesions, too. But there are now more direct ways to treat the cervix. Laser therapy is one such method, says Ruth Schwartz, M.D., a Rochester, New York, gynecologist and member of the American College of Obstetricians and Gynecologists Task Force on Hysterectomies.

EXPLORE OPTIONS

The bulk of hysterectomies (an estimated 80 percent) are used to treat uterine problems such as fibroids, uterine prolapse, endometriosis, or abnormal menstrual bleeding—conditions for which there may be appropriate nonsurgical remedies or less extensive surgical procedures. If you suffer from any of these and a hysterectomy has been suggested, you owe it to yourself to first explore other options with your gynecologist—or seek a second opinion. There are more alternatives to hysterectomy than ever before. Only you and your doctor can decide if they're right for you.

Fibroids, those troublesome hard knots of muscle fiber that sprout from the muscular wall of the uterus, are the most common reason for hysterectomies. Although they rarely develop into cancer, fibroids can cause pain and excessive bleeding. And the larger they get, the more they can affect other organs like the bladder and kidneys.

"What we're leaning toward now in younger women who still want to bear children are myomectomies, which remove just the fibroids," says Dr.

Schwartz, who is also a clinical professor of obstetrics and gynecology at the University of Rochester School of Medicine. But if a woman is done with childbearing and experiences abnormal bleeding and pain or has a rapidly growing fibroid, a hysterectomy may be wise.

If a woman whose uterus has prolapsed—slipped down because of weakening muscular support—still wants to have children, there are ways to resuspend it. But if she's past her childbearing years, such alternatives to hysterectomy usually aren't worth the effort, Dr. Schwartz says.

Hysterectomy for endometriosis is a totally individual choice, says Dorothy Barbo, M.D., professor of obstetrics and gynecology at the University of New Mexico School of Medicine. In this often painful condition, the endometrial tissue lining the uterus can implant itself on the ovaries, bladder, bowels, or outer wall of the uterus. It, too, swells and bleeds during the menstrual period. Endometriosis can sometimes be controlled by medicine and sometimes by a procedure known as laser laparoscopy, in which a laser cauterizes the tissue through a tiny incision. The mode of treatment depends upon how extensive the condition is, says Dr. Barbo, who is also medical director of ambulatory services at the school's Women's Health Center.

In cases of abnormal bleeding, hormonal treatments may be able to create a more normal menstrual period and regulate flow. But for the woman "who floods every month" and/or becomes anemic, a hysterectomy may be necessary, says Dr. Barbo.

IF SURGERY LOOMS

If you and your doctor decide to go ahead with the surgery, determine whether your doctor intends to remove the ovaries, too. If your ovaries are removed and you haven't begun menopause, you'll begin it after the hysterectomy.

Removing the ovaries will eliminate your chances of getting ovarian cancer, a disease that's both difficult to detect until it is advanced and difficult to treat. The downside is that you'll lose the sex hormones estrogen, progesterone, and androgens. Estrogens can be replaced with a pill or a skin patch. But androgens, which the ovaries would normally continue to secrete even after menopause, "are much more difficult to replace," says Sadja Greenwood, M.D., assistant clinical professor of gynecology at the University of California Medical Center, San Francisco. Androgens contribute to sexual responsiveness and muscular strength. "Loss of the androgens is the reason why some women don't find their sex drive and energy restored completely after the operation," says Dr. Greenwood.

The operation is likely to require a hospital stay of three to five days. You might be able to return to normal activities within six weeks, but "don't expect to have all your zip back," says Dr. Barbo. Depending upon your general health, it may take you six months or longer to fully recover.

Possible complications of the operation include excessive blood loss, infection, and damage to surrounding organs.

If you're about to undergo a hysterectomy, Dr. Greenwood advises you to bank at least two units of your own blood in advance. And, if you're anemic, ask your doctor about taking iron supplements to build you up before the surgery.

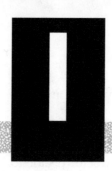

ibuprofen (eye-BOO-pro-fen *or* eye-byu-PRO-fen) It used to be simple. "Take two aspirin and call me in the morning," your doctor might say. But choosing a painkiller has gotten more complicated these days. Your doctor might still recommend aspirin, of course. Or she might suggest ibuprofen, an analgesic approved for over-the-counter sales in 1984.

You could think of ibuprofen, the active ingredient in products such as Advil, Motrin, and Nuprin, as an aspirin substitute. It does many of the same things aspirin does.

Like aspirin, ibuprofen kills pain, cools fevers, and eases headaches. Ibuprofen reduces swelling. And it relieves dysmenorrhea, the painful menstrual cramps some women get every month.

You might wonder, who needs an aspirin substitute? Why not take the real—and so much less expensive—thing?

FEWER SIDE EFFECTS

The reason is simple: Aspirin may be a great pain reliever, but it doesn't come without side effects. Gastroin-testinal problems, even ulcers, commonly accompany long-term aspirin use. However, small doses of ibuprofen appear to work as well as larger doses of aspirin. That means equal pain relief with fewer side effects.

Ibuprofen belongs to a relatively new class of drugs known collectively as NSAIDs—nonsteroidal anti-inflammatory drugs. The NSAIDs now are among the most widely prescribed drugs in the world. Aspirin, strictly speaking, is an NSAID, although the term usually refers to drugs such as ibuprofen, indomethacin, and fenoprofen.

Ibuprofen, like aspirin, kills pain by inhibiting your body's production of prostaglandins, chemicals responsible for triggering pain and inflammation. When you have an infection, a hurt knee, or a sudden flare-up of rheumatoid arthritis, prostaglandins push the panic button. Pain rushes to your brain; white blood cells rush to your injury. The result: painful swelling.

Ibuprofen, then, acts like an "off" switch. It switches off the prostaglandins, which turns off pain and swelling.

Aspirin's side effects, for many

292

people, make it a tough pill to swallow. Most people seem to tolerate ibuprofen quite a bit better. In one study, people with rheumatoid arthritis took several different NSAIDs—aspirin, ibuprofen, fenoprofen, naproxen, and tolmetin. Ibuprofen was preferred second only to naproxen, a prescription drug. (Aspirin, incidentally, scored last.)

How strong is ibuprofen? In one study, 107 dental patients took either ibuprofen, acetaminophen, or a nontherapeutic placebo prior to having a tooth extracted. The people taking ibuprofen reported less pain than people taking the placebo or acetaminophen.

Ibuprofen is so strong, in fact, that it's been found to equal methylprednisolone, a powerful steroid, for pain relief. Ibuprofen even has been found to work as well as a combination of acetaminophen and codeine. Better yet, it's a lot cheaper than prescription painkillers!

INHIBITS CLOTS

Aspirin, you may remember, grabbed headlines when a Harvard Medical School study suggested low doses (one tablet every other day) may help prevent heart attacks in healthy people. Could ibuprofen compete?

Perhaps. Ibuprofen, like aspirin, "thins" your blood by inhibiting clot-producing cells in your bloodstream from clumping together. In any case, the idea is simple: If you keep your blood flowing smoothly, you might reduce your risk for heart attacks.

Sometimes, of course, you *want* your blood to clot—when you cut

yourself, for example. Your doctor may ask you to refrain from taking ibuprofen or aspirin before surgery. In addition, women who take ibuprofen may bleed more heavily during their periods.

On the other hand, ibuprofen helps reduce uncomfortable intrauterine pressure and the frequency of uterine contractions, which may reduce menstrual discomfort.

British researchers have suggested that ibuprofen, aspirin, and other NSAIDs may protect regular users from cataracts. What's more, ibuprofen has been found to improve cerebral blood flow in dogs following cardiac arrest—a promising sign that the drug may aid neurological recovery after heart attacks.

As you may have guessed, ibuprofen isn't without side effects. Like aspirin, it may cause some gastrointestinal discomfort. Ibuprofen also may interfere with the action of some antihypertensive drugs. And in fact, ibuprofen actually may slow the time it takes you to heal. Here's how.

Ibuprofen, you'll recall, reduces swelling by inhibiting your body's production of prostaglandins. However, wounds *need* swelling. That's why your body creates inflammation in the first place. All that swelling helps clean things up; white blood cells crowd into the area and gobble up impurities. So when you stop the swelling, you also interfere with healing.

In a dramatic case described in the *Journal of the American Academy of Dermatology,* a man's wounds just wouldn't heal after surgery. The doctors' conclusion: "When the drug [ibuprofen] was discontinued [he was taking 1,800 milligrams a day], no further wound complications were experienced."

Most people who take ibuprofen aren't likely to have problems with healing. If you do experience side effects, of course, you should consult your doctor. However, for the occasional cold, hurt, or headache, ibuprofen works well—and with fewer side effects than aspirin. *See also* **anti-inflammatories; painkillers**

ileal bypass (IL-ee-al) Years ago, long before effective drugs were available, battling cholesterol occasionally meant undergoing major surgery.

During the procedure, called a partial ileal bypass, surgeons rerouted the digestive tract around about 7 feet of the ileum, the segment of the small intestine that absorbs most of the cholesterol from the foods we eat.

But today, most doctors believe the surgery, first done about 25 years ago, is a radical step needed only in rare cases.

BYPASSED BY DRUGS

"In those days, the drugs that were available for reducing cholesterol were often difficult for people to tolerate. So back then, the surgery was a better approach for some people," says Basil Rifkind, M.D., chief of the lipid metabolism and atherogenesis branch of the National Heart, Lung, and Blood Institute. "That's no longer the case with our new drugs. They're very good at reducing cholesterol. They're as good as, if not better than, a partial

ileal bypass, and they're easy to take. So it's seldom that we even think of surgery as an option." While most doctors prefer drugs over surgery, more natural techniques are the choice over drugs. A low-fat, high-fiber diet and an exercise program have been proven effective when it comes to lowering cholesterol.

IMPRESSIVE RESULTS

Henry Buchwald, M.D., a surgeon at the University of Minnesota, however, is one doctor who prefers surgery. "If you want the most effective way to lower cholesterol, then it's the partial ileal bypass," says Dr. Buchwald. "It's as safe as, if not safer than, many of the drugs to lower cholesterol that are available today."

Dr. Buchwald offers evidence to support his position.

In a study of 838 patients followed for an average of ten years, he concluded that the partial illeal bypass was more effective in lowering blood cholesterol than a low-fat diet.

Another study at the Royal Postgraduate Medical School in London found that cholesterol levels in 11 patients fell by an average of 26 percent in the month following surgery. Two years later, their cholesterol levels were still 20 percent below what they were before the bypass.

Dr. Buchwald admits that not everyone with high cholesterol is a candidate for the operation. "A 65-year-old man who has a blood cholesterol level of 260 but no evidence of cardiovascular disease might be treated with drugs and diet," he says. "On the other hand, a 32-year-old man with the same cholesterol level, but who recently had a heart attack, might be a prime candidate for the surgery." In either case, Dr. Buchwald says, the aim is the same: to get cholesterol down so heart disease risk is reduced.

Like all surgeries, partial ileal bypass can result in complications. Some patients suffer from diarrhea and bowel obstruction. The surgery also increases the likelihood that patients will develop kidney stones and gallstones.

imagery After nine months of languishing in a hospital bed battling multiple sclerosis, Carlton was not a pretty sight. Three bedsores, each about 4 inches deep, had slowly eroded his buttocks and infected surrounding muscle and bone.

"He was in a lot of pain and was very depressed. Surgeons actually had to remove several inches of both femurs [thigh bones] that were severely infected. Basically, it was becoming a potentially lethal situation," says Dennis Gersten, M.D., a San Diego psychiatrist.

It seemed little could be done to help, but Dr. Gersten had an idea. He suggested that Carlton *imagine* his wounds were healing.

"In three days, the patient said that he could feel the sores healing. In seven days, a surgeon said he could see the wounds healing, and in two months two of the sores had healed. In four months, all of the bedsores were gone," Dr. Gersten says.

Was Carlton some sort of psychic

wizard? "I don't think there was anything special about him," Dr. Gersten says. "His belief was just very strong." After all, Carlton isn't the only patient who has successfully used imagery to cure an ailment. In fact, many researchers and doctors now believe that imagery or visualization techniques can definitely enhance the body's ability to heal itself.

"We know the circuitry is there. There are nerves everywhere in the body, and where there are nerves, there is mind. If you can learn how to activate the switches, you can use the nervous system to convey healing messages to the body," says Andrew Weil, M.D., author of *Health and Healing.*

For example, one man successfully destroyed a wart by visualizing that a steam shovel was scraping off its surface each evening, Dr. Weil says.

PAIN FLEW AWAY

In another instance, Dr. Gersten helped a 40-year-old musician overcome neck pain and spasms following an automobile accident.

"I asked him to imagine that his pain was some type of animal. The first thing that popped into his head was a bird. So I asked him to imagine that in the distance there was a beautiful nest. Then I asked him to imagine the bird flying off to that nest. When the bird flew off, his pain dropped to zero," Dr. Gersten says.

If you're like most people, you probably have at least 3,000 random images flit through your mind daily, says Dr. Gersten. Any one of those images might affect what's happening in your body, *your physiology.* Visualization techniques simply give you a way to shape some of those images to achieve a desired result.

In fact, Gerald Epstein, M.D., author of *Healing Visualizations,* believes that imagery can be a powerful, specialized tool in battling many diseases. He says the use of healing images can help patients fight at least 80 physical and psychological disorders, including high blood pressure, cataracts, diabetes, cancer, acne, premenstrual syndrome, arthritis, and colds.

That contention is supported by intriguing research. Researchers at Southern Methodist University found that 30 people who used imagery to envision neutrophils and lymphocytes—two types of disease-fighting white blood cells—affected the number of those cells in their bloodstream over a six-week period.

CANKER SORES COATED

In another study, researchers at Pennsylvania State University concluded that imagery was an effective method of relieving the symptoms of recurrent canker sores in the mouth. At least three of the seven participants in the study had suffered from the ailment for more than ten years, and all had had at least one canker sore every two weeks during the previous year.

The cause of recurrent canker sores remains a mystery, and no consistently successful method of treatment has been discovered, says Howard Hall, Ph.D., Psy.D., a coauthor of the study who is

now with Case Western Reserve and Rainbow Babies' and Children's Hospital, Cleveland. But imagery certainly helped.

"We asked them to imagine that a coating of white blood cells was covering and soothing the sores. The results were even more positive than we originally expected. Every one of the subjects had significant relief," Dr. Hall says.

But some researchers aren't so sure that people can consciously direct their immune systems to attack specific trouble spots in their bodies. An understanding of how imagery works is still elusive.

"The extent that they may be guiding lymphocytes to the site of a tumor or activating hormonal pathways is unknown," says Nicholas Hall, Ph.D., director of the Division of Psychoimmunology at the University of South Florida.

Dr. Hall believes guided imagery to be at least a behavioral placebo. A placebo is an inert, nontherapeutic substance given to some patients instead of a drug. Occasionally, the placebo works for those patients simply because they believe it will relieve their symptoms.

"I firmly believe guided imagery works, and I don't mean to use the term placebo in a negative way," he says. "I see placebo as a very powerful phenomenon, one that provides very convincing evidence that there is a connection, a mechanism of action, between one's expectations and health." In other words, if you believe imagery will heal you, then it probably will, Dr. Hall says.

Dr. Gersten agrees that belief is an important factor in the successful use of imagery. He remembers treating a 15-year-old boy whose right leg was ¼ inch shorter than the left. The boy and his mother asked if imagery would help the right leg grow so it was even with the left.

"That was a tall order. But I said if they believed we could do it, then we'd probably have a good shot at it," Dr. Gersten says. "I completely suspended my doubt and so did they. Six months later, his legs were exactly even."

During those six months, the boy spent about 10 minutes of each day visualizing a machine creating new bone within his right leg.

IMAGINE THIS

So how can you get visualization to work for you? Dr. Weil says for imagery to work, you need to select an image that has a strong emotional impact on you. Drawing those specific images out of your mind may require the help of a therapist or counselor.

But Dr. Gersten suggests several more general imagery exercises that may help relieve pain, stress, and anxiety. You may have to adapt some of them to your own needs, but he says many of his patients who use these exercises get relief from their symptoms in less than 5 minutes.

If you feel tense, for example, close your eyes and imagine yourself sitting on your favorite beach. As the waves slip onto the shore, image them roll-ing up to your neck. Then as the waves recede, picture them pulling all the tension out of your body.

Another stress-relieving possibility is to imagine that you are a feather gently floating to the ground. When you reach the ground, picture youself being fully relaxed.

For pain, Dr. Gersten suggests that you imagine that your pain is a ball of mercury. After you can "see," "feel," and "touch" the mercury ball, imagine it rolling down the nearest arm or leg and tumbling out of your body. Watch it roll across the floor and out of the room. Or kick it far into outer space. Dr. Gersten says that image has helped some of his patients relieve their chronic pain completely in just one session. *See also* **meditation; placebo; Relaxation Response**

Imodium (ih-MO-dee-um) The only good thing you can say about diarrhea is that it rarely sticks around. In most cases, diarrhea makes people miserable for a day or two and then clears right up. In fact, many doctors don't even treat diarrhea, preferring to let it run its course.

But there are times when people just can't wait for diarrhea to disappear. And that's when an over-the-counter drug called Imodium (loperamide hydrochloride) can help.

"Loperamide interacts with the nerve endings in the intestinal muscles and shuts them down, so you slow down the propulsion of contents through the intestine," says Howard Rodenberg, M.D., assistant professor of emergency medicine at the University of Florida College of Medicine and medical director of ShandsCair, an emergency-medicine flight program in Gainesville, Florida.

Imodium is also thought to bind to receptors in the brain that inhibit the motility (movement) of the bowel. That may be why the drug reduces both the frequency of bowel movements and the sense of urgency—or panic—that may precede them.

Imodium begins working in about 45 minutes, and its action continues for about 6 hours. Taken in large doses, it affects the central nervous system, so some people feel sleepy or nauseated. It also may cause constipation. "If you shut things down too much, you may get a little bloating, and you just won't feel good," Dr. Rodenberg warns.

In most cases, it's best to leave diarrhea alone so the gastrointestinal tract can purge itself. "If you stop the diarrhea, then you leave bad stuff in the GI tract, and that prolongs the duration of the illness," Dr. Rodenberg says.

"On the other hand, people don't want to ruin their vacation by staying in the hotel room for two days. When it's reached the point where your fluid intake is not going to be equal to what you're losing through the stools, you want to shut diarrhea down to avoid dehydration," he says. *See also* **bismuth; Kaopectate**

inhalers   Years ago, if you suffered from asthma attacks, your doctor might have urged you to smoke cigarettes—special *botanical* cigarettes that helped open the windpipes. Today, asthma patients are puffing a different kind of medicine. And a special delivery device called an inhaler helps them do it more efficiently.

"There is impressive evidence showing that inhaling asthma medicine gets it quickly and directly into the airways with less of the side effects associated with swallowing medicines," says Allan Weinstein, M.D., assistant professor of medicine at Georgetown University and author of *Asthma: The Complete Guide to Self-Management of Asthma and Allergies.*

Today's inhalers are as portable as those botanical cigarettes of yesterday. The pocket-sized metered-dose inhaler, or MDI, is the most commonly used device. The MDI is a sealed canister containing an asthma medicine suspended in a liquid aerosol propellant mixture. The canister is inserted into a mouthpiece apparatus. A metered valve releases a dose of medicine in a fine spray when the canister is activated.

RELIEF IN TWO PUFFS

No matter where you are, should you suddenly experience a bout of wheezing, you can whip out your inhaler, take two slow puffs of the asthma medicine (usually, a bronchodilator such as albuterol), and begin breathing normally again within minutes. "You can also use your MDI to *prevent* an asthma attack due to exercise," adds Dr. Weinstein. Two prerace puffs from your MDI, for example, could help you breeze—not wheeze—past the finish line.

Inhalers aren't just for immediate, emergency relief, though. They can also prevent and control symptoms on a routine basis. Inhaled steroids, for example, are sometimes used to open up swollen, inflamed airways over time.

With a few exceptions, MDIs require a doctor's prescription. "Prescription brand inhalers have the advantage over over-the-counter inhalers in that they're longer acting and have less potential effect on the heart," says Dr. Weinstein. An added advantage of having your doctor prescribe an inhaler is that you can get some hands-on instruction in its proper use.

Researchers have found that about half the people using inhalers do not use them correctly. That's not so surprising, considering that these gadgets require some coordination. "The spray comes out with great force, traveling at a speed of 70 miles an hour. It takes monumental coordination to synchronize pressing the device with inhaling something that is traveling at such high speed," says Bernard Berman, M.D., chief of pediatric allergy at St. Elizabeth's Hospital in Boston. Poor technique can mean that less of the drug gets into your lungs, so more medication may be required to control your asthma.

Mastering Your MDI

"With a little practice, it's possible to master the proper technique for using an MDI and get the most out of your asthma medication," assures Dr. Weinstein. For starters, shake the inhaler vigorously to mist the suspension. Then position the device two finger-widths away from your open mouth and tilt your head back. Next, exhale as much as possible. Then as you begin to breathe in, press the device, slowly inhale, and hold your breath for a count of ten. "If you see a foggy mist floating out of your mouth, your breath wasn't deep enough," says Dr. Weinstein. Try again. Then slowly exhale. "For best results, wait at least 2 minutes, then take a second puff," he says. "The first puff opens the airways and allows further penetration by the second."

Don't make the common mistake of putting the device between your closed lips. Research has shown that the open-mouth technique can deliver twice as much medication to the lower respiratory tract as the closed-mouth technique. "The idea is to direct the jet stream of medicine into your breath stream and into your air tubes rather than hitting the back of the throat," says Dr. Weinstein.

If your middle name is Butterfingers, take heart. Your doctor can prescribe a relatively inexpensive tube-like apparatus called a spacer or extender that attaches between the mouthpiece and canister of your MDI and helps channel the spray to your mouth.

Add-on devices can do more than improve your aim. One type of extender, the Aero Chamber, has a valved holding chamber that traps the large droplets of medicine and allows time for them to decelerate and evaporate. What finally arrives in your breathstream are smaller and slower-moving aerosol particles. That means you have less of the medicine deposited in your throat, where it may cause hoarseness and—in the case of a steriod spray—a fungal infection known as thrush. A

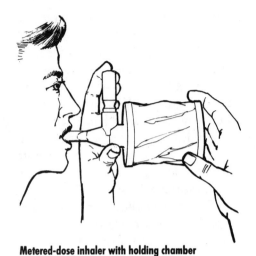

Metered-dose inhaler with holding chamber

large holding chamber can also dilute the unpleasant taste of some inhaled medicine.

"Add-on devices are an absolute must for children and others who can't master the technique of the MDIs, as well as anyone who must take inhaled steroids or frequent puffs of asthma medicine," advises Dr. Berman. "You simply shake the canister, press the device to fill the reservoir with spray, and slowly inhale. No special synchronization is required."

A less bulky alternative than add-on spacers is the newer breath-activated inhalers, or BAIs. A study conducted in Scotland has shown that BAIs are just as effective as MDIs but are a lot easier to use. A capsule of powdered medicine is inserted into a pocket-sized inhaler device that you place between your lips. You twist the inhaler to puncture the capsule, take one quick, deep breath, and presto! The powder is swiftly sucked into your lungs. "BAIs are ideal for people who may be irritated by the MDI aerosols' fillers. They're also good for managing chronic asthma," reports Jerry Dolovich, M.D., clinical professor of pediatric medicine in the Department of Pediatrics at McMaster Medical Center in Hamilton, Ontario.

MORE MASSIVE MISTER

If your asthma is acute and you are unable to effectively use a pocket inhaler, your doctor may recommend a wet aerosol, also called a compressor-driven nebulizer. This machine works by forcing air past a solution containing asthma medicines, producing a fine mist. The mist is inhaled through a mouthpiece or mask while you breathe normally. Airways open almost immediately. "Nebulizers may be cumbersome and costly, but they're a better alternative than the hospital emergency room if you have unpredictable or severe asthma flares," says Dr. Weinstein.

Whatever device you use, be sure to have your technique checked periodically by a doctor.

Also be sure that your inhaler has plenty of medicine when you need it. A float test will determine if your MDI is nearly empty. Remove the mouthpiece and place the inhaler in a container of room-temperature water. "The higher the inhaler floats, the more empty it is," says Dr. Weinstein. To be on the safe side, keep a spare MDI at work or at the gym. If you are using a nebulizer machine, be sure to have enough asthma solution on hand. If you are using a plugless model, make sure the batteries are recharged. *See also* **bronchodilators**

interferon   (in-ter-FEER-on) Named for its ability to interfere with viral infections, this natural protein—which virus-infected cells secrete to protect healthy cells—shimmered with promise in the first decade following its discovery in 1957. Although short supply hampered initial research efforts, the wave of excitement created by interferon crested again in the early 1980s, when a major breakthrough in genetic engineering made it the first naturally occurring substance in the human body to be cloned and mass-produced as a drug. Could interferon wipe out the major cancer killers?

There were good reasons to suspect that it might. First, certain cancers are viral-induced. And interferon was found to be effective against not just one kind of virus but a wide range of them. Second, interferon revealed a talent for slowing down the rate at which cells multiply—which might account for its ability to make certain tumors regress. Third, interferon was shown to increase the effectiveness of other naturally occurring cancer fighters, such as macrophages and natural killer cells.

But practical uses for the drug have been slow in coming. To date, interferon—which is given by injection because digestive enzymes would inactivate it if swallowed—is an approved treatment in the United States for only a limited number of conditions.

For sufferers of hairy cell leukemia, a rare and once deadly disease, interferon is a literal lifesaver. (The disease is so named because hairlike projections extend from the diseased white blood cells.) It brings complete remission or marked improvement for many patients who use it.

"I think it produces remarkable results with this disease," says Sidney Pestka, M.D., chairman of the Department of Molecular Genetics and Microbiology at the University of Medicine and Dentistry of New Jersey–Robert Wood Johnson Medical School and a 20-year researcher in the field. "How many drugs can put people with cancer into complete remission? People with this condition used to die within a few years. Now they can be put on this drug and maintained on it for virtually the rest of their lives."

As an approved treatment for Kaposi's sarcoma, the AIDS-related cancer, interferon can reduce the size of tumors and slow their growth, although it doesn't eliminate them entirely.

Injected into genital warts, interferon does a much better job of preventing them from coming back than freezing, burning, or chemical peels. (However, it is also more expensive and time-consuming than the other therapies.)

The drug is also approved for chronic hepatitis C, where it is thought to work by stimulating resistance in the noninfected cells in the liver. It may also offer a successful nonsurgical alternative in the treatment of certain skin cancers. But it is not yet approved for the latter use by the Food and Drug Administration.

RALLYING THE DEFENSE

How does interferon work? Researchers have a long way to go to definitively answer this question. They do know that once interferon is injected into the body, it "activates virtually all the cells it reaches," says Dr. Pestka. Although its strategy differs from virus to virus, it changes these healthy cells in ways that frustrate the virus's attempts to reproduce itself. Interferon doesn't protect against all viruses, however, he says.

Even though interferon drugs are modeled on a protein the body makes itself, they do produce some side effects. The most typical ones are flulike symptoms: fever, chills, muscle aches, and stomach upset. Many people seem to develop a tolerance for these symptoms as treatment continues.

Exactly how interferon injections complement the interferon the body makes is not well understood. Do people who benefit from the drug have too little interferon in their bodies—or do they simply need more than normal to stop the progression of their disease? Researchers can't say for sure.

Perhaps as researchers learn more about the various jobs this family of proteins performs in the body, interferon drugs will prove to have many more uses. Dr. Pestka says he has not given up on it as a cancer combatant.

"While it is disappointing that we haven't learned to make interferon effective against the most common cancers, I'm encouraged by studies which show that the drug can produce small but real effects in people in the late stages of cancer," he says. (Because the drug is considered experimental for all cancers except hairy cell leukemia and Kaposi's sarcoma, it is only given to patients whose cancers have not responded to more proven treatments.)

These limited results "show something is working," Dr. Pestka says. "Whatever interferon is doing in these cases, it is doing it quite effectively. We just have to learn to use it better. I'd like to see it tried at earlier stages before the tumors are so advanced, and also in situations when patients have relapsed. In my opinion, we should also try interferon to eliminate the residual cancer cells left after the bulk of the tumors are removed by surgery, radiation, and chemotherapy."

The other intriguing possibility is that interferon may one day help wipe out the common cold. In preliminary studies at the University of Virginia Medical School, an interferon nasal spray proved effective against colds caused by the rhinovirus but not the influenza virus. The big drawback of the spray is that it caused painful nosebleeds in some of the people who used it.

"The pain it produced was probably worse than the misery of the cold," Dr. Pestka says. "I don't think many people would be willing to use the spray to prevent a cold under these circumstances. We need to find a better form of delivery."

interpersonal psychotherapy "No man is an island," said a famous English poet a long time ago. In keeping with this notion, interpersonal psychotherapy examines personal relationships and how they affect your state of mind.

Barely ten years in use, interpersonal psychotherapy (IPT) was initially developed by Gerald Klerman, M.D., a psychiatrist at Cornell Medical School, as a brief therapy for major depression. IPT differs from psychoanalysis and many other mind therapies in that you concentrate only on the present. The therapy is also short, usually lasting just 12 to 16 weeks.

A basic tenet of IPT is that while problems in your relations with other people may not always be the cause of your depression, your moods and the shape of your current relationships are intimately entwined, says Myrna M. Weissman, Ph.D., professor of epidemiology in psychiatry at Columbia University College of Physicians and Surgeons.

BLUES BUSTER

IPT was a star player in a big study on depression by the National Institute of Mental Health. Two hundred fifty depressed people were divided up and given one of four different treatments, IPT among them. After 16 weeks, IPT had a success rate equal to that of both cognitive therapy and drug therapy, two blues busters with long, impressive track records. For those who came into the study severely depressed, IPT and drug therapy worked; cognitive therapy didn't do as well.

The fact that not everyone can—or wants to—take drugs for depression makes IPT an exciting and growing development, says Stanley D. Imber, Ph.D., professor of psychiatry and psy-

chology at the University of Pittsburgh School of Medicine, one of the places where therapists are trained in IPT techniques.

What are these techniques? Your interpersonal therapy program might begin with a look at what changes in your relationships may have occurred around the time you started feeling down. "We'll explore things such as major losses, perhaps a death that you're still grieving over. We'll look particularly at role transitions, such as the loss of a job or a promotion (which can be as stressful as losing a job), or a relationship split-up," says Dr. Imber.

Together with your therapist, you'll decide which interpersonal issues you want to work on. In the course of your treatment, typically one session a week for no more than 20 weeks, "not all of your problems will be resolved, but you'll start to recognize which interpersonal issues are most affecting you, and how you are going to deal with them," says Dr. Imber.

SPOTTING PATTERNS

A very important part of the therapy is learning to recognize patterns in relationships. For instance, last week John mentioned that whenever he gets criticism from his supervisor he boils. The week before, he talked about how he can't stand it when his wife says anything critical. In such a case as this, "I might say something like, 'It seems interesting that the same kinds of things are happening at work and at home,'" says Dr. Imber. John may then begin to see he is a little too thin-skinned.

"IPT is not a coaching kind of therapy—you don't instruct the patient," says Dr. Imber. Rather, the therapist's role is to help clarify, to guide, and to push for greater exploration on the part of the patient, he says.

Where else, other than the treatment of depression, might IPT be useful? Small studies have so far pointed to IPT's usefulness in marriage counseling and the treatment of bulimia (the binge/purge disorder), says Dr. Weissman. And research is continuing to look at IPT's effectiveness for different kinds of depression, particularly among adolescents, the elderly, and some terminally ill patients. IPT has been shown to be *ineffective* as a treatment for drug abuse.

Where do you find an IPT practitioner? Because IPT is new and limited in what it can treat, few if any psychologists, psychiatrists, or social workers carry business cards that read "IPT practitioner"—although a growing number are familiar with the practice. To find someone, you may have to dig, says Dr. Imber. A good place to start would be your state psychological association or your local university, particularly if it has a medical school with a psychiatry department.

iodine   It's a bright, sunny day. Everyone in the neighborhood seems to be out bike riding. Before you know it someone is pedaling straight into your path. You brake and skid. You taste gritty gravel and feel the searing sting of a scraped knee—flashbacks to bike-riding wounds incurred as a kid.

Don't bother reaching for tincture of iodine, the familiar antiseptic wound dressing your mom used to clean your boo-boos. Experts now say that, compared with iodine, you'd probably be better off not using any wound dressing at all.

It's true that tincture of iodine is a strong germ fighter. But using it for skin wounds is the equivalent of dropping a bomb on enemy forces in occupied territory. It wipes out germs but also the innocent bystanders—the skin cells that regrow at the gap of your wound.

"Iodine has been in first-aid kits for years. But it's a step backward to use it," says Peter Lynch, M.D., professor and head of the Department of Dermatology at the University of Minnesota in Minneapolis. "Iodine simply doesn't work as well as antibiotic ointments for treating fresh wounds."

Studies show that iodine actually *slows* wound healing. In a study from the University of Pennsylvania, two different antibiotic ointments were tested against iodine and other traditional antiseptic treatments. In the interests of science, 47 volunteers submitted to six minor wounds (three on each arm), which were later infected with a mild strain of staphylococcus bacteria. One wound out of six was left untreated for comparison purposes.

The results: Each untreated wound healed by itself in an average of 13 days. Both the antibiotic ointments healed wounds in an average of 9 days. But the tincture of iodine preparation actually slowed healing time to 16 days.

"There is no longer any reason to use a tincture of iodine for any wound.

It's just too caustic," says Daniel Dire, M.D., director of the emergency medicine residency program at the Darnall Community Hospital in Fort Hood, Texas. The best way to treat a wound, he says, is to use a little soap and water and a bit of antibiotic ointment.

DISINFECTS WATER

If you really want to use iodine, take it with you on your outings to the backwoods. Iodine can help kill giardia and other parasites that often lurk in even the clearest mountain streams, rivers, and lakes. These microbes are responsible for gas, bloating, abdominal pain, diarrhea—and putting a definite kink in a camping trip.

If you can't disinfect water by boiling it, using iodine is the next best thing, according to experts. Three drops of tincture of iodine added to 1 quart of water kills bacteria and amoebae within 15 minutes. Frigid water should sit for at least ½ hour to 1 hour before drinking. You can buy iodine water disinfectant in tablets or crystals from camping supply stores.

ion generator   According to Longfellow's legend, a waterfall inspired Hiawatha to choose the cheerful nickname Minnehaha (laughing water) for his sweetheart.

It's no joke that cascading water, the pounding surf, the cool mountains, and other natural settings can make people feel positively cheerful and energized, some experts say. The air in these environs is brimming with negative ions, tiny charged air molecules that supposedly enter your lungs, boost your body chemistry, and give you a mental lift.

Unfortunately, many of us live and work in smoggy cities and tightly sealed, air-conditioned homes and offices with stale air and tons of electronic equipment. These settings are overloaded with *positive* ions that, theoretically, at least, should make us feel tired and prone to respiratory problems and other ailments.

Personal ion generators are supposed to change all that. These small appliances are designed to artificially provide air charged with negative ions, whether you are sitting at home, in the office, or in your car.

Environmental scientists have confirmed that ion generators do a good job of scrubbing the air clean of odors, aerosols, smoke, soot, and small dust particles. And, as one user puts it, the air ionizer "makes a New York City office smell as pristine as a park in the mountains of Vermont."

But whether these high-tech air fresheners do anything to improve your mood or health is a cloudy issue. The evidence showing a link between negative ions and positive effects on the body is unconvincing. And without good evidence, the Food and Drug Administration does not allow these negative ion generators to claim health benefits.

Despite the lack of official endorsement, many ion generator users swear that the devices do more than clean the air. A Denver father uses one to help control his son's asthma. A New York psychiatrist switches on his ion generator to help him sleep. And a

Tucson man uses his machine to reduce anxiety when the hot, dusty wind blows across the Arizona desert.

"Some of the Arizona Indians called this the winds of sickness," says Frank Gray, a retired lecturer in psychiatry at the University of Arizona Health Sciences Center who has been involved in research on the effects of negative ions and anxiety levels. "The hot wind kicks up positively charged sand particles, and you feel like staying in bed. But the generator makes me feel more energetic," he says.

Researchers around the world have long observed that people report more fatigue, irritablity, insomnia, asthma, and arthritis flare-ups when positive-charged, dry winds such as the Santa Ana in California, the Sirrocco in Italy, or the Sharav in Israel start blowing.

RESULTS UNCONFIRMED

In the 1960s and 1970s, the late Albert Krueger, M.D., biometeorologist and founder of the now-defunct Air Ion Research Laboratory at the University of California at Berkeley, conducted scientific investigations to shed some light on just how ions affect the body. Among Dr. Krueger's most important findings was that negative ion exposure seemed to increase the level of serotonin in humans. Serotonin is a brain hormone that plays a positive role in sleep, mood, pain control, and even breathing.

Over the years, other studies have suggested that a high concentration of negative ions could help relieve everything from headaches to hay fever.

Unfortunately, researchers have tried and failed to duplicate earlier results. In an exhaustive review of the existing data, Jonathan Charry, Ph.D., president of Environmental Research Information in New York City and past president of the American Institute of Medical Climatology, found that most of the studies were scientifically unacceptable.

"The best we can say about the data is that there probably are some minor effects of negative and positive ions," says Dr. Charry. "But the effects are subtle, difficult to prove, and likely to affect some people more readily than others."

"Don't expect the ion generators to solve your allergy or asthma problem," adds Harold Nelson, M.D., senior staff physician in the Department of Medicine at the National Jewish Center for Immunology and Respiratory Medicine in Denver. In a study conducted by the Fitzsimmons Army Medical Center outside Denver, asthmatics who sat in a room with a negative ion generator did not breathe easier or feel any better than when there was no ionizer in the room.

Another expert says that, until scientists show us otherwise, using an ion generator is about as "beneficial as sitting beside a fountain." Or maybe Hiawatha's waterfall.

iridology (ear-ih-DOLL-uh-jee) If a mechanic told you he could troubleshoot all of your automobile's woes simply by looking at the steering wheel, would you believe him?

Well, you should be just as wary of people who tell you that they can locate sites of disease within your body by studying the markings and texture of your eyes.

That's exactly what a small group of practitioners called iridologists claim they can do. They say that in some cases they have successfully spotted serious ailments simply by examining their clients' irises.

In the iridologist's world, the colored part of the eye, known as the iris, is divided into sections that correspond to various parts of the body. For example, an iridologist may tell you that an irregularity near the bottom of your left iris could mean you have kidney problems.

In the scientific world, that is considered to be nonsense.

"It's full of bull. It doesn't work," says James Lowell, Ph.D., vice-president of the National Council Against Health Fraud. "Iridology is outdated and flies in the face of science. These people are using antiquated ideas as if there have been no advances in science in the last 100 years."

In fact, Dr. Lowell feels some iridologists may be con artists. "It's identical to the old snake oil pitch except that iridologists have updated the lingo," Dr. Lowell says. "I like to call it biobabel. They've put together some technical-sounding terms that really don't mean anything."

There is only one degree-granting school—the Oriental Medical Institute in Honolulu, Hawaii—teaching iridology in the United States, says Don Bodeen, D.C., Ph.D., an iridologist in Poughkeepsie, New York. Most iridologists are informally trained by other iridologists, and the technique is not officially licensed as a profession in any state.

"Many practicing iridologists have little or no formal training in health care or health care–related fields," Dr. Lowell says.

Inspired by an Owl

Iridology was concocted by Ignatz von Peczely, a 19th-century Hungarian homeopathic physician who, as a child, helped nurse an owl with a broken leg back to health. While he was caring for the bird, Peczely noticed that it had a small spot in one of its eyes. It was probably just a coincidence, but as the owl's limb healed, the spot faded from its eye. Based on this observation, Peczely concluded that the spot had corresponded to the bird's broken leg. From there, he reasoned that all diseases could be diagnosed by looking at specific parts of the iris.

Iridologists still support Peczely's theory.

"The iris is a direct extension of the brain. It's actually brain tissue. It's the only part of the brain that we can see without doing surgery," Dr. Bodeen says. "The iris can mirror changes the brain receives from remote parts of the body. Therefore, by looking at the iris we can tell what is going on in other parts of the body."

But vision experts say that is a misconception. The iris isn't brain tissue—it's a membrane composed of circular muscle fiber—and there is no evidence that it interacts with the brain in the way that Dr. Bodeen and other iridologists claim.

It is true that symptoms of some diseases such as syphillis, diabetes, and atherosclerosis can be detected in the eyes. But those diseases are systemic, meaning they affect every part of the body, says Russell Worrall, O.D., an assistant clinical professor of optometry at the University of California at Berkeley. There is no evidence that diseases affecting specific body organs can be determined by examining the eyes, he says.

Dr. Bodeen agrees, to a certain extent. He says that iridologists can't diagnose specific diseases, but they can tell if a person is likely to have some type of problem with a particular body part.

But in dozens of studies of that purported ability, the overwhelming majority of researchers have concluded that iridologists might more accurately confirm the presence of health problems if they simply flipped a coin.

Ailments Overlooked

In Holland, for example, researchers asked five iridologists to examine photographs of the irises of 78 people and determine which of them had gall-bladder ailments. The iridologists were right only 56 percent of the time.

In another study conducted by Dr. Worrall, four iridologists were shown photos of the irises of University of California athletes taken before and after an injury. Mixed in with those images were photographs of the eyes of healthy athletes.

The iridologists were asked to simply determine if a bone was broken, and if so, indicate which side of the body it was on. They didn't even have to state which bone was broken.

To be fair, Dr. Worrall asked ten optometrists and two University of California art students to do the same thing. "We figured if there was an obvious change in the iris because of a broken bone, then even an untrained person would be able to spot it," he says.

So how did they do? Well, as you might suspect, the optometrists and art students didn't do well. But the iridologists didn't do any better.

The accuracy of both groups hovered around 50 percent, and the best iridologist was right only 52 percent of the time. "They might as well have been guessing," Dr. Worrall concludes.

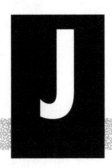

journal writing Confronting your thoughts and feelings and putting them into words, on paper, can help you feel unburdened and renewed. Perhaps you've experienced that feeling of catharsis after writing an angry letter complaining about poor service or shoddy merchandise. Or perhaps you wrote a love letter to someone you secretly admired, but never sent it.

Keeping a diary or personal journal is more than just a means of catharsis, though. It's also a valuable tool for self-understanding, according to psychologists. Journal writing helps you to explore your fears, worries, and concerns at your own pace in order to understand yourself and find a solution to problems. Better yet, writing enables you to open up about personal problems without baring your soul to others. In one study, people who wrote about their problems day after day gradually changed their perspectives. One woman who had been molested in her childhood, for example, went from embarrassment and guilt to anger and finally to acceptance.

A COPING TECHNIQUE

A researcher at Southern Methodist University has come up with what looks like concrete evidence that, when used as a way to cope with stress, journal writing may help you stay healthy. In his third large-scale study of journal writing, psychologist James W. Pennebaker, Ph.D., compared two groups of freshman students. One group spent 20 minutes a day writing about how they felt about the transition to college life. Common themes included isolation, loneliness, homesickness, worries about their studies or their future, problems with their girlfriends or boyfriends, and similar concerns. A second group kept a simple log of their daily activities—what they did when they woke up, where they went, their plans for the day—without mentioning their emotions, feelings, or opinions.

After four or five months, the students who kept a journal of their deepest feelings were rated healthier—they had visited the college health center less frequently than students who

309

simply logged in their day's activities. Also, blood samples showed that the journal writers benefited from an enhanced immune response.

Journal writing is a safe, convenient way to cope with upsetting experiences, concludes Dr. Pennebaker in his study, published in the *Journal of Personality and Social Psychology.* "Writing about traumas or other stressors has positive physical and long-term psychological benefits," he says. "Above all, writing may provide an alternative form of preventive therapy that can be valuable for individuals who otherwise would not enter therapy."

HERE'S HOW

If you decide to keep a journal, plan to spend about 20 minutes a day writing. Focus on anything that upsets or angers you, especially topics you don't discuss with others. (This may be painful at first. But remember, nobody will be reading this but you.) Feel free to write about either one traumatic event or several different topics. And don't worry about grammar, spelling, or sentence structure. The idea is to express your innermost thoughts and feelings, not to produce a literary masterpiece. Hopefully, you'll begin to see things in a new light. And who knows? You may even come down with fewer colds! *See also* **poetry therapy**

juniper You wouldn't think James Bond, after all these years, could keep up the pace. He fills his days with car chases, shoot-outs, and miscellaneous mayhem. Worse, he drinks altogether too many martinis—shaken *or* stirred.

Fortunately, there's *one* ingredient in all those martinis that might actually be doing him some good: juniper. The principal flavoring agent in gin, juniper traditionally was used as a diuretic and to treat problems of the kidneys and bladder. No wonder Mr. Bond takes an aisle seat.

The diuretic action stems from the volatile oil found in the juniper plant's berries—specifically, from the constituent in the oil called terpinen-4-ol—which increases the rate at which the kidneys filter fluids.

For many years, tea made from juniper berries was recommended to help ward off cystitis and other urinary tract infections. "I think juniper does contain urinary antiseptics, although bayberry and cranberry are more famous for that," says James A. Duke, Ph.D., a botanist and toxicol-

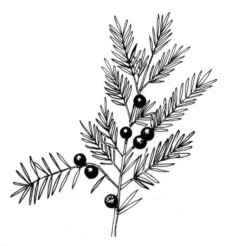

Juniper

ogy specialist with the U.S. Department of Agriculture in Beltsville, Maryland.

A survey of the herbal literature suggests juniper, while effective, may be too dangerous for unsupervised use. For one thing, it stimulates uterine contractions that would be hazardous for expectant mothers. And while juniper may work as a diuretic, it also stimulates the kidneys. That's bad news for someone who *already* has kidney problems.

According to the editors of *Herbal Medicine Past and Present,* it's unlikely juniper ever was widely used. And in today's world, they argue, using juniper as a healing agent is, in many instances, "hardly prudent in the light of the availability of less toxic products." And you can also forget taking your juniper in the style preferred by James Bond. The alcoholic bang of a martini probably outweighs any therapeutic value that may be contained in the juniper of its gin.

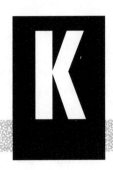

Kaopectate If diarrhea has beset you, Kaopectate "is a good choice for relief," says Samuel Klein, M.D., associate professor of gastroenterology at the University of Texas Medical Branch in Galveston.

"Kaopectate is an over-the-counter treatment for minor diarrhea," says a spokesman for The Upjohn Co., which markets the product.

The company first introduced Kaopectate in 1936. "Its origins go back to ancient times," he says. "The original active ingredient, a type of clay called kaolin, was used to stop diarrhea by the ancient Chinese and also by the Cherokee Indians when they inhabited what is now Georgia."

Kaolin — and the product's other original diarrhea-fighting ingredient, pectin — gave Kaopectate its famous name. But by 1984, the company gradually started to phase out kaolin and pectin, a process it completed in 1989.

The new active ingredient in Kaopectate liquid, caplets, and children's chewable tablets is attapulgite. "Attapulgite is a pharmaceutical grade of adsorbent clay — a natural mineral," the Upjohn spokesman says.

USE WITH CARE

Taken as directed at the first sign of diarrhea and after each bowel movement, Kaopectate works quickly and with very few adverse effects, according to the company spokesman. "Consumers observe some relief after the first dose. As an adsorbent, Kaopectate changes the consistency of the diarrheal stool, making it less liquid."

Because the product is an adsorbent, however, it should not be taken simultaneously with other drugs. It could conceivably adsorb other medications, rendering them ineffective.

Kaopectate is not for serious or severe cases of diarrhea. If the malady lingers on, people need to see a doctor to identify the cause.

But uncomplicated diarrhea can safely be treated with Kaopectate for about three days, says Dr. Klein. Because it treats the symptoms instead of the cause of diarrhea, he warns against taking the medication if there is colitis or other inflammatory disease in the intestines. People should also see a doctor if they have such severe diarrhea that they're losing lots of fluid, he says. Symptoms that demand medical treatment include light-headedness or dizziness.

Kaopectate isn't the only readily available remedy for simple diarrhea. Imodium A-D, a product whose active ingredient is loperamide, is a fast-acting, over-the-counter antidiarrheal medication, says Charles D. Ericsson, M.D., professor of medicine at the University of Texas Health Sciences Center in Houston. Pepto-Bismol (bismuth subsalicylate) is another. *See also* **bismuth; clay; Imodium**

Kegel exercises (KAY-gel) These exercises, which involve consciously tightening the pubococcygeus muscles stretching across the pelvic floor, can be completed in seconds without stress or sweat, providing relief for what can be embarrassing and uncomfortable physical problems.

Kegel exercises, developed in the late 1940s by gynecologist Arnold H. Kegel, may be used to relieve incontinence, interstitial cystitis (a painful bladder condition), and irritable bowel syndrome. They can also improve both men's and women's sexual response and are helpful during pregnancy, says Kristene E. Whitmore, M.D., chief of urology at Philadelphia's Graduate Hospital and clinical assistant professor of urology at the University of Pennsylvania. Some doctors also recommend them for a prolapsed uterus.

The two most common reasons for doing Kegel exercises are to control either stress incontinence (involuntary escape of urine during moments of stress) or urge incontinence (inability to hold back urine when feeling the urge to go to the bathroom), explains Dr. Whitmore, author of *Overcoming Bladder Disorders.*

You can develop an awareness of where the pubococcygeus muscles are by stopping the flow of urine when you go to the bathroom. This tightens the target muscles, which are actually sphincter muscles around the urethra, vagina, and anus. It's important to contract these muscles and not the abdominal muscles during Kegel exercises, Dr. Whitmore says.

"What I have my patients do is put one hand over the lower part of the abdomen so they can feel that that part is relaxed while they contract the pubococcygeus muscles," Dr. Whitmore explains. "Most people can learn to do it that way."

DAILY DRILLS

Dr. Whitmore says that you may begin the exercises with sets of five to ten contractions at a time, several times per day. After three or four weeks, you may increase the number of contractions in each set. It's best to start doing the exercises while lying down, but you may try sitting or even standing once you're comfortable with the technique, she says.

Kegel exercises vary for different types of incontinence. For stress incontinence hold the contractions for 3 to

10 seconds, with a short rest phase in between. "These are slow exercises and you do many repetitions per day," Dr. Whitmore says. For urge incontinence, you perform 10 to 15 quick contractions to learn to inhibit bladder contractions, she explains. You should see results in three to six weeks, she says, adding that Kegel exercises are effective in about 70 percent of urinary incontinence cases.

Dr. Whitmore says she prescribes a special drill for her patients with interstitial cystitis. "They do Kegel exercises when they feel the urge to go. They do 10 to 15 real quick and strong Kegel contractions and then they wait 15 minutes before they go to the bathroom," Dr. Whitmore explains. "People with irritable bowel syndrome can do the same thing in order to turn off the urge to go and to increase the interval in between bowel movements. It's very effective."

Kegel exercises also can increase the strength of orgasm for some women and can give some men firmer erections, stronger orgasms, and more control over premature ejaculation.

Pregnant women may benefit by doing Kegel exercises, especially during the last two months before delivery, to increase muscle tone and lessen muscle trauma. The exercises also may hasten recovery after delivery, Dr. Whitmore says.

kelp If you use a health food store like a supermarket, kelp may be as familiar to you as cornflakes. But the majority of Americans don't know that kelp is edible—or that it may have healing potential.

Kelp is a water plant, a form of algae—not that slimy stuff that floats on lakes in big green globs but a large, dark brown seaweed that grows in ocean waters.

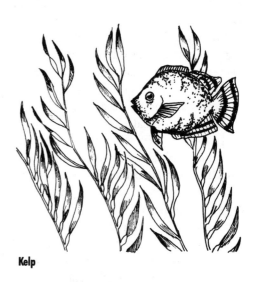
Kelp

Some people like it because of its taste. Kelp is used in Japanese dishes such as sushi, for example, and also made into tea and broth. And in powder form, it is used as an alternative to regular table salt because its sodium content is much lower.

RICH IN IODINE

Kelp's reputation as a healing food goes back to the days when it was used to help cure goiter, a disease characterized by an excessively large thyroid gland due to lack of iodine in the diet. Kelp is rich in iodine. Since the inception of iodized salt, however, most Americans get plenty of this mineral in their daily diet and don't need the additional iodine kelp provides.

Some people use kelp powder or tablets as a laxative, explains herbalist Varro E. Tyler, Ph.D., professor of pharmacognosy at Purdue University. Dr. Tyler says that a nondigestible substance in kelp creates the laxative effect.

Still others use kelp as a diet "pill," perhaps believing that the iodine in kelp will help speed up their metabolism and burn more calories. The problem is, this only works in people with a thyroid problem caused by iodine deficiency. And that's a somewhat rare condition.

But there are *real* theraputic uses for kelp.

Bandage manufacturers in Britain have taken the calcium alginate in kelp and spun it into a soft, extremely absorbent fiber that is used as a surgical dressing for wounds. In addition to increasing the speed of coagulation, the calcium alginate dressing is able to absorb up to 20 times its weight in fluids, explains microbiologist David Marshall, director of the University of Miami Wound Care Information Institute.

"This high absorbency means kelp can more quickly absorb fluids and excess pus from wounds," says Marshall.

The *British Journal of Plastic Surgery* reports that these alginate wound dressings, sold in U.S. medical supply stores under the brand names Kaltostat and Sorbsan, help manage chronic and bleeding wounds, including skin graft donor sites.

Another long-touted potential benefit of the alginates in kelp relates to the Nuclear Age. Sodium alginate is believed to decrease the body's absorption of radioactive strontium-90, linked to a variety of cancers. Animal studies have found that alginate supplements can reduce strontium-90's absorption rate by about 80 percent.

Back in the 1960s, kelp was first used as a protection against radiation poisoning due to fallout from nuclear testing. But since the nuclear test ban treaty, there's not as much scientific interest in nuclear poisoning from fallout.

L

lactase This enzyme produced in the intestine breaks down lactose (milk sugar) into two simple sugars, glucose and galactose, which the body can absorb.

"The purpose of the enzyme is to make milk sugar available to the body for use," says Theodore Bayless, M.D., a gastroenterologist and professor of medicine at Johns Hopkins School of Medicine.

Lactase becomes a concern, though, if you don't have enough of it. If you are lactase deficient (lactose intolerant), you get gas, bloating, cramps, and maybe diarrhea several hours after drinking milk because your intestine can't break down the milk sugar. The sugar then stays in the intestine and ferments in the colon, causing the uncomfortable feelings in your gut, Dr. Bayless explains.

It is believed that, with the exception of adults with northwestern European and Scandinavian backgrounds, most people's lactase levels start to fall after weaning. The lactose intolerance symptoms usually appear during the early teen years, Dr. Bayless says.

Certain groups are more susceptible to lactase deficiency because of heredity. Many American Indians and Orientals have deficient enzyme levels within a year or two of birth, and some blacks also lose the enzyme as they get older, Dr. Bayless says. Some Jews also have low lactase levels. A person may also become lactase deficient following a viral or parasitic infection, which temporarily knocks out the enzyme.

"If lactase levels are high, you can drink three or four glasses of milk without any symptoms," Dr. Bayless says. If lactase levels are low, you may have gas and bloating from drinking even one glass of milk.

ADD DROPS TO MILK

If you think milk is cramping your style, he offers a simple test: Skip milk for two or three days. Then test yourself with two glasses of skim milk on an empty stomach. If you still have symptoms with this self-administered test, see your doctor.

If you are lactase deficient, there are products you can buy at your supermarket or drugstore for help. There are lactase drops you may add to milk and lactase pills you can take with meals. There also are lactase-enhanced milks available, which already have 70 percent of the lactose broken down, Dr. Bayless explains. If you need more lactose breakdown, you may add drops to the milk, he says.

Is one form of the enzyme best?

The drops may be the top choice, Dr. Bayless explains, because you add them yourself, then let the milk sit overnight. "If you add enough drops, you could get 90 percent of the lactose broken down," he says.

Overall, how best to add lactase is up to you. But if you are deficient in the enzyme, you'll find the effort worth your time.

laser surgery   Imagine a beam of light so concentrated it produces power totaling *millions* of watts—many times the energy of the sun's surface. Imagine, too, the ultimate in precision, a beam of light that can be focused down to one ten-thousandth of a meter.

Science fiction? Nope—laser surgery.

Many doctors in all specialties are laying down their steel scalpels for scalpels of light that instantaneously cut, clean, and cauterize—all with incredible speed and efficiency.

Although Albert Einstein developed the concept of high-powered light some 75 years ago, it wasn't until the 1960s that doctors started using real lasers on real people. Now, more than one million laser surgeries are performed

in the United States every year, says Ellet Drake, M.D., secretary of the American Society for Laser Medicine and Surgery.

A laser puts its energy right where the doctor wants it, Dr. Drake says. The searing heat seals small blood vessels, so there's little bleeding. The heat reduces the risk of infection, too.

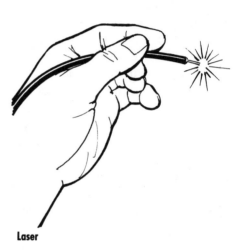

Laser

"Lasers have tremendous power, concentrated in one place," Dr. Drake explains. "It's like a woman who wears high heels on your tar roof—the heels go right through."

PRECISION EXCISION

Dermatologists use lasers to vaporize warts, remove birthmarks, and blast away tattoos. Because lasers may be adjusted to precise specifications—to cut no deeper than $\frac{1}{10}$ millimeter, for instance—doctors may remove a birthmark without touching underlying tissue. Lasers generally produce less scarring than conventional techniques, Dr. Drake says.

Lasers affect only the tissues they're aimed at. Highly reflective (or transparent) tissues scarcely are touched at all. "Lasers can be extremely precise," Dr. Drake says. "Neurosurgeons can vaporize certain kinds of tumors and do very little damage to the surrounding cells." If you have the vision-threatening condition called diabetic retinopathy, for example, your doctor may shoot laser light right *through* your cornea. Your eye won't be affected, but the tumor will be corrected.

Lasers are also being used for abdominal surgery—most recently, for gallbladder surgery, Dr. Drake says. With laser laparoscopy, your gallbladder may be removed through incisions much smaller than those used for conventional surgery. There's less pain and bleeding than with traditional surgery, and some people go home the same day.

Gynecologists use lasers to remove tumors, vaginal warts, and endometrial tissue. Some neurosurgeons are using lasers to excise herniated (slipped) disks, and oral surgeons use lasers for some types of soft-tissue surgery.

ARTERIES UNCLOGGED

Lasers even appear poised on the cutting edge of heart disease, Dr. Drake says. Since blocked coronary arteries lead to heart attacks, surgeons now are looking to lasers to "canalize" plaque-clogged vessels. Unlike balloon angioplasty, which merely compresses plaque against the arterial wall, lasers actually eliminate some types of plaque.

Laser angioplasty still is in its infancy, but doctors hope it someday will reduce the high rate of restenosis—that is, the return of arterial plaque that sometimes follows balloon angioplasty. In early trials, however, restenosis still is a problem with laser angioplasty.

Laser angioplasty also is limited to the peripheral arteries, except for approved trials. "There still is the danger of perforation," Dr. Drake says. "In the leg vessels, that isn't a big deal. In the heart vessels, it's a tremendously big deal."

Nearly everything a scalpel is used for, lasers also will do. Doctors are using lasers to remove ingrown toenails. And in vascular surgery, lasers have been used instead of sutures to weld together blood vessels.

Since lasers often do their work with less pain and trauma than conventional techniques, they're much in demand these days by doctors *and* patients. Of course, lasers can present complications as well. For example, what happens to a vaporized wart, or vaporized arterial plaque? All that smoke goes *somewhere.*

Doctors now are taking a hard look at laser hygiene, Dr. Drake says. "Are you going to scatter cancer cells all over the operating room? Are you going to scatter virus and bacteria all over? In the case of the blood vessels, what happens to this particulate matter [the small particles of plaque] that goes downstream?"

Thus far, laser debris isn't thought to present serious problems. Dr. Drake says surgical "vacuum cleaners" are used to trap smoke and prevent it from circulating.

Lasers also are expensive, costing anywhere from $50,000 to $150,000. To pay for that shiny, high-tech gadget, your doctor must perform a lot of procedures. As one saying goes: "When you have a new hammer, everything looks like a nail."

Laser surgery generally costs more than conventional surgery, but it probably saves money in the long run, Dr. Drake says. People spend less time in the hospital. They have less pain and discomfort. In most cases, they return to work sooner.

"There are procedures that are better done with the laser than with conventional methods," he says. "That's the only excuse for this technique to exist." *See also* **cauterization; endoscopy**

laughter   In a hospital rec room, the TV is tuned to a special humor channel where stroke patients watch videos ranging from Bob Hope to Bugs Bunny. In a cancer ward, therapists wheel "comedy carts" alongside pill carts and dole out cartoon books and silly toys. Patients in a postoperative unit are visited by a psychotherapist dressed as a clown and carrying balloons.

Is this some kind of joke? Yes and no. Today a growing number of health professionals—in and out of hospital settings—are dispensing laughter and humor to help patients cope with surgery, strokes, cancer, and other life-threatening conditions.

The reason is simple. Studies have begun to affirm that laughter could very well be the best medicine.

A hearty laugh causes huffing and puffing similar to aerobic exercise, according to William F. Fry, Jr., M.D., emeritus associate clinical professor in the Department of Psychiatry at Stanford Medical School in Palo Alto, California. It speeds up the heart rate, temporarily raises blood pressure, accelerates breathing, and increases oxygen consumption. That's not all. A good laugh also gives the muscles of the face, shoulders, diaphragm, and abdomen a vigorous workout. As laughter subsides, your heart rate slows, blood pressure drops, and tension drains from your muscles. You feel calm and refreshed all over.

IMMUNE BOOST

At this point no one can say for sure that a good chuckle will help you overcome illness. What scientists have found, however, is that experiencing positive emotion, whether it's a giggle, a grin, or a guffaw, can perk up the immune system.

In a study conducted by Kathleen Dillon, Ph.D., a psychologist at Western New England College, Springfield, Massachusetts, students who reported using humor as a coping device had higher levels of virus-fighting immunoglobin A than their more serious-minded counterparts.

Here's another intriguing finding. Dr. Fry and his colleague Lee S. Berk, director of clinical laboratories of Loma Linda University Medical Center in

California, measured blood samples of students who had viewed a humorous film. They discovered increased immune cell activity and decreased levels of blood cortisol, a hormone that has an immune-suppressing capability. The punch line: Laughter dramatically cut the effects of everyday stress on the immune system.

What many caregivers are particularly interested in, however, is laughter's ability to alleviate emotional pain and stress.

"Cancer can be debilitating and dispiriting, and we believe laughter could reverse these negative emotions," says Felix Scardino, a psychotherapist with the Stehlin Foundation for cancer research at St. Joseph's Hospital in Houston. Cancer patients are encouraged to visit a special area of the hospital dubbed The Living Room, which features games, toys, and movies on a large-screen TV. "Whether our humor program helps boost patients' immune system remains to be seen. Our primary aim is to boost their moods," says Scardino.

Other health-care experts are finding that humor creates a bonding between patient and staff that can help motivate healing. At Sunnyview Hospital in Schenectady, New York, a physical therapist dresses in army fatigues, calls himself a "physical terrorist," and assists stroke victims to walk. "When the patient laughs, it gets his mind off of his illness, it builds trust with the therapist, and the patient becomes more willing to participate in his treatment," says Connelly Todt, coordinator of the hospital's Humor Program, which also offers a humorous evening entertainment and a "first-aid kit" containing joke books, rubber noses, and windup toys. "We've found that while humor may not speed recovery, it can improve the quality of life for our patients."

Research findings concur. In a Swedish study a group of patients with painful musculoskeletal disorders and depressive moods participated in a humor group that used funny books and videos. After 13 weeks, the group had less symptoms, prompting the researchers to conclude "humor therapy can improve the quality of life for patients with chronic problems."

SELF-HELP HUMOR

Laughter can improve the quality of your life, even if you are not seriously ill. Annette Goodheart, Ph.D., a psychotherapist in Santa Barbara, California, suggests that laughter is part of nature's coping mechanism, just like crying. "Laughter can help you reframe a distressful event, and it can serve as an agent for change," says Dr. Goodheart. "We don't have to be happy to laugh. Indeed, we *become* happy because we laugh."

You don't have to be a Joan Rivers to experience the healing power of laughter. Start by opening yourself up to the possibility of humor. Learn to become a comic observer. Maddening or threatening situations lose their negative impact if you can manage to see them in a humorous light. For example, picture the cop who's writing you a ticket wearing a silly dress.

Or put together your own humor

kit. Collect funny videos, books, and cartoons. Keep a funny hat and goofy glasses to wear when you're having a crisis—then go look in the mirror. Try to be around people who make you laugh.

"The idea is to be aware of the things that make you laugh so you can increase your exposure to them," says Joel Goodman, Ed.D., director of the HUMOR Project.

If you would like a free information packet telling how to use laughter, play, and humor to help yourself or someone else, contact the HUMOR Project, Department R, 110 Spring Street, Saratoga Springs, NY 12866.

lavender Its stately purple stalks and silvery leaves make lavender the perfect visual complement to a flagstone walk. Its heady scent, though, is what people remember. Nothing else smells like French lavender, and perfumers around the world gladly pay top dollar for their share of the season's harvest.

The same essential oils that give lavender its distinct odor also have healing properties, says James A. Duke, Ph.D., botanist and toxicology specialist with the U.S. Department of Agriculture in Beltsville, Maryland. There may be effects on the brain as well. In the United States, lavender is frequently used in aromatherapy, a treatment that employs various scents to affect mood.

A member of the mint family, lavender contains a long list of biologically active compounds, some proven to kill bacteria and viruses, including the germs that cause typhoid, staph

infection, diphtheria, and strep throat. Roman soldiers carried it with them in their medical kits to use as a disinfectant, an application that carried over into the Middle Ages.

Even today in some parts of Europe, particularly France, lavender oil is dabbed on wounds as a disinfectant. "It seems to work particularly well for minor burns," says Judith Jackson, aromatherapist and author of *Scentual Touch.* "It has an immediate soothing effect." Lavender oil is also massaged into the skin for a variety of muscle and joint aches and pains.

Rubbed into the temples, lavender oil is said to help relieve headaches, perhaps because its scent helps people to relax or revive. Some aromatherapists claim the scent of lavender helps lift depression, although there are no convincing studies to confirm it has that effect.

AFFECTS NERVOUS SYSTEM

Lavender scent does have a long history of use as a pick-me-up. Proper Victorian women, prone to swoon from too-tight corsets, often carried lavender oil–scented handkerchiefs. "Lavender and other mints do contain compounds that are known central nervous system stimulants," says Dr. Duke. Inhaled, their odors stimulate olfactory nerves that alert the brain with a message: "Hey, check this out."

Used on the skin or inhaled, lavender is considered to be a safe herb. But, like any essential oil, lavender oil should not be used internally except in consultation with a doctor knowledgeable in its use, warns Dr. Duke.

Unfortunately, some of those same compounds that kill germs are poisonous if eaten in large amounts. *See also* **aromatherapy**

laxatives You know you've got trouble when you read Shakespeare in the bathroom—and finish two plays and a sonnet in one visit. You need a laxative, all right, but which kind? After all, there are bulk-forming laxatives and stimulant laxatives, saline laxatives and lubricating laxatives. And, doctors warn, not all are created equally safe.

Some laxatives, for example, simply work too well, and that's not necessarily good. Stimulant and saline laxatives may "cure" constipation with cramping and explosive diarrhea. What's more, some people get hooked on laxatives: The colon simply becomes sluggish without them.

The best laxative—and one you may use every day—is a natural one: a high-fiber diet. Dietary fiber acts like a sponge in your lower intestine, soaking up water and making stools larger, softer, and easier to pass. Of course, you have to drink a lot of extra water with your high-fiber diet. Otherwise, all that fiber could clog you up.

If you must reach for medication, a bulk-forming laxative such as Metamucil is your best bet, say doctors. These usually contain psyllium seed, a natural stimulant filled with fiber. Like all high-fiber foods, bulk-forming laxatives swell stools and get them moving. They don't have the nasty side effects of the chemical stimulants. Look for bulk-forming laxatives containing flaxseeds or psyllium seeds. All add bulk to stool. You can even buy these seeds in health food stores and grind them up yourself. Flaxseeds have a nutty flavor. You can even put them on soups and salads.

Stimulant and saline laxatives should be used sparingly, doctors warn. That goes for herbal stimulants as well. Senna, for example, is a very strong laxative that has to be treated with a lot of caution.

Lubricant laxatives like mineral oil help hard stools slip right out. However, mineral oil hinders the absorption of vitamins A, D, and E. It also can leak out and stain your clothes. *See also* **bran; castor oil; kelp; mineral oil; prunes; psyllium**

leeches In *The African Queen,* Humphrey Bogart spoke for many people when he reviled these segmented, blood-sucking, hermaphroditic worms. "If there's anything in the world I hate, it's leeches—the filthy little devils!" Bogey cried.

Indeed, there are many things about leeches—not least is their penchant for blood—that make people feel a little squeamish. However, plastic surgeon James W. Wade, M.D., says that unsuccessful operations make him feel a lot more squeamish than leeches do. And so he opts for leeches. By removing congested blood after some procedures, leeches can help improve blood flow, speeding the entire healing process.

During some operations—for example, when a severed finger is reattached—damaged veins are simply too small to repair, says Dr. Wade, a clinical assistant professor of plastic surgery at Louisiana State University Medical Center in New Orleans. That means blood may not circulate efficiently through the reattached part—precisely where it's needed most.

"If that congestion is not relieved, blood in the artery will clot, the transferred muscle or reattached finger will die, and the operation won't work," Dr. Wade explains.

Enter *Hirudo medicinalis,* the medicinal leech. Usually less than 1½ inches long, it quickly attaches to the wound and goes to work. Leeches do more than suck congested blood, Dr. Wade says. They also release a chemical called hirudin, which widens blood vessels and prevents blood from clotting. This ensures a drained wound *and* a full leech.

"In microsurgery, even a very small clot can block blood flow," Dr. Wade says. "The leech not only prevents new clots from forming, it even dissolves existing clots."

A leech may feed for as little as 5 minutes or as long as 4 hours. When it's sated, it simply drops off, Dr. Wade says, leaving a Y-shaped bite mark that looks like the hood ornament on a Mercedes-Benz.

Leech saliva, researchers have discovered, is packed with medically useful compounds. Along with anticoagulants, vasodilators, and clot dissolvers, leeches may even secrete an anesthetic, which allows them to bite

without being noticed. They may contain antibacterial agents, as well.

A MEDICAL COMEBACK

From antiquity nearly to the present, leeches were used for bloodletting—the elimination of supposedly harmful substances from the body. In fact, some people used leeches to reduce the swelling of a black eye.

Medically out of favor for nearly 100 years, leeches now are making a comeback, says Marie Bonazinga, president of Leeches U.S.A., which sells some 10,000 leeches a year to doctors and hospitals in the United States.

When Dr. Wade first started using leeches—he now uses about 12 a year—he worried that his fellow surgeons might not approve of this ancient practice. "Once they understood the nature of the treatment, it was very well received," he remembers. "Of

L

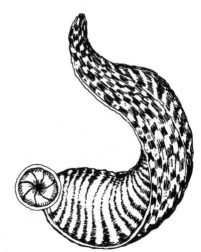

Leech

course, we also took some good-natured ribbing."

While leeches have come and gone on the medical stage several times, they soon may be taking their final bow, Dr. Wade says. As scientists isolate and synthesize the chemicals now found in leeches, there will be little medical use for the creatures themselves.

In the meantime, Bonazinga says, there is a special relationship that develops between patients and leeches. "People realize that if it weren't for the leech, they might be without whatever part of their body was being reattached," she says.

levodopa This drug, commonly called L-dopa, is used to treat the symptoms of Parkinson's disease as well as related movement disorders that may occur as a result of encephalitis or carbon monoxide poisoning.

Levodopa helps to relieve virtually all symptoms of Parkinson's, including tremors, muscle rigidity, and hesitancy to begin movements. (People with Parkinson's often can't begin moving until someone helps them.) But the drug does not stop the progress of the disease, and it may have side effects.

Parkinson's disease is caused by low levels of dopamine, a chemical neurotransmitter produced by certain brain cells that lets the brain process and send messages regarding muscles and movement.

L-dopa boosts brain levels of dopamine. It is a "metabolic precursor" of dopamine, which means that the body can convert it to dopamine.

Large dosages of L-dopa must be taken to have an impact on symptoms, and these large amounts often cause nausea and vomiting. That's why now, in most cases, an additional form of the compound, carbidopa, is prescribed. Carbidopa lets L-dopa cross into the brain at lower dosages. It reduces the amount of L-dopa people need to take to one-tenth to one-fourth the amount they would need if they were taking L-dopa alone.

L-dopa alone is available under the trade name Larodopa. The most widely used Parkinson's drug, Sinemet, is a combination of L-dopa and carbidopa.

When it was first used in the 1960s, L-dopa was considered something of a miracle drug. "In fact, it was the first drug prescribed for a neurological disorder that actually replaced a missing brain chemical," says Franz Hefti, Ph.D., professor of gerontology at the University of Southern California School of Medicine in Los Angeles. Except for a few antiseizure drugs, until L-dopa came along, treatment for neurological disorders had mostly been hit-or-miss.

BENEFITS WEAR OFF

There's no doubt that L-dopa can produce dramatic improvements. But it does have some possible side effects. Involuntary movements, nausea, confusion, and visual hallucinations have been noted in a small percentage of Parkinson's patients, says Thomas Hutton, M.D., director of the Parkinson's Disease Center at St. Mary's Hospital in Lubbock, Texas, and author of *Caring for the Parkinson's Patient.*

The trick for any doctor is to try

to balance the benefits of the drug with its side effects, providing the patient with the best possible quality of life, Dr. Hutton says.

Typically, L-dopa therapy is begun when muscular rigidity or slowness of movement starts to significantly impair everyday performance. Usually, once treatment is started, slowed or reduced movement, rigidity, and tremor are so improved that a person may almost be unaware of his symptoms. This "L-dopa honeymoon" usually lasts from two to five years, Dr. Hutton says. During that time, the person usually does not feel any wearing off of the medication.

But many Parkinson's patients eventually begin to experience the wearing-off phenomenon, or "end of dose" failure. When they awake first thing in the morning, their symptoms may be particularly prominent. Their symptoms may return prior to the next scheduled dose. They become aware of when a dose is "kicking in" and become acutely aware of the need to take the medication regularly. Doctors treat these symptoms by breaking the daily dose into smaller, more frequent doses or by giving a timed-release version of Sinemet.

They may also add other drugs. These days, there are several types of drugs that help to minimize the side effects of L-dopa or allow the dosage to be reduced. One drug, selegiline hydrocholoride (Eldepryl), is thought by some researchers to actually delay the death of brain cells involved in Parkinson's disease. (Preliminary research suggests vitamin E may do the same thing.)

People taking L-dopa are advised to "start low and go slow," says Marie Saint-Hilaire, M.D., director of the Parkinson's Day Program at University Hospital in Boston. It's important for your doctor to know exactly what symptoms you have and when during the day you have them, she says. Your dosage of L-dopa and other drugs can be customized, and it will probably need to be adjusted occasionally, too, she says.

Librium.   *See* **antianxiety drugs; tranquilizers**

licorice.   *See* **Chinese herbs**

light therapy   Imagine a single substance that can boost the disease-fighting power of your white blood cells, melt tumors, banish depression, and clear the scales of psoriasis. That substance is light. Medicine keeps finding new — and increasingly exciting — ways to use it to heal.

LOW-LIGHT DEPRESSION

One area where light has the potential to help many people is in the treatment of seasonal affective disorder (SAD), a form of wintertime depression that can become so severe it renders people incapable of working or maintaining relationships. This condition and its milder variant, the winter blues, affect 35 million Americans every year. (In Alaska, where levels of natural sunlight are unusually low for many months, SAD can set in as early as August.)

SAD is characterized by a tendency to sleep too much (as many as 14 hours a day), by cravings for carbohydrates or sweets, and by increased irritability. In the past, it's been treated with antidepressant drugs. These can take several weeks to bring relief, and they don't always work. Encouraging results are now being achieved in as little as two to four days with special light boxes, which supply the extra light SAD sufferers seem to be lacking. People sit in front of the lights for an hour or more each day. Morning and noon are considered the best times, says Karl Doghramji, M.D., director of the sleep disorders center at Jefferson Medical College in Philadelphia.

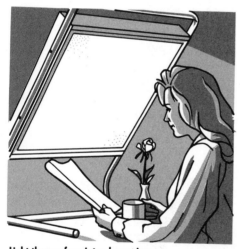

Light therapy for winter depression

In the future, visors equipped with two bright bulb lights may be available as a second option. Currently being tested for effectiveness, these are more portable, which could make them popular with people who travel. Since they deliver light more directly, they require only 30 minutes' use a day, says Charlotte Brown, coordinator of sea-

sonality studies at the National Institute of Mental Health.

How do these light supplements help? Researchers aren't sure, but theories abound. They do know that nerve impulses created by light waves reach the hypothalamus, a brain center responsible for controlling vital functions such as sleeping, eating, sex drive, and mood. SAD sufferers are thought to have some biochemical abnormality in the hypothalamus that becomes aggravated by lower levels of light. Whatever the exact problem, light therapy seems to compensate for it.

Just how bright the light needs to be to reverse SAD is still debatable. Boxes now on the market use a type of light measured in units called lux. "To be effective, a box has to generate at least 2,500 lux at a distance of 3 feet," Dr. Doghramji says, "but 4,000 lux is probably better." In his opinion, the best units offer full-spectrum light (which closely matches natural light) and a timer, which allows them to gradually increase in brightness. Many people set these to turn on just before they wake up.

PSORIASIS THERAPY

Ultraviolet light has proven to be a boon to sufferers of psoriasis, a chronic skin condition in which patches of cells multiply rapidly, creating raised, itchy areas called plaques. Patients treated with ultraviolet B light (or UVB) require a total of about 40 sessions, scheduled daily or several times a week, to clear their plaques. This form of ultraviolet radiation is thought to work by inhibiting the mechanisms the speeded-up cells use to reproduce themselves.

"I often treat patients who have extensive psoriasis with UVB," says John H. Epstein, M.D., a clinical professor of dermatology at the University of California at San Francisco. It's simpler than a related therapy called PUVA, which combines a light-sensitizing drug and ultraviolet A (UVA) radiation. (One disadvantage of ultraviolet B is that it requires more treatments per week than PUVA.)

The *P* in PUVA stands for a drug called psoralen, which makes the body more sensitive to ultraviolet A and in turn is activated by the light. A growing number of drug/light therapies work this way.

Patients take psoralen up to 2 hours before they're treated with light. Most take it by mouth, although some treatment clinics add it to bathwater, a plus for people who are nauseated by ingesting it. Either way, psoralen inserts itself into the DNA, the genetic material in the body's cells. Then ultraviolet A activates the psoralen, causing it to damage the DNA in a way that impairs the rapidly dividing skin cells' ability to proliferate.

PUVA can clear psoriasis in four to five weeks. Three treatments a week are considered standard at the beginning. Once the plaques clear, most people need two to three treatments a month to stay clear. Eczema and vitiligo, a skin disorder that marks its victims with smooth white spots, also respond to PUVA.

Like ultraviolet B treatments, PUVA can increase the risk of certain skin cancers. Studies show that men's genitals are particularly at risk if they're not protected during treatments.

AN OUT-OF-BODY EXPERIENCE

An emerging therapy called photopheresis also teams psoralen with ultraviolet light—but the action occurs *outside* the body. The treatment is currently approved for cutaneous T-cell lymphoma, a rare and usually deadly form of leukemia. "Some cases are being completely cured by it," says Peter Heald, M.D., assistant professor of dermatology and director of photopheresis at Yale New Haven Hospital. Trials are now under way to see how well photopheresis works against autoimmune diseases like rheumatoid arthritis and scleroderma, a progressive condition characterized by the buildup of fibrous tissue on the skin and internal organs. In autoimmune diseases, certain disease-fighting cells become traitorous and begin attacking the body.

Patients take psoralen 1 hour before they arrive at the treatment center. There, they spend 90 minutes hooked up to an intravenous line, which feeds blood into a centrifuge. The centrifuge separates the red from the white cells, taking about 10 percent of the white blood cells out of circulation. These are treated with ultraviolet light for another 90 minutes, Dr. Heald says. Then they are returned to the patient, now altered in a way that stimulates them to fight the "traitor" cells.

A different light-sensitizing drug, dihematoporphyrin, or DHE for short, is proving useful as part of an exciting—and still experimental—treatment for cancer. DHE is known to accumulate in cancer cells and become lethal when activated by light of a specific wavelength.

The combination of DHE and light has disintegrated tumors—in full or in part—in a matter of days, leaving most normal tissue intact, according to Thomas Dougherty, Ph.D., head of the Division of Radiation Biology at Roswell Park Memorial Institute in Buffalo, New York. Exactly how the treatment kills the tumor is not yet known.

The technique is being used experimentally against cancers of the lung, esophagus, and bladder, in studies designed to compare its effectiveness with that of standard treatments. It is also being tried against skin cancers, certain breast cancers, and recurring gynecological tumors. Studies show it can clear enough tumor mass, for example, to allow people with esophageal cancer to eat and people with advanced lung cancer to breathe better. Dr. Dougherty says studies show the DHE/light treatment particularly effective in controlling a lethal form of bladder cancer.

"By and large, DHE does not cause toxic side effects," Dr. Dougherty adds. But it does have one major drawback. Take it and you'll be sensitive enough to the sun for the next four to six weeks to get a sunburn very easily if you don't cover up or stay away from sunny windows. "The drug is activated by visible light. Sunscreens won't protect you," he says.

liposuction (LIP-o-suck-shun) Determined to lose weight, you give up your favorite foods, drink oceans of water, and sweat through months of aerobics. After all that work, you peek in the mirror for a glimpse of the new, svelte you.

Sigh! You lost weight all right, but those *bulges* in your thighs didn't shrink one bit.

You're not alone. Many people have fat deposits somewhere on their body that simply won't go away. A surgical procedure, called liposuction, lipoplasty, or suction-assisted lipectomy, may be able to quickly remove those deposits so they don't come back.

"We're genetically programmed with more fat in certain areas, and these *mis*programmed areas do not respond well to exercise and dieting," says Peter Bela Fodor, M.D., clinical instructor of reconstructive plastic surgery at Columbia University and president of the Lipoplasty Society of North America. "Liposuction is devoted primarily to treating those areas: under the chin, the back of the arms, the thighs, the abdomen, the waist."

Liposuction is by no means a substitute for dieting or exercise, Dr. Fodor emphasizes. Nor will liposuction work for someone who is seriously overweight. Doctors may remove, in one operation, a *maximum* of 4 to 8 pounds of fat, he says.

VACUUMS AWAY FAT

People first are given a local or general anesthetic, Dr. Fodor explains. The surgeon then makes a small incision—frequently less than ½ inch long. Into the incision goes a cannula, a blunt-tipped, hollow instrument that works like a vacuum cleaner wand. Fat particles are dislodged with the blunt tip, then sucked up by the wand.

Many procedures take less than an hour, although that depends on how many body areas are being worked on. Dr. Fodor says there's generally little discomfort after the operation. Some people report significant pain, but that's highly unusual.

You may not notice changes in your appearance until several weeks after the operation. Postsurgical swelling, called edema, puffs up the flesh where fat was removed. "In two or three weeks, you'll lose most of the swelling," Dr. Fodor says.

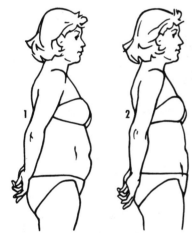

Before (1) and after (2) abdominal liposuction

According to statistics from the American Society of Plastic and Reconstructive Surgeons, liposuction is big business. In 1988, member doctors performed more than 100,000 lipectomies. By contrast, they performed only 71,720 breast augmentations, 68,880 collagen injections, and 48,480 facelifts.

Women most frequently undergo liposuction to remove "saddle bags"—fat deposits that cling to the outsides of the thighs. Men worry about their chin and "love handles." Liposuction also may be used to remove fat pads from male breasts, a condition called gynecomastia.

THINGS TO CONSIDER

It's important that people have realistic expectations about the outcome of the surgery, Dr. Fodor says. Most people would enjoy looking like a dancer, weight lifter, or model, but liposuction can only do so much.

"If you were to try to suction morbidly obese people who weigh 300, 400, or 500 pounds, then you see immediately that this procedure does not work for them," Dr. Fodor says.

"Also, if someone has a lot of irregularities in her skin and fatty tissue, and she says, 'I want you to remove the fat and make my skin look 20 years younger'—obviously, that's not possible," Dr. Fodor says. "The physician's job is to determine if the person is a good candidate for surgery—not just physically and anatomically, but emotionally."

Liposuction has been performed on people of all ages, but regardless of age, those with elastic, healthy skin will show the best results.

As with all types of surgery, liposuction isn't without risks. When properly carried out, however, it is the safest aesthetic surgical procedure performed today, Dr. Fodor says. It's also quite costly. People may expect to pay, on average, about $1,000 for each body part they have worked on, he says.

That's the doctor's fee; other expenses are extra. And since some body parts—such as knees, thighs, and buttocks—come *only* in pairs, the costs quickly multiply.

There is a hidden benefit of liposuction, though, according to Dr. Fodor. People who've undergone the procedure want to maintain their new looks. So after surgery, they tackle their diet and exercise programs with renewed vigor—and usually with success.

lithium It's been more than 40 years since lithium was first used in psychiatry, and today it's still the drug of choice for relieving symptoms of manic-depression—a terrifying mental roller coaster that hurls people from uncontrollable peaks of excitement to devastating troughs of despair.

Lithium doesn't cure manic-depression—clinically called bipolar disorder—but it does help level the alternating highs and lows as long as the patient continues to take it, says psychiatrist Carol North, M.D., assistant professor of psychiatry at Washington University in St. Louis. For many people lithium has relatively few side effects, and some people take it for their entire lives.

A MOOD NORMALIZER

"If you're manic, it will bring you down to baseline," Dr. North says. "If you're depressed, it should help bring you up to baseline. And if your mood is okay to begin with, it really shouldn't affect you."

Doctors agree lithium is most effec-tive at relieving the manic half of manic-depression, a condition thought to afflict some two million Americans. Manic behavior, described by one medical reference book as a "social emergency" because of the way it can disrupt a person's life, demands quick medical attention, Dr. North says.

Left untreated, people going through a manic stage become highly excited and may lose all control over their behavior. They quit sleeping, stop making sense. They lose touch with reality. Often, depression follows—and sometimes suicide.

"Mania often comes on very quickly, and it can get quite severe within hours or days," Dr. North says. "Some people in a manic state may think the president hired them for a special mission, or the FBI is following them—they get totally psychotic. People who've had more than one manic episode often are advised to go on lithium."

Doctors aren't sure how lithium works. Because the drug generally takes four to ten days before subduing manic-depressive symptoms, it's often combined with a tranquilizer in the early days of treatment. After a week, lithium alone is sometimes used, Dr. North says.

In therapeutic doses, lithium is considered quite safe, although in certain circumstances it may accumulate in the body. In that case, the gap between lithium *therapy* and lithium *toxicity* becomes quite narrow, Dr. North says. Close monitoring by the doctor is essential. (Lithium toxicity may cause diarrhea, vomiting, and other symptoms.)

It's also important to keep the water pitcher filled. "Lithium causes people to urinate a lot, so they have to keep replacing their fluids," Dr. North warns.

While lithium isn't thought to impair mental activity, some people complain it makes them less creative and less alert. Also, people with manic-depression often don't believe they're sick, Dr. North says. It's tough to convince them even to *try* lithium—and harder to convince them to keep taking it.

"They think they're just fine, they think they're okay, they think they've never been better," Dr. North says. "Then they quit taking their medication, and they get sick again."

lithotripsy (LITH-o-trip-see) This new noninvasive procedure uses shock waves to disintegrate kidney stones and—more recently—gallstones. The shock waves are created underwater and pass from a water bath or water-filled cushion into the body's soft tissue and to the stones themselves.

Several variations of lithotripsy exist. One method delivers the waves from outside the body. It's called extracorporeal shock wave lithotripsy (ESWL), and offers the advantage of no incision and minimal postoperative discomfort. Often it is performed on an outpatient basis, allowing you to return to your regular routine within 48 hours. In some cases, the procedure requires a hospital stay of a day or two.

A new shock wave machine called the Dornier HM 3 can deliver this treatment without the need for anesthesia. In this procedure, you're secured to a padded metal chair, which is lifted into a stainless steel tub of water. During the 30 to 45 minutes you remain in the water, you're bombarded with up to 2,000 separate electrode-generated waves. The pressure crumbles the kidney stone into sandlike particles, now small enough to be passed in the urine.

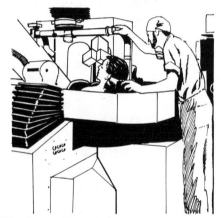

Lithotripsy machine and tub

The good news is that this technique may be safer than surgery or other forms of lithotripsy. In a review of 700 patients with urinary stones, postprocedural complications, requests for painkillers, and length of hospital stay were reduced for those treated with ESWL compared with other methods. In another study, 83 percent of 2,035 patients who had ESWL were stone free three months after having the procedure.

The procedure doesn't always work perfectly, however. In up to 15 percent of the cases, the stones don't disintegrate enough, so patients need to undergo the procedure a second time or try an entirely different procedure. Patients may experience colic for a few days afterward, or nausea, vomiting, and pain during the two to four weeks it will take to pass the stone fragments. Infections are another possible complication, although some doctors head this problem off by prescribing antibiotics before the procedure is done.

Doctors generally don't recommend this technique to people who have atherosclerosis, heart valve disease, or myocardial insufficiency.

Gallstone Buster

In percutaneous ultrasonic lithotripsy, a more invasive technique than the one described above, the shock wave approach is applied to gallstone destruction. Doctors insert a thin tube called an endoscope into the gallbladder. The tube has a wire probe attached. Doctors locate the gallstone, then send an electrical charge down the wire along with some salt solution to act as a conductor. The electrical spark is converted into a shock wave that breaks up the stone. The fragments are removed through the scope with tiny wire baskets.

Recovery time is much shorter than for traditional surgery, which removes the gallbladder altogether; three to four days versus three to six weeks, says Desmond Birkett, M.D., chief of the Section of Surgical Gastroenterology at University Hopsital, Boston University School of Medicine. And it's less risky than major surgery, an important consideration for people with other problems such as heart disease.

The drawback: The procedure is only effective for people with moderate-size stones that have not calcified. And, because the gallbladder isn't removed, stones can recur (about a 10 percent chance per year). Still, many people may be willing to take that chance.

Lovastatin. *See* **cholesterol-lowering drugs**

low-fat diet "Reducing dietary fat isn't just a health tool, it's an entire health tool chest," says Bryant Stamford, Ph.D., director of the Health Promotion and Wellness Center at the University of Louisville. "By reducing dietary fat, most people could reduce their risks of virtually every major degenerative disease suffered in this country today."

That may sound like a pretty fat promise, but the evidence doesn't lie. Reducing dietary fat—and saturated fat, especially—has been shown to reduce risks not just of our number one killer, heart disease, but also of strokes, high blood pressure, diabetes, gallstones, and cancers of the colon, prostate, and breast. Add the unparalleled weight-loss benefits of cutting back on fat and you can see why many health experts believe that next to quitting smoking, reducing dietary fat is the single most important health effort most people could make.

Where's the proof? In some very convincing pudding.

Research shows that reducing dietary fat encourages the liver to decrease its production of cholesterol—

especially LDL cholesterol, the bad kind that can lead to heart disease and strokes by sticking to artery walls. There's also evidence that reducing dietary fat may help the body resist cancer, possibly by giving the immune system a boost. This was demonstrated in one study that found an increase in the activity of cancer-killing cells when dietary fat was reduced.

Factor in equally exciting evidence from hundreds of other diet and disease studies from around the world, and it becomes clear why so many doctors are now recommending the low-fat route as such an advisable path to higher health. "The human body simply wasn't designed to handle the 90 grams a day of fat that most Americans now eat," Dr. Stamford says. "That's an increase of approximately sixfold over what anthropologists estimate our intake was for the hundreds of thousands of years our digestive systems were evolving."

How Low to Go

So what is an optimal amount of fat to consume?

Many experts feel the less, the better. A scant 14 grams a day (approximately 7 percent of total calories on a 1,800-calorie-a-day regimen) would be enough to satisfy the body's basic needs, says Dean Ornish, M.D., an assistant clinical professor of medicine at the University of California, San Francisco, School of Medicine and author of *Dr. Dean Ornish's Program for Reversing Heart Disease*. Dr. Ornish doesn't recommend that amount, because it's a level most people would simply find too

difficult to stick to, but he is calling for a percent-of-calories-from-fat ceiling of about 20 percent—a good ten points lower than the 30 percent figure recommended by the American Heart Association.

Thirty percent is certainly better than the current American average of about 40 percent, Dr. Ornish says, but research indicates that deposits on artery walls still can continue to accumulate in some people even after fat is reduced to the 30 percent level. Such accumulation seems to stop when fat is reduced to 20 percent, however, and at a level of 10 percent, the accumulation can actually begin to disappear. How low you go, therefore, should depend on how much heart disease protection you want—and how readily your cholesterol level responds to dietary changes.

How It's Done

What would these diets actually look like on your plate? Dr. Stamford says that most people could achieve a 30-percent-fat diet simply by cutting back on the obvious no-no's—fatty cuts of beef and pork, foods that have been deep-fried, butter and margarine, salad dressing, ice cream, cheese, and eggs. These foods tend to derive 50 percent or more of their calories from fat, so they should be enjoyed sparingly at best. As for the specific arithmetic of a 30-percent-fat diet, it should include no more than about 66 grams of fat a day based on an average caloric intake in the 2,000 calorie range.

A 20-percent-fat diet becomes a bit more difficult but is still achievable without major dietary overhaul, Dr.

Stamford says. Grams of fat a day need to be cut to approximately 44 based on a 2,000 calorie intake, a goal best accomplished by switching from animal foods to plant foods for the majority of calories consumed. That means more potatoes, pasta, beans, rice, vegetables, cereals, fruits, and bread. Animal products should be restricted to the leanest cuts of beef and pork, poultry with skin removed, low-fat or nonfat dairy products, egg whites, and fish.

As for lowering fat intake to 10 percent of calories—and fat grams to a scant 20 a day, based on a 2,000 calorie intake—both Dr. Stamford and Dr. Ornish say you would have to eat plant foods almost exclusively. The only exceptions might be nonfat milk, nonfat yogurt, and egg whites. All oils must be excluded, as well as high-fat plant foods such as avocados, seeds, and nuts. Most people find it best to work into this sort of strict, low-fat diet gradually, but once they do, changes in their blood chemistry and even in their arteries can be remarkable. Some of Dr. Ornish's patients have experienced drops in cholesterol of over 400 points. And arterial blockages have regressed to the point that blood flow increased by as much as 270 percent.

WEIGHT-LOSS BENEFITS

Heart health aside, weight control may be the most compelling reason to go on a low-fat diet. People who trim fat from their diet frequently find that they also trim pounds, even though the number of calories they consume may remain the same. This is because fat's calories are actually more fattening than the calories in carbohydrates or protein. Dietary fat is very similar to body fat even before the process of digestion begins, so very little digestive "energy" is needed to make the conversion from dietary fat to body fat. Only about 3 calories of energy is needed for every 100 calories of fat consumed. Compare this to the 23 calories of energy required to convert 100 calories of carbohydrate to body fat and you can see why dietary fat really does tend to "stick to the ribs," after all. Worse yet, studies with animals suggest that weight gain from excess dietary fat tends to occur more in the area of the abdomen than elsewhere on the body. That's bad not just for cosmetic reasons but for health reasons as well. Some studies suggest that people who carry their excess weight in the stomach area may be at the greatest risk of developing cardiovascular disease.

And last but not least—weight-loss maintenance. A study reported in the *Supplement to the Journal of the American Dietetic Association* found that people who lost weight by reducing dietary fat gained much less of it back 9 to 12 months later than people who had lost weight by cutting calories. On average, people in the low-calorie group gained over half of their weight back, while people in the low-fat group gained back only about 25 percent. Weight loss was achieved in the low-fat group by cutting fat intake to approximately 30 grams a day. *See also* **vegetarian diet**

low-sodium diet Imagine 1 teaspoon of salt. Sprinkle it into your hand, the fine grains white against your palm. That's it.

That's all the sodium you can eat if you're on a typical low-sodium diet. You're holding roughly 2,000 milligrams of sodium, your daily allotment.

Some low-sodium diets can run even lower, allowing only 500 to 1,000 milligrams of sodium daily, says Kim Galeaz Gioe, a registered dietitian and spokesperson for the American Dietetic Association. Your doctor will fill you in on the sodium plan that might be best for you. Get ready for what may be a sizable sodium cut, though, because the average American consumes anywhere from 4,000 to 10,000 milligrams of sodium per day, Gioe says.

Even people without high blood pressure, heart disease, or kidney problems (the leading problems requiring low-sodium intakes) should take in no more than 3,000 milligrams daily, the American Heart Association recommends. And that's still considerably more than the body actually *needs*— about 180 milligrams of sodium per day, says Alicia Moag-Stahlberg, a registered dietitian and research nutritionist at Northwestern University Medical School in Chicago.

How can a low-sodium diet help control high blood pressure?

"Hypertension [high blood pressure] is such a complicated disease that no one knows the exact mechanism," Moag-Stahlberg says. "But simply put, when people consume a lot of sodium, it acts like a sponge, causing the body to retain fluids. That makes the heart pump harder, raising blood pressure."

While cutting back on sodium is

prudent for everyone, not all people with hypertension who do so will see a corresponding drop in blood pressure, researchers have found.

"The problem is that a low-sodium diet does work for some hypertensives, even for some normotensives [people with normal blood pressure], but not for everyone," says Judy Z. Miller, Ph.D., an associate professor of medicine and medical genetics at Indiana University's Hypertension Research Center in Indianapolis.

The challenge doctors struggle with is finding out who is sodium sensitive, who will respond to a salt cut. "That's not been an easy thing to tack down, though there's been a lot of work in the area," Dr. Miller explains.

Most doctors ask their high blood pressure patients to follow a low-sodium diet and see if their blood pressure drops. "The low-sodium diet is the standard first line of treatment for blood pressure problems," Dr. Miller says. Medication may also be needed, she adds, especially if there is no response to the salt cutback.

If you've been told to follow a low-sodium diet, you're not alone. High blood pressure occurs in more than 20 percent of adults aged 25 to 74, affecting about 60 million American adults.

"It may be a big change for some people who are used to eating a lot of high-salt foods and to salting their food at the table before they even taste it," Gioe says.

Ways to Halt Salt

What does it take to cut back successfully?

Cutting back on visible salt from the shaker isn't enough. Many foods—including items you wouldn't normally think of as being salty, such as salad dressing and catsup—are significant sources of "hidden" salt. Most nutritionists agree that reading labels is a key. "A lot of the foods that people select for convenience are high in sodium and high in fat," Gioe says.

"An easy way to remember is, if a food is packaged in any way, there has probably been sodium added to it," Moag-Stahlberg explains. "Seventy-five percent of the sodium in our diet is added to food during processing and manufacturing."

Both nutritionists agree you should select fresh foods first, then frozen, while avoiding regular canned foods and selecting low-sodium canned foods instead. In the snack department, replacing salty chips or pretzels with fruit saves not only sodium but fat and calories as well.

When you cook, reach for garlic, onion, celery powder, and other herbs and spices instead of salt. Don't add salt when cooking noodles, rice, and hot cereals. Watch out for condiments such as soy and steak sauces, Worcestershire sauce, mustard, and salad dressings, which are hidden sodium sources. Check ingredient lists for sodium word combinations such as monosodium glutamate and sodium benzoate, as these all count in your daily sodium tally. Try to purchase low-salt products whenever possible, but be sure you understand what you're getting.

"The nitrates and nitrites in luncheon meats are sodium compounds," Dr. Miller explains. "So it's almost impossible to get a low-sodium bacon. They label it 'less salt.' They took the salt out. But they didn't take the sodium out. It's still a very-high-sodium product."

Any product with 140 milligrams of salt or less per serving is considered "low-sodium," Gioe says. Check for that first. With frozen entrees, which tend to be high in salt, she recommends going no higher than 800 or 900 milligrams per serving and only eating them occasionally.

A formula offered by Moag-Stahlberg may aid you in planning: Divide the total milligrams of sodium you're allowed to eat daily by the number of meals you'll eat in a day. That gives you an idea of how much sodium you can eat at each meal. (For an example of how basic food choices can affect sodium intake, look at the sodium content of the two sample meals in the table on the opposite page, with figures supplied by the American Heart Association.)

These food choice changes are important to make and take to heart. Simply shoving aside the salt shaker and reaching for salt substitute is not the answer, Dr. Miller says. In fact, many doctors discourage the use of salt substitutes because they may contain potassium chloride, which may be harmful.

If diet changes aren't enough, there are other sources of sodium you should know about, including water softening systems and plain drinking water. Look for water softeners that don't use

SODIUM COMPARISON

Your food choices *can* make an impact. The two sample meals below are poles apart in terms of their sodium content.

Food	Portion	Sodium (mg)
HIGH-SODIUM MEAL		
Salted peanuts	3 oz.	418
Baked ham	4 oz.	1,027
Green peas, canned	½ cup	294
Scalloped potatoes	½ cup	430
Baking powder biscuit	1	272
Margarine	2 tsp.	92
Spinach salad	1 cup	39
French dressing	2 Tbsp.	438
Instant pudding	½ cup	161
Skim milk	8 oz.	126
Total		**3,297***
LOW-SODIUM MEAL		
Unsalted peanuts	3 oz.	15
Broiled halibut	4 oz.	152
Broccoli	½ cup	28
Boiled potatoes	2	4
Italian bread	2 slices	118
Margarine	3 tsp.	138
Lettuce salad	1 cup	trace
Oil	4 tsp.	trace
Vinegar (cider or distilled)	2 tsp.	trace
Sherbet	½ cup	5
Coffee	6 oz.	2
Total		**462**

SOURCE: Reproduced with permission from *Salt, Sodium, and Blood Pressure,* copyright © 1986 by American Heart Association.
*Sodium content is calculated without added table salt. Adding 1 teaspoon of table salt would increase sodium approximately 2,000 mg.
Sodium content is calculated without added salt at table or in cooking.

the sodium exchange system, Moag-Stahlberg advises. And if you're limited to 1,000 milligrams of sodium a day, have your tap water checked. If there are more than 24 milligrams of sodium per liter, consider buying bottled water, she says.

Once you've committed to the low-sodium way of eating and drinking, make it stick. The bright spot is that by following a low-sodium diet, you may not have to take as much blood pressure medication. "We've shown that a lot of people can get away with taking less medication if they comply with the low-sodium diet," Dr. Miller says. "And that's the goal." *See also* **antihypertensives**

lozenges When you have a sore throat, letting a medicated lozenge dissolve in your mouth is like having a fireman and anesthetist on hand: It douses and dulls the pain at the same time.

For starters, the sugar (or sugar substitute) stimulates saliva flow that gushes over your fiery membranes and coats your throat with a soothing, liquid blanket. You no longer feel as if you're guzzling ground-up gravel each time you swallow.

Next, as the lozenge slowly dissolves on the back of your tongue, the local anesthetic (usually benzocaine, hexylresorcinol, or dyclonine hydrochloride) is gradually released directly on irritated tissues. This numbs the nerve endings and deadens the pain.

Menthol, another anesthetic often found in throat lozenges, is a fooler. It does seem to freeze out the pain. Ironically, though, menthol produces this cooling sensation because of its counterirritant effect on the nerve endings, says Branton Lachman, Pharm.D., clinical assistant professor at the University of Southern California School of Pharmacy in Los Angeles. "The nerve endings become supersensitive to air and you experience this sensitivity as coolness," he says.

To get pain relief without clobbering your throat tissues, you may be better off choosing a sugar-free, fruit-flavored throat lozenge, says Dr. Lachman.

FOR MAXIMUM RELIEF

You can make a lozenge super-soothing if you first gargle with salt-water. The salt helps cut through excess mucus in the throat, which is a major source of irritation, says Dr. Lachman. Once you remove the mucus, you have a clear path so the anesthetic from the lozenge can flow directly onto the mucous membrane and do its job deadening the pain.

Don't chew your lozenge. Let it sit on the back of your tongue and slowly dissolve. "The longer the ingredients are in contact with throat membranes, the greater the relief," says Dr. Lachman.

The labels on the longer-lasting, maximum-strength lozenges may recommend that you wait 2 hours before you take the next one. That's so you won't swallow too much of the medicine and overdose on the disks—it's not because the effect lasts that long.

"Most medicated lozenges' effects last about 15 minutes after they have completely dissolved," says Dr. Lachman.

To douse your pain between lozenges, candy is dandy. Lemon and other sour flavors seem to be especially helpful in stimulating the flow of saliva, says Thomas Gossel, Ph.D., chairman of the Department of Clinical Pharmacy at Ohio Northern University in Ada. "Plain, hard candy adequately coats the rough area of your throat and may be all you need for temporary pain relief," says Dr. Gossel.

ZINC FOR COLDS?

You may suck on an ordinary lozenge to soothe a scratchy throat. But how about dissolving a special kind of lozenge—a zinc lozenge—to ward off a bad cold? Evidence from a study at the University of Texas at Austin suggests that you shouldn't sneeze at that idea.

Researchers there found that, after the end of a 7-day trial, 86 percent of cold sufferers who were given zinc gluconate lozenges had no remaining cold symptoms, compared with only 46 percent of the people who had been given a placebo (an inactive substance). The zinc group's colds averaged just 3.9 days, while the placebo-treated group reported colds averaging 10.8 days—a difference of 7 days.

And in a British study, researchers found that dissolving a zinc gluconate tablet (containing 23 milligrams of zinc) every 2 hours reduced cold symptoms by a third.

Other studies do not show such a favorable zinc link to the common cold. Researchers at the University of Penn-

sylvania School of Medicine, for example, found that zinc lozenges did not reduce the duration of cold symptoms. In fact, half the participants in their study suffered side effects such as nausea and altered taste. The previous favorable findings, these researchers theorize, may have more to do with zinc's horrible taste than with its ability to stop the virus.

The zinc supporters, on the other hand, say that zinc zaps colds because it keeps the virus from multiplying. "If you use zinc gluconate at the first sign of a runny nose, by the end of the second day, your cold will be gone," says William Halcomb, M.D., a coresearcher of the Texas study who is currently in private practice in Mesa, Arizona.

Dr. Halcomb recommends that his patients dissolve (not chew) 23 milligrams of zinc every 2 hours on the first day, and half that amount every 4 hours on the second day. "I rarely see cold sufferers because they know to use zinc," says Dr. Halcomb.

Check with your doctor before *you* try zinc. If you get his consent, you can find zinc gluconate lozenges at health food stores.

But keep in mind this warning from the British researchers: Large intakes of zinc may inhibit your immune system. And never use the tablets for more than two days without your doctor's advice, says Dr. Lachman.

By the way, that's good advice for taking *any* medicated lozenge. If your sore throat persists beyond two days, see your doctor. *See also* **sore throat remedies**

lumpectomy   Since 1960, the incidence of breast cancer in the United States has increased 45 percent. One out of every ten American women will be afflicted by it. But those cold, bleak numbers hide signs of hope. Yes, breast cancer has become increasingly common, but thanks to new diagnostic techniques, tumors are being detected earlier. Because of that, women not only are more likely to survive the disease, they also have more surgical options that allow them to retain their breast while the tumor is eradicated.

One of the most promising of those breast-conserving surgeries is the lumpectomy, a procedure that removes the tumor, some surrounding tissue, and the lymph nodes under the arm. It is almost always followed by daily radiation therapy lasting more than a month. But the breast is saved, and studies indicate that the long-term survival rate is similar to that for a breast-removing mastectomy.

In a study of more than 1,800 women who had lumpectomies or mastectomies, researchers found that when the cancer hadn't spread to the lymph nodes, 77 percent of the lumpectomy patients were still alive eight years after surgery, compared with 79 percent of mastectomy patients. Women who had lumpectomies and radiation therapy did even better. Nearly 83 percent of those women were still alive at the conclusion of the study.

"In selected patients whose breasts are the right size and whose tumors have the right characteristics, there is no reason not to offer breast-conserving surgery because there is absolutely no difference [when compared with mastectomy patients] in their chances of being cured," says Ralph Broadwater, M.D., an assistant professor of surgery at the University of Arkansas College of Medicine in Little Rock.

"Today, with early-stage disease, no patient need leave the operating room without a breast," asserts Michael P. Osborne, M.D., head of the Breast Cancer Research Laboratory at the Memorial Sloan-Kettering Cancer Center in New York City. In fact, researchers estimate that nearly two-thirds of women who develop breast cancer are good candidates for lumpectomy.

FACTORS TO CONSIDER

Women who choose to have the procedure can look forward to shorter hospital stays—a lumpectomy can be done as an outpatient procedure, while a mastectomy often requires up to a five-day hospitalization.

Unfortunately, while the radiation following a lumpectomy helps prevent recurrence of the cancer, it also is a drawback for some patients, says Richard Perry, M.D., a Phoenix, Arizona, surgeon. Many patients, particularly elderly women who live in rural areas, opt to have mastectomies because they would have difficulty traveling to hospitals for the daily radiation treatments. Others simply fear radiation or cancer more than they do losing their breast, Dr. Broadwater adds.

Of course, some patients aren't good candidates for a lumpectomy. Women who have tumors larger than 2 to 2½ inches in diameter, have a large tumor in a small breast, or have an intraductal tumor (a tumor that is limited to a breast duct without invasion of surrounding tissue) probably should consider other surgeries and treatments, Dr. Perry says.

But for the vast majority of the 95,000 women who are diagnosed each year with early-stage breast cancer, lumpectomy is just as good an option as mastectomy. Often, that choice simply is a matter of which procedure is most appealing to the patient's psyche.

ATTITUDE ASSESSMENT

Researchers are still sorting out evidence about that. In a University of Pensylvania study, women who had lumpectomies had a more positive attitude toward their recovery. About 87 percent of them felt "cured," while only 36 percent of the mastectomy patients felt that they were free of cancer.

But in other studies, researchers found it more difficult to assess if a lumpectomy was more psychologically satisfying than a mastectomy. For example, in a study of 235 breast cancer patients in Quebec City, Canada, researchers found that women who had lumpectomies were more likely to have high levels of anxiety three months after surgery than women who had mastectomies. That study, however, also concluded that lumpectomies apparently helped women under age 40 cope with their disease better.

Out on the front lines of the cancer battle, surgeons say studies like these are of limited value. In reality, it just depends on the individual.

"I think you can say that women who have breast-conserving surgery are happy with their results and they have a good self-image. On the other hand, you can't say that women who have mastectomies all have problems with their body image," Dr. Broadwater says. *See also* **mastectomy**

lysine   Many medical experts are paying more than lip service to lysine when they praise it as a treatment for the prevention and alleviation of canker sores. In fact, this amino acid—which occurs naturally in foods but is used therapeutically in the form of concentrated supplements—may have been the nicest thing to happen to a pair of lips since the invention of the kiss.

Treatment with lysine results in rapid recovery and decreased recurrence not only of canker sores but also of shingles and genital herpes as well, says Richard S. Griffith, M.D., professor emeritus at the Indiana University School of Medicine in Indianapolis. All three conditions are caused by a herpes-type virus.

Amino acids are the building blocks of protein. Although there are 21 amino acids in all, lysine is one of 10 deemed "essential" because it has to be taken in through diet; the body can't manufacture it.

Lysine treatment of canker sores and genital herpes works best in conjunction with abstinence from another amino acid called arginine, according to Dr. Griffith. Arginine—found in chocolate, nuts, and seeds—is actually a growth stimulant for the herpes virus. Lysine works by blocking the virus's ability to absorb arginine.

SYMPTOMS REDUCED

In a study conducted by Dr. Griffith and others, 27 people given lysine tablets reported slightly fewer herpes outbreaks, as well as "significantly diminished" symptoms and much faster healing time. During the study, subjects were also instructed to avoid those foods known to contain large amounts of arginine, because previous studies had shown that arginine restriction may reduce herpes occurrence.

"Lysine may not be effective without strict arginine restriction," emphasizes Barbara North, M.D., a Laguna Niguel, California, physician. You may be able to take 1 to 3 grams daily of a lysine supplement and successfully put a lip lock on cold sores if—and this is a mighty big if—you are careful to avoid all arginine-rich foods, she says.

Significantly, experiments conducted by Dr. North showed that eating arginine-rich peanut butter is a bad move for people with a history of herpes infections. Eating 2 to 3 tablespoons of peanut butter was shown to raise arginine levels in the bloodstream, which could help stimulate a new outbreak of oral or genital sores, she says.

Unfortunately, lysine hasn't been taken as seriously as it should by the medical community for two basic reasons, according to Dr. Griffith.

First, the earliest lysine studies were not as rigidly conducted as they might have been, causing some doctors to dismiss the results as anecdotal. Second, because lysine is a relatively inexpensive product found in most health food stores and drugstores, the substance did not get the media attention and research funding that the synthetically derived antiherpes drug acyclovir got, he says.

"We compared our early studies with studies done with acyclovir, and lysine appeared to be equally effective," reports Dr. Griffith. He predicts that lysine will find greater acceptance in the future as more studies are done.

During his more than a decade of lysine research, Dr. Griffith says he has seen many people successfully fight formerly debilitating herpes infections.

One nurse, for example, had such painful and irritating genital herpes each month that she couldn't report to work, he recalls. On the verge of being dismissed for her absences, she began taking lysine in desperation. Her symptoms disappeared entirely—except when she lapsed and indulged in eating peanut butter, he says.

"We followed her case for five or six years, and she remained symptom free as long as she didn't have any food containing arginine and stayed with a supplement of 500 milligrams of lysine twice a day," says Dr. Griffith. (Lysine is found in such foods as meat, eggs, milk, and beans, but not in sufficient amounts to combat herpes, he notes.)

Many people with herpes infections have had similar success stories with lysine under her care, says Dr. North. Her impression is that a patient who doesn't do well on acyclovir often will do well on lysine, and vice versa. "It should at least be available to people as something they can try," she concludes. *See also* **acyclovir**

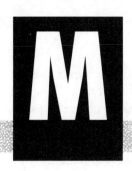

macrobiotic diet As a philosophy, a lifestyle, and a diet, macrobiotics is primarily concerned with how people can live in harmony with nature. According to macrobiotics advocates, you can recover your natural good health when you maintain a grain- and vegetable-based diet.

The standard macrobiotic diet is composed of 50 to 60 percent whole grains, 20 to 30 percent vegetables, and 5 to 10 percent beans and sea vegetables. Fish, seasonal fruits, nuts, condiments, and beverages are included as supplementary foods.

The diet was brought from Japan in the 1960s by the late George Ohsawa and refined by its chief proponent, Michio Kushi, head of The Kushi Foundation in Brookline, Massachusetts. Michio and his wife, Aveline, believe that macrobiotics can prevent—or even help treat—a host of diseases, including cancer, heart disease, diabetes, and allergies.

There is little scientific evidence for those claims. And some of the studies that have been done are almost two decades old. More recent studies, however, do suggest these health benefits from a very-low-fat diet—though not specifically a macrobiotic diet.

In the 1970s, for instance, Harvard University's Frank Sacks, M.D., studied 210 Boston-area macrobiotic practitioners. He found that their blood pressure readings averaged about 10 points below those of people following a nonvegetarian diet. In another study, Dr. Sacks and epidemiologist William Castelli, M.D., of the Framingham Heart Study, found that blood cholesterol levels among followers of macrobiotics averaged just 125, compared with 185 in a nonmacrobiotic group. Reducing cholesterol levels is regarded as a prime deterrent of heart disease.

CANCER CLAIMS

The link between this diet and heart health hasn't received nearly as much attention as macrobiotics' reported power to help treat cancer. One of the more startling anecdotal reports was a book titled *Recalled by Life*, written by a Philadelphia medical doctor, Anthony Sattilaro, who claimed that macrobiotics helped cure him of cancer. Viviene Newbold, M.D., a Philadelphia emergency room physician, says she has documented six cases in which medically incurable forms of cancer disappeared completely in patients who followed the macrobiotic approach to healing. "The evidence is irrefutable," she claims. (The medical community has refused to publish her data.) What linked the six, she says, is that the families of the cancer patients were very supportive and usually adopted the diet, too. Plus, the patients had an exceptional mental outlook.

But the American Cancer Society isn't impressed. In a position paper, it urges cancer patients not to adopt the macrobiotic diet as a treatment. The society says it has found no objective evidence that adherence to macrobiotics can help people with cancer, and the diet may in fact be too low in protein and calories for people recovering from surgery or chemotherapy.

A more recent study looked at the impact of a macrobiotic diet on men with AIDS. Boston University Medical School researchers found that men who began the regimen soon after they were diagnosed with Kaposi's sarcoma (an AIDS-related condition characterized by purple skin nodules) maintained higher lymphocyte counts than could be expected from studies of comparable patients. (Lymphocytes are infection-fighting white cells. They generally diminish in number in people who test positive for AIDS. Their decline is a strong indicator of the progression of the disease.) The counts continued to increase for three years after the date of the disease's diagnosis.

Elinor Levy, Ph.D., a microbiologist who participated in the study, says the men were monitored for four years. Eventually, the white cell counts dropped.

CAUTION ADVISED

What do researchers like Dr. Levy and Dr. Sacks think of the macrobiotic diet, in general? Both consider it safe, provided, as Dr. Levy says, that people recognize the basic nutrients required for good health and select foods that provide those nutrients.

There are some concerns about children, however. A Dutch study and an earlier Boston study found that children on macrobiotic diets were smaller and lighter in weight than children fed more mainstream diets.

"I think adults can get what they need from the macrobiotic diet," says Dr. Sacks. "It offers a wide range of foods. I also think you can raise healthy children on a macrobiotic diet, but you've got to realize that this regimen doesn't stress scientific nutrition. I'd advise parents to consult a dietitian or pediatrician to make sure their children are getting the necessary nutrients." See also **vegetarian diet**

massage   Few things are as soothing and uplifting as the touch of another human being. Perhaps that's why therapeutic massage has become so popular in the 1990s.

Practitioners say a good basic massage can stretch and loosen muscle and connective tissue, improve blood flow to the heart and the rest of the body, and allow more oxygen and nutrients to reach the cells.

"Massage strokes improve circulation, increase nutrient supply, and remove metabolic waste, thus helping the repair of damaged tissue," according to Robert Edwards, president of the New Jersey chapter of the American Massage Therapy Association. "By doing this, the massage therapist facilitates the body's ability to heal itself."

Massage can also "wake up" sensory receptors in the skin, bringing new awareness to areas that have been deadened by chronic tension. It can also relieve pain by stimulating the release of endorphins, the body's natural painkillers.

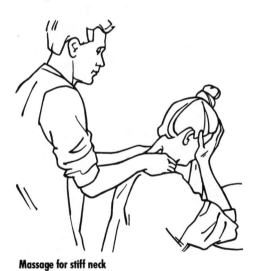

Massage for stiff neck

DIFFERENT STROKES

Specialized forms of massage promise even more. Sports massage can help repair tears and knots that heavy exercise inflicts. Eastern energy-based systems like shiatsu aim to revitalize the weary and relieve pain. And some bodywork therapies, which bill themselves as neuromuscular reeducation, claim to rewire the nervous system so that the flexible, tension-free state people experience on the massage table is always available to them.

The problem is trying to sort out what's out there. Here are some general guidelines. But be aware that many massage therapists mix and match techniques to create a style uniquely their own.

Muscle movers. Swedish massage, developed by 19th-century educator and athlete Peter Heinrik Ling, is the purest version of massage the West has to offer. It kneads the muscles, helps the lymph circulate, and relaxes tension. Deep muscle or connective-tissue massage goes a little deeper. It employs slow strokes and deep finger pressure to release chronic patterns of tension in the body.

Frame jobs. Rolfing is the best known of the techniques that aim to help you realign your body frame, supposedly by softening the hardened connective tissues that have twisted the bones in a less than ideal relationship to each other and gravity. Hellerwork is said to be a gentler variant of the technique.

Point pressers. East and West have their own versions of pressure-point massage. The West works with "trigger points," painful irritated areas in muscles, in order to break the cycle of spasm and pain. Myotherapy is another word for this style of massage. The East works with acupuncture points to stimulate the body's internal energy. Shiatsu, polarity, and reflexology (foot massage) are examples of this style.

Sport support. Sports massage incorporates techniques from acupressure and Swedish massage, but it tends to emphasize deeper, more vigorous manipulation than relaxation-style massage. The more forceful maneuvers are used both for regular fine-tuning in conjunction with races or hard workouts and for injury rehabilitation.

Self-massage. If you've got a tense or sore spot that needs attention now, and your schedule or budget won't allow for a professional massage, you can achieve some of the benefits on your own. To make the most of your self-massage, keep these pointers in mind. First, when you rub, gently move the skin over the underlying tissue, using a circular motion. Then occasionally rub toward the heart in long sweeps. Also try direct pressure on the muscles, using your fingertips, knuckles, whatever it takes.

"The important thing to remember is to stay within your own comfort zone. Applying too much pressure or holding pressure too long may be detrimental, not beneficial," says Edwards. "Take your time and cover the sore areas a few times with appropriate breaks in between to allow the muscles to recover. No massage should be painful."

And rub smart. Don't massage a serious injury or inflamed area. Don't massage if you have phlebitis or other vascular problems. When in doubt, seek out a qualified massage therapist. *See also* **acupressure; reflexology**

mastectomy She has a lump in her breast and it scares her to death. As she sits in the doctor's office waiting for the results of a biopsy, she tries to convince herself it's not cancer.

After all, four of five breast lumps are not cancer, the doctor had told her. If it's a fluid-filled cyst, it can be drained by fine-needle aspiration. If it's a benign tumor, it can be removed with no further problems. If it's cancer . . . she didn't want to think about it.

But then the doctor enters the room and gently tells her the bad news—she has cancer.

Now she and her physician must make an important decision. They need to choose the type of breast cancer surgery that is best for her. The options available depend on several factors, doctors say.

"It depends on the type of cancer, where it's located, how big the tumor is, and the size of the breast," says Ralph Broadwater, M.D., an assistant professor of surgery at the University of Arkansas College of Medicine in Little Rock.

Some patients, if their cancer is detected early, can opt for a lumpectomy, a surgical procedure that removes the lump and the lymph nodes under the arm. The surgery is followed by extensive radiation therapy, but the breast is preserved.

If the tumor is large or the cancer is difficult to control, however, the patient may have to undergo a mastectomy, a type of breast cancer surgery that removes all or part of the breast, the lymph nodes, and surrounding tissue.

"Both lumpectomies and mastectomies take about the same amount of time to do," says Richard Perry, M.D., a Phoenix, Arizona, surgeon.

SIMILAR SURVIVAL RATES

Doctors have been doing mastectomies since the late 19th century. The first mastectomies were performed by Dr. William S. Halsted, a Johns Hopkins surgeon, who removed the breast, chest muscles, all of the lymph nodes under the arms, and some additional fat and skin. The surgery, now called a radical mastectomy, is still used occasionally, but doctors have learned that less extensive operations are often just as effective for very early breast cancer.

In fact, five-year survival rates for those undergoing less drastic surgeries are virtually the same as with radical mastectomy. Other factors, such as tumor size or presence of cancer cells in the lymph nodes, are more important in determining long-term survival than the type of surgery done, says Lynn Hartmann, M.D., an oncologist at the Mayo Clinic in Rochester, Minnesota.

Today, the most common form of the surgery is the modified radical mastectomy. During this procedure, the surgeon removes the breast, the lymph nodes, and the lining over the chest muscles.

A simple mastectomy removes just the breast. Many surgeons dislike it because the lymph nodes aren't removed at the same time.

"It's not advisable to do it without removing the lymph nodes because you need to check at least some of the nodes in order to determine how far the cancer has spread and if any other treatment such as chemotherapy is necessary," Dr. Perry says.

Another surgical option is the partial or segmental mastectomy. The surgeon removes the tumor and a section of normal tissue around it. The lining of the chest muscle underneath the tumor and the lymph nodes also are usually removed. Examples of this type of surgery include the lumpectomy and the quadrantectomy, which removes one-quarter of the breast surrounding the tumor. The surgery preserves most of the breast and is appealing to many women.

Of course, this type of mastectomy isn't possible in many cases. Women who are pregnant, have tumors larger than 2 to 2½ inches in diameter, or have recurrent cancer probably aren't good candidates for breast-conserving surgery.

Even if a breast needs to be removed, however, the surgery isn't necessarily disfiguring because of advances in reconstructive surgery.

"In today's world, most women should be able to have a normal-appearing breast even if they have had breast cancer," Dr. Broadwater says. "Many surgeons are offering the possibility of mastectomy followed by immediate reconstructive surgery. That eliminates the possibility of the woman having a cosmetic deformity." *See also* **lumpectomy**

mattresses and beds When Shakespeare called sleep "Nature's soft nurse," he knew — as usual — what he was talking about. Anything you spend roughly a third of your life doing is bound to have some impact on how you feel, mentally as well as physically.

And yet the Better Sleep Council reports that as many as a third of us in the United States may not be getting the quality of sleep we need, with everything from bad backs to bad attitudes being the result. In many cases, our beds are responsible. "We tend to take our beds for granted, but they're very crucial for our overall sense of well-being," says Willibald Nagler, M.D., chief of physiatry at the New York Hospital–Cornell University Medical Center in New York City. "Some health ailments can be not only prevented by the proper bed but also treated."

BACK PAIN RELIEF

Dr. Nagler also believes that "99.9 percent of the population would sleep better on a firm mattress than a soft one. This holds true for back pain sufferers especially. A soft mattress allows the back muscles to become overextended, which prevents them from getting the rest they need. A firm mattress, on the other hand, allows the back

muscles to keep the spine in a more restful alignment."

Best of all for most backaches are adjustable beds, Dr. Nagler says, the "hospital" type that can be adjusted to raise the head and also elevate the knees. "Most low back pain responds well to an elevation of the knees, which can be done in a normal bed by using pillows, but the pillows usually slip out during the night. An adjustable bed prevents this."

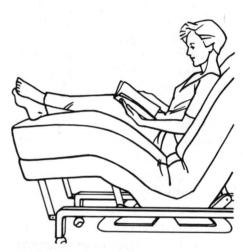

Bed adjusted for aching back

Would a futon — one of those Japanese-style beds that sits low to the floor and touts firmness to the point of forgoing a box spring — be advisable for chronic back pain?

"They're good for support, but getting in and out of them can be a problem for back pain sufferers," Dr. Nagler says. "This tends to be true for older people especially. A mattress that's at roughly the same level as the hips makes getting in and out easiest of all, which is another plus for adjustable beds. They tend to be higher than conventional beds and hence easier to enter and exit."

But more than just an aching back can find comfort in an adjustable bed, Dr. Nagler says. They can help alleviate the discomforts of gastric reflux (those unpleasant little "burps" in the night), hiatal hernia (a condition in which the upper portion of the stomach extends partially into the chest), and even snoring. "Not only does elevating the upper body in an adjustable bed tend to keep the stomach's contents where they belong, but it helps keep the windpipe straight and hence less likely to become kinked in a way that can cause snoring."

Edema (swelling) of the legs is yet another condition that frequently responds well to the elevation possible with an adjustable bed, Dr. Nagler says. "The adjustable beds offer a lot of therapeutic options, and for older people especially."

WATER BED WONDERS

Also overflowing with therapeutic potential is the increasingly popular water bed. "They can be good for people with bed sores or varicose veins, because their ever-changing contour helps minimize the discomfort caused by the pressure of surface contact on sensitive areas," Dr. Nagler says.

Relief from back pain, muscular aches, insomnia, and even arthritis also has been attributed to the fluid softness of water beds. One nationwide survey of water bed owners found that 60 percent reported back pain relief while 50 percent reported relief from muscular aches and/or arthritis. Moreover, the comforts of a water bed appear to be lasting. One study found that 90 out of 100 back pain sufferers continued to get relief from their beds over a five-year period. Water beds bestow their comfort in two ways, says Steve Garfin, M.D., professor of orthopedics at the University of California School of Medicine at San Diego. They provide uniform support at an infinite number of points, and the firmness can be adjusted for your individual needs.

"You need to let your comfort be your guide, however," warns Dr. Nagler. "Some people do not sleep better on water beds, and if the bed is not filled firmly enough, back pain can actually be made worse because of a lack of proper support. There also is some research to suggest that gastric reflux may be exacerbated by water beds."

But water beds have come a long way since they used to feel like bowls full of jelly. The wavelike action has been significantly reduced by way of stabilizing inserts. There are even water beds now called "softsides," which resemble conventional coil mattresses in every respect except that instead of springs, vinyl bags of water provide the cushioning. This style also allows for individual temperature control for the bed's users. Another water bed innovation has been the cylinder bed, which uses several individual cylinders of water for cushioning instead of just one large bag. Cylinder beds allow softness control to be "split" in order to accommodate differing preferences of couples.

PADS TO THE RESCUE

If a water bed seems a bit radical, much of the same gentle softness can be achieved by way of a good foam mattress pad, Dr. Nagler says. Made of convoluted foam approximately 2 inches thick, the pads can provide softness to a mattress without sacrificing firmness. "This can reduce the amount of fidgeting a person may do during the night, because the sleeper may not need to change positions as often to relieve pressure on the heaviest parts of the body such as the shoulders and hips," he says. "The pads also can be helpful in preventing bedsores in people who need to be confined to bed for long periods."

The convoluted pads, which are available through most outlets that sell mattresses, can be used under a traditional mattress pad or simply placed directly beneath the bottom sheet. Mattresses with foam pads permanently embedded in them also are available. Prices for mattress pads, as with mattresses themselves, can vary significantly depending on size, thickness, and density. (One drawback to expect with a mattress pad, however: Don't hope to be able to pop it in the washer for cleaning. The pads need to be spot washed or washed in a bathtub by hand.) *See also* **pillows**

meat tenderizers It may sound as hard to swallow as the cuts of beef they're designed for, but these tenderizing treasures can make mincemeat of the pain caused by a wide variety of stings and bites.

"Meat tenderizers degrade protein—that's how they tenderize meat," says Arthur Jacknowitz, Pharm.D., professor and chairman of the Department of Clinical Pharmacy at West Virginia University. "And since many venoms are protein in nature, the bites or stings from those insects and marine animals can be alleviated with meat tenderizer."

That's a lot of critters, including many of the more noticed backyard pests, such as bees, yellow jackets, and fire ants; it also includes jellyfish and other venomous sea dwellers likely to come in contact with beachgoers. However, this is not a recommended treatment for toxic poisons such as those from snakebites. And people prone to severe sting or bite reactions, as well as anyone whose symptoms persist, should seek medical treatment.

"If you apply a paste of meat tenderizer within a minute or two of the sting, you may actually be able to degrade enough of the venom to reduce the chance of any allergic reaction as well as the inflammatory reaction," adds David Golden, M.D., assistant professor of medicine at Johns Hopkins University in Baltimore. That means at the least, your backyard barbeque or beachside holiday won't be such a painful experience; at the most, it could help prevent a trip to a hospital emergency room for serious medical care.

ENZYME ACTION

So how did meat tenderizer go from the spice rack to the medicine chest? "Actually, meat tenderizer itself isn't the cure; it's the enzymes in it—particularly one called papain that breaks down the protein in venom the same way it breaks down the protein in meat," explains Dr. Jacknowitz.

Allergic to papain? Don't fret. Some meat tenderizers, like McCormick's, use another protein-busting enzyme—bromelain—which is just as effective.

No matter the enzyme or brand of meat tenderizer, it's applied the same way: Mix with water to make a thick paste and place directly on the affected area. Although fresh water is used in most instances, Dr. Jacknowitz says that saltwater must be used when treating jellyfish stings (which is convenient, since you'll be at the beach anyway). "Fresh water causes jellyfish tentacles to explode," he says.

Of course, since the folks at Adolph's or McCormick's aren't trying to rank up there with Albert Schweitzer in the Healing Hall of Fame, don't think of meat tenderizer as supermarket armor against *all* that lurks in your lawn. Meat tenderizer provides *only* temporary relief. "And you're not necessarily going to eliminate all the effects of the sting," adds Dr. Golden. "But if you apply it quickly enough—and the key is to apply it in the first couple of minutes—you'll likely get some relief."

meditation   Years ago, in the heat of a tight pennant race, a baseball player confessed that he would like to sit in a laundry bag. He thought if he sat in the bag and pulled it taut over his head, he could find relief from the stress of the season.

Unfortunately, there probably aren't enough laundry bags in the world for all of us to try that approach to stress reduction. But doctors say there is an even better way to quiet our mind and get relief from our physical and emotional wounds. It's called meditation.

Practitioners describe meditation as a form of inward concentration that allows you to focus on your senses, step back from thoughts and feelings, and perceive each moment as a unique event.

MIND/BODY BENEFITS

"Many people have used meditation as a way of reducing stress, lowering blood pressure, and putting the nervous system into a relaxed state. Others have used it as a way of gaining control over difficult thoughts and feelings. It can be used to provide emotional solace or relieve anxiety," says Mark Epstein, M.D., clinical instructor in psychiatry at Cornell University Medical College in New York City.

That opinion is supported by research conducted by Stephen DeBerry, Ph.D., assistant clinical professor of psychiatry at Albert Einstein College of Medicine in New York City, who compared the short-term effects of meditation and psychiatry on 32 elderly people who complained of anxiety, nervousness, tension, fatigue, sadness, and insomnia. During the 12-week study, the people were divided into three groups. One group was taught meditation and imagery techniques. A second group received assertiveness training and was taught ways to think more positively about their problems. A third group was given information, but no formal training, about meditation and psychiatry techniques.

Those in the first group, which was taught meditation and imagery techniques, were better able to cope with certain types of anxiety caused by such things as illness than those in the other two groups, Dr. DeBerry concluded.

"Rather than give people medication or get them involved in more intensive analytical therapy, it may behoove us to try meditation first. It can definitely make a change in their lives," says Dr. DeBerry.

Other studies indicate that meditation may have some influence on our immune system. For example, researchers at the University of Arkansas College of Medicine challenged 28 meditators by injecting into their skin the viral antigen that causes chickenpox and shingles. (By checking later for a reaction at the site, doctors use such skin tests to gauge immune response.) Then they randomly divided the meditators into two groups. One group was asked to attempt to suppress their immune response to the test. The second group was told they should try to enhance their immune response.

At the end of two days, the enhancer group had a more significant reaction to the antigen than the inhibitor group.

"I think this tells us there is a definite connection between the nervous system and immune response," says G. Richard Smith, M.D., author of the study. "What is unclear is if there is any *conscious* connection between the two. I think the results point in that direction: that you can modify, to some extent, your immune response."

But meditation may do much more than that. Evidence from a small preliminary study hints that it actually might extend your life span.

In a study of 73 residents in eight nursing homes, researchers from Maharishi International University in Iowa found that those who practiced Transcendental Meditation (TM) for 20 minutes twice a day felt younger, were better able to cope with inconvenience, and scored higher on mental tests than their peers.

Some of the nonmeditators played word games, and others used a relaxation technique that involved repeating a verse, phrase, or song with their eyes closed. A fourth set of residents received no instructions and were simply told they would be used as a comparison group.

Three years later, all 20 residents who had practiced TM were still living. In contrast, 13 percent of those who played word games, 23 percent of those in the comparison group, and 35 percent of those who had practiced the relaxation technique had died.

TRAIN THE MIND

Although there are many types of meditation, they can be classified into two broad categories.

Concentrative meditation uses an object, picture, keyword (mantra), or activity such as breathing to focus the mind in a one-pointed way. When your mind begins to wander, continuing to repeat the mantra, for example, should guide your attention back to your focus, Dr. Epstein says. Mindfulness meditation is more sophisticated. Instead of focusing on a single sensation or object, this approach allows you to pay attention to thoughts, desires, and moods. As these feelings and images float through your mind, you view them as if you were an outsider nonjudgmentally eavesdropping on a conversation. Some forms of meditation use a combination of concentrative and mindfulness techniques.

"Meditation can't really stop life from being stressful," Dr. Epstein says. "It can't stop your spouse from getting sick or make the pressures of your job go away, but it can alter how you respond to those things."

If you suffer from arthritis, for example, meditation may help you separate yourself from the pain so it doesn't bother you as much, he says.

"You learn to stay with the pain longer and notice how it changes. It might become a burning sensation, or you may be able to distinguish it as 10 or 11 different pains that flair and subside. Over time, your tolerance of the pain may grow," Dr. Epstein says.

Getting to that point may take time and practice, but proponents say meditation is easy to learn.

FOCUS ON THE BREATH

"The simplest form of meditation is concentrating on your own breathing," says Jon Kabat-Zinn, Ph.D., director of the University of Massachusetts stress reduction clinic in Worcester.

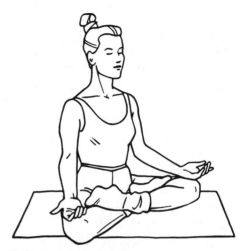

Meditating in the lotus position

To do it, he suggests that you stand or sit in an erect, dignified posture. Closing your eyes may help you concentrate. Let any thoughts or outside distractions drift into the background and focus on the sensation of your breath. Don't think about breathing. Instead, just feel the sensation of your breath flowing in and out of your body without manipulating or judging the breath at all.

"Meditating like this can be profoundly centering and relaxing, and it's something you can do with your eyes open or closed, walking, standing on your head, or sitting at your desk," says Dr. Kabat-Zinn. "You can do it for 30 seconds or you can do it for 5 minutes at lunch. The longer you do it, the more you will cultivate concentration and calmness." *See also* **Relaxation Response**

menthol The pink-flowered peppermint plant is the natural source for this common pain-relieving ingredient, which soothes as it cools. Suck on a menthol cough drop when your throat is scratchy or rub a mentholated balm on your sore muscle, and the effect is the same: A delightful cool sensation rushes in to temporarily ease your discomfort. Menthol does this in two ways: It stimulates the nerve endings that perceive cold, making them so sensitive that even a stirring of room-temperature air feels like an Arctic breeze. It also mildy numbs the nerve endings that register pain.

"A lot of folk remedies substitute one sensation for another," says Arthur I. Jacknowitz, Pharm.D., professor and chairman of the Department of Clinical Pharmacy at West Virginia University. "Menthol substitutes coolness for pain. Agents like these are called counterirritants because they produce a mild irritation to counter a more severe pain usually adjacent to or underlying the skin surface being treated."

This talent accounts for menthol's use in many over-the-counter products. You'll find it in certain brands of sore throat lozenges and cough supressants, in liquids like Vicks Vaposteam that you add to hot steam vaporizers, and in topical creams, lotions, and gels such as Therapeutic Mineral Ice. Some dandruff shampoos and mouthwashes include it, too. Often, topically applied products combine menthol with ingredients like camphor, eucalyptus, and methyl salicylate—other plant-derived substances that also relieve pain by producing mild stimulation. The combination of such ingredients is thought to enhance the pain-relieving effect.

But camphor, eucalyptus, and methyl salicylate aren't considered safe for internal use the way menthol is. Menthol is sometimes even used in small quantities as a flavoring agent.

SOOTHE THAT COUGH

Cough and cold remedies that contain menthol have been around for years. Vicks VapoRub, which combines menthol, eucalyptus, and camphor, was developed back in 1890 by a pharmacist who wanted to cure his son's "croupy cough." But it was only in the last decade that the Food and Drug Administration (FDA) added menthol to the list of cough suppressants it considers safe and effective. By law, these cough drops, sprays, syrups, and inhalants can only claim to bring temporary relief to coughs caused by colds or by inhaling irritants like dust.

"Mentholated vapors in hot steam do make people feel better," says Jerome Goldstein, M.D., an ear, nose, and throat specialist who is executive vice-president of the American Academy of Otolaryngology (Head and Neck Surgery) in Alexandria, Virginia. The steam helps thin out the thicker-than-normal mucus that can trigger coughs. But if you're coughing because you've got a bacterial infection, such as bronchitis, "these menthol cough and cold remedies don't take the place of the appropriate antibiotic," he says.

There is some evidence that menthol cough drops may bring fast relief to a stuffy nose. A study in Wales found that cold sufferers who took lozenges containing menthol noticed significant improvement in their ability to breathe freely. The menthol lozenges took effect within 2 minutes and relief lasted up to 30 minutes, long after the lozenges had dissolved. Cold sufferers who took a placebo lozenge experienced little relief.

Although menthol is currently not approved as a decongestive agent by the FDA, it is under review. "That cooling effect does seem to give people a feeling that nasal passages are being opened," says Dr. Jacknowitz. But it's not known whether menthol actually clears a stuffy nose or just creates the perception of greater air flow, he says.

MUSCLE UP TO MENTHOL

Menthol is also popular as an active ingredient in sports ointments, creams, and gels you rub on to relieve muscle aches and pains caused by overexertion.

"You'd do okay using these for minor sports injuries," Dr. Jacknowitz says. "They do have a soothing, cooling effect." If your pain comes from bursitis or tendinitis, however, the use of topical preparations might not be as helpful as taking an oral analgesic like Advil or Nuprin, which work more effectively from inside to combat pain throughout your body.

With products like Ben-Gay Original ointment, which Dr. Jacknowitz says contains 16 percent menthol, you're likely to feel a surge of warmth following that initial blast of coolness. That's because your body reacts to the

coolness by sending additional blood to the area to bring skin temperature back to normal. It is possible that the extra oxygen supplied by that fresh blood could speed healing of the injured muscle, Dr. Jacknowitz says. But don't count on such products for anything more than short-term relief. They can help you get by while the muscle heals on its own, he says.

"If the problem doesn't get better within seven days, or it gets worse, or it gets better and then worse within a few days, you should discontinue use of the product and consult your physician," he says.

Menthol also may temporarily ease the urge to itch, depending upon the cause of the itching. Anti-itch creams, such as Medicone Derma Ointment, have less menthol in them than the sports rubs, as little as 0.1 to 1 percent, Dr. Jacknowitz says. In this concentration, menthol actually depresses rather than excites skin receptors.

And such creams aren't always your best bet. Cortisone-containing creams might be better for itching accompanied by swelling, and plain old calamine lotion is good for itchiness over large areas of the body, Dr. Jacknowitz says. Menthol's slight irritating action rules it out when you've got lots of skin to cover.

In general, menthol is considered safe in small doses. But you can hurt yourself with it. Never use menthol-containing products with a heating pad because it can substantially increase the rate at which your body absorbs menthol, Dr. Jacknowitz says. (You could potentially take in enough to inflame the cells in your kidneys, which can cause kidney damage.)

Similarly, if you're using mentholated cough drops, nasal sprays, or liquids, never use more in any 24-hour period than recommended on the product label. And get your doctor's okay before you give menthol cough drops to children. The less a person weighs, the more potent this central nervous system stimulant is. Be aware too that sensitive individuals have been known to have allergic reactions to menthol-containing preparations. *See also* **eucalyptus; oil of wintergreen**

methyl salicylate. *See* **oil of wintergreen**

milk   Well known for its culinary roles, there's evidence that this drink also may help us avoid some health problems: high cholesterol, osteoporosis, and perhaps even cancer.

One of milk's chief benefits is the calcium it contains, says Arun Kilara, Ph.D., a food science professor at Pennsylvania State University. Most experts agree you need an average of 1,000 milligrams of calcium per day, which you'll find in just over three 8-ounce glasses of milk. Some people need more calcium and some need less, depending on age and other health considerations. Ask your doctor or a dietitian how much you need.

In his research, Dr. Kilara found that drinking 1 quart of milk daily may lower cholesterol levels, because some of milk's compounds seem to inhibit the synthesis of cholesterol in the body.

"We found that drinking milk lowered cholesterol levels by an average of 8 percent in those individuals whose cholesterol level was high. And it didn't raise the cholesterol levels of those with normal or below normal levels," he explains, adding that the type of milk didn't matter.

Researchers at the Chicago Medical School reported that men who drank 1 quart of 2 percent milk a day increased the proportion of good to bad cholesterol (HDL to LDL) in their blood by almost 20 percent after three months. After six months, the ratio was even more favorable, increasing by 31 percent.

BONE PRESERVER

On other fronts, milk is considered important in helping people add calcium to their diet to protect against osteoporosis. Milk and other calcium-rich foods, along with exercise and sometimes estrogen therapy, may help women fend off this bone-weakening disease, researchers have found.

In a study at the University of Massachusetts Medical School, premenopausal women who consumed 1,500 milligrams of calcium daily from low-fat, calcium-rich foods lost none of their bone mass after three years. Another group of women, who consumed only 800 milligrams of calcium, lost about 3 percent of their bone mass.

"With regard to osteoporosis, the calcium in milk is a beneficial thing," Dr. Kilara says.

Finally, milk has been studied as a way to possibly lessen the chances of getting cancer. Researchers at Buffalo's Roswell Park Memorial Institute interviewed almost 5,000 patients with and without cancer, asking them, among other things, how many glasses of whole, 2 percent, and skim milk they drank each day. What did they learn?

First, people who drank 2 percent milk had a much lower risk of cancer than those who drank whole milk. Second, they found that the cancer risk for those who drank low-fat milk also was lower than for those who drank no milk at all.

The first finding is consistent with other research, which has linked dietary fat to certain types of cancer. Whole milk has four times the fat of skim milk; 2 percent has twice as much fat as skim. The second finding is more difficult to explain, but it is known that some of milk's nutrients, such as vitamins A and C and riboflavin, have been associated with reduced risk of certain cancers, the scientists report.

"It's possible that milk drinking is associated with other health habits," says Curtis Mettlin, Ph.D., chief of epidemiologic research at the institute and one of the study's authors. "It's difficult to say it has therapeutic or preventive properties. But there is an association."

MAKING THE SWITCH

Dietitians strongly advise adults to consume low-fat milk and dairy products. The recommendations are to go as low on fat as the palate will allow.

Whole milk is one of the largest sources of fat in the American diet and the second leading source of saturated fat, the Roswell Park researchers report. Since various studies link dietary fat to heart disease and various types of cancer, it makes sense to try to lower your overall fat intake, something you can begin by switching to low-fat or skim milk.

"If you shift to skim, that has a major effect in reducing animal fat, while giving you the same nutrients," Dr. Mettlin says.

Try the step-down approach to drop from whole to 2 percent to skim milk. Start by mixing a carton of whole milk with a carton of 2 percent. Drink the mixture until you become used to the taste. Then start decreasing the proportion of whole milk until you like 2 percent alone. Then gradually add skim milk to the 2 percent milk, working your way down to pure skim.

In a few months, you can drop from whole milk, which gets over 50 percent of its calories from fat, to skim, which derives slightly under 5 percent of its calories from fat. (Two percent milk gets about 35 percent of its calories from fat.)

"It's a simple change," Dr. Mettlin says. And one that may mean a big difference to your health, while letting you enjoy the benefits of milk. *See also* **lactase**

mineral oil   When you're bothered with constipation, you may be tempted to try anything—including taking a swig of mineral oil—to get things moving again. Mineral oil is an old-fashioned laxative, made from refined petroleum, that is sold right along with the newer laxative products. The drawback is that mineral oil may clean out more than you bargained for.

Mineral oil is a lubricant-type laxative. It acts by softening the stool and lubricating the lining of the intestine. The problem is this: Mineral oil is a fat that, when swallowed, can cause fat-soluble vitamins to dissolve within it instead of being absorbed by your body. "Ingesting mineral oil may interfere with the absorption of vitamins such as A, D, E, and K," explains Philip Miner, M.D., director of the Division of Gastroenterology at the University of Kansas Medical Center. "If you have a borderline deficiency in these vitamins, taking mineral oil could potentially cause a more severe deficiency," says Dr. Miner. "There's also the possibility that mineral oil could stay in the esophagus, or migrate up and be aspirated to cause an active inflammation in the lungs."

In light of these concerns, if you want to do something about constipation, try increasing the fiber in your diet—eating more whole grains, fruits, and vegetables—and drinking lots of fluids, suggests Dr. Miner. If that doesn't do the trick, ask your doctor about the prescription drug lactulose. It's a nonabsorbable sugar that pulls water into the colon, softens the stool, and gently stimulates the bowel. "There are better choices for constipation than consuming oils," says Dr. Miner.

If you are often constipated, talk to your doctor before heading for the drugstore. "You need to get at the cause of your constipation as well as the proper course of treatment," says Dr. Miner.

MOISTURIZES THE SKIN

Swallowing mineral oil may not be advised, but smearing mineral oil on your body is often recommended for relieving dry skin and for managing conditions triggered by dryness. If you have psoriasis, for example, the National Psoriasis Foundation suggests using mineral oil as a low-cost alternative to the expensive moisturizers sold specifically for this problem. Soak first in a warm bath so your skin is fully hydrated. Then apply the oil. "Mineral oil provides an even seal over the skin surface and prevents evaporation of moisture,"says Bill Fuegy, registered pharmacist and pharmacy consultant for the National Psoriasis Foundation. "Moisturizing with mineral oil helps control the dryness and cracking that can worsen psoriasis. It can also help reduce the maddening itching associated with this condition." There are no perfumes, preservatives, or additives in mineral oil, so it is ideal for supersensitive skin. "Mineral oil is the purest sealant available,"says Fuegy.

For treating everyday dry skin, though, pure mineral oil can be sticky, messy stuff. Mixed with water, it can also be very slippery, so be careful using it in the bathroom and especially around the tub. Because it is so messy, mineral oil is often combined with other ingredients in moisturizing products

for better spread and feel. *See also* **laxatives; moisturizers**

minoxidil (mi-NOKS-i-dil) Baldness
has always been a hair-raising experience for men. So scary, in fact, that it's
spooked countless men enough to
endure laughable cheap toupees, costly
yet questionable snake oil remedies,
and painful hair transplants—just to
hide the bald truth about themselves.

Then along came Rogaine Topical
Solution—minoxidil to the masses—
viewed by many as *the* answer to the
Great Recession suffered by 55 million
American men: Just two applications
a day of this liquid, containing a safe
and effective animal protein that helps
thicken hair, and . . . *voilà*! That hair
today *won't* be gone tomorrow. No
pain, no hassles. Just a full head of
hair—*forever.*

Sigh! If only it worked that easily.
"There are a lot of advantages to
minoxidil, but there also are several
disadvantages," says Douglas D. Altchek, M.D., a dermatologist and assistant clinical professor of dermatology
at Mount Sinai School of Medicine in
New York City.

First, the good news. . . . Minoxidil
is painless, unlike hair transplants.
Minoxidil is effective, unlike other
creams, sprays, and ointments (usually
advertised on matchbook covers). And
unlike so many toupees or parts used
to hide baldness, no one has to know
you're using it. "It's odorless, colorless,
and as easy to use as mousse or styling
gel," says Dr. Altchek. "And it's superior to other treatments for baldness."
But there are some drawbacks to this

miracle from The Upjohn Co., the
only company allowed to sell Rogaine.

LONG-TERM COMMITMENT

The bad news about minoxidil is
once you commit to using it, you commit for life. That's *every* morning and
every night for *every* day of your life.
"If you miss a day, or one application a
day, you'll lose some of the progress. If
you miss a few days, you lose the hair
you've grown back," says Dr. Altchek.
"Once you commit to it, it's forever or
you'll lose what you've gained."

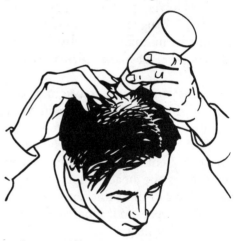

Applying minoxidil

And it's an expensive commitment:
One bottle of minoxidil—a one-month
supply—costs between $48 and $98,
depending on where you live. Insurance companies and health plans usually *don't* cover its cost. And since it's
available only by prescription, you must
also add the cost of a doctor's visit.
"Figure you'll need at least $1,000 a
year for it—for every year of your
life," adds Dr. Altchek.

Now, the *really* bad news: Minoxidil is a treatment—not a cure. Using it

doesn't guarantee you'll grow hair. Upjohn says only about one-third of men who use it grow hair after 4 months (those statistics improve substantially after 12 months of use). And only about 8 percent of men experience "substantial" hair growth.

"Like any prescription medication, it doesn't work for everyone," says Brent Schillinger, M.D., a Boca Raton, Florida, dermatologist who has appeared in an Upjohn Co. video on Rogaine. "The degree of success varies greatly from patient to patient." Translation: Don't expect miracles from this "miracle" drug. In fact, most experts agree that minoxidil is really better at slowing (baldness) than growing (new hair).

But you can expect *some* improvement—if only a slowdown in your male pattern baldness. If you're already a full-fledged chrome-dome, however, forget it. Remember, it can't grow new hair on your head where there is none—it can only thicken what you already have, even if what you have is only "peach fuzz."

And that peach fuzz doesn't have to be on your head. "Some people have used minoxidil successfully to grow eyebrows or chest hair," says Dr. Altchek. "It's also been used by women to grow hair on their heads or other body parts."

Sometimes—albeit rarely—this growth gets out of hand. "In two cases I know of, men who have used minoxidil on their head had hair growing from the base of the spine, resembling a tail," says Dr. Altchek. "Others have

gotten hairy cheeks or *really* bushy eyebrows from using it." Usually, however, side effects only include itching or mild irritation on the scalp.

Other things to remember: It's most effective on men under age 30 whose hair loss is not severe and has started in the past five years. And Rogaine *shouldn't* be used by heart patients or those with high blood pressure because it's an antihypertensive drug as well as a hair-loss treatment.

mint. *See* **peppermint**

moisturizers Your skin is exposed to desert-dry indoor air, harsh winds, hot showers, strong soaps—all factors that strip away protective skin oils and deplete natural moisture. As a result, your skin may become so dry and rough that it itches and splits, inviting further irritation, eczema, or even an infection.

A moisturizing product can help quench your skin's thirst in two ways: It puts water into the top layers of the skin, and it also provides a protective barrier to prevent moisture loss. Because the new breed of supermoisturizers trap and hold water better than ever, they can help prevent or relieve even the most stubborn dry skin problems.

There's more good news. The daily use of moisturizers can play an important part in managing eczema, psoriasis, and other skin conditions accompanied or triggered by dry skin, according to Nelson Lee Novick, M.D., associate clinical professor of dermatology at Mount Sinai School of Medicine in New York City and author of *Super Skin: A Leading Dermatologist's Guide to the Latest Breakthroughs in Skin Care.*

Selecting from among the hundreds of moisturizing products available can be a mind-boggling experience. There are products formulated for the hands, body, feet, eye area, even the neckline. There are lotions for daytime use, creams for nighttime use. "The thing to remember is that all moisturizers serve the same basic function—the main difference is in the packaging," advises Paul Lazar, M.D., clinical professor of dermatology at Northwestern University in Chicago and author of *The Look You Like.*

Technically, all moisturizers are really emollients, substances that soothe and soften the skin. "The term 'moisturizer' has become popular because it implies that the product somehow changes the skin structure. That's not so," says Dr. Lazar.

The standard moisturizer only penetrates as far as the thin, lifeless top layer of the skin, called the stratum corneum. It does not seep into the deeper, living layers of the skin.

The most important ingredients in moisturizers are oil and water. The water is absorbed into the stratum corneum, making it supple and soft. The oil sits on the skin surface and locks in the moisture. The oil component may be some sort of mineral oil, vegetable or animal fat, wax, or even a synthetic oil compound. "The heavier the oil, the more effective the product is in trapping water," says Dr. Lazar.

"The best water-trapping agent is petrolatum [petroleum jelly]—it's thick and allows very little water to escape from the skin."

SUPER SOLUTIONS

If you really want to help your dry skin, look for one of the newer "supermoisturizing" products with added humectants, says Joseph Bark, M.D., chairman of dermatology at St. Joseph's Hospital in Lexington, Kentucky. Humectants are substances that bind water from the atmosphere or draw it up from the body tissues and hold it next to the skin. Glycerin is one humectant that's being used increasingly in moisturizers.

Another humectant, lecithin, is a soybean-derived substance with super water-holding abilities. Scientists refer to it as a phospholipid. According to Dr. Bark, each molecule of a phospholipid is capable of holding 15 molecules of water. "Phospholipids soak into the dead layer and bind water in, making your skin softer," he says. "Skin tests have shown that the use of a phospholipid moisturizer such as Complex 15 will keep the skin moisturized for up to ten days after using it."

Lactic acid, urea, and glycolic acid are also humectants. They, too, help bind water to the skin surface, but with an added bonus: Because they also help remove dead skin cells, they may be more effective than regular moisturizers at treating very dry, flaky skin.

"Extremely dry skin becomes thick and cannot be effectively taken care of with simple moisturizing products," says Eugene Van Scott, M.D., clinical professor of dermatology at Hahnemann University Hospital in Philadelphia. "Lactic acid penetrates the thick armor, thins the skin, and makes it softer, more pliable, and less prone to cracking."

You can purchase over-the-counter moisturizers containing lactic acid (LactiCare and Lac-Hydrin V are two examples). But for severely dry skin—especially in thick areas like the heels, feet, hands, and arms—you might ask your doctor for a prescription for Lac-Hydrin 12%, which contains more than twice the amount of lactic acid as over-the-counter products. Unlike cosmetic moisturizers, Lac-Hydrin 12% is a topical moisturizing drug approved by the Food and Drug Administration—which means it had to demonstrate safety and also efficacy. "Studies revealed that Lac-Hydrin works at the skin's deeper levels and helps alleviate dry skin conditions," says Dr. Van Scott. Lac-Hydrin's effects were observed to last for up to two weeks after application.

USING A MOISTURIZER

In general, you should be able to use the same moisturizer on your eyelids as well as your heels, says Dr. Bark. The key is to find a light, all-purpose product that's powerful enough to work all over your body but mild enough that it doesn't irritate your face.

If you have sensitive skin, avoid products containing perfumes, preservatives, or colors. If your skin is very oily or acne-prone, look for water-based rather than oil-based products, suggests Dr. Novick. To determine the difference, rub a small amount on your arm. Water-based lotions feel cool on the skin as the water evaporates. Oil-based products feel warm, he says.

Drugstore brands are as good or better than higher-priced moisturizers found in department stores, Dr. Bark says. "The more expensive the brand, the more additives it may contain, with more potential for irritation," he says. "Buy the cheapest moisturizer that feels good to you."

And be sure to apply the product two to four times a day, depending on whether you buy a lotion or a thick cream. For best results, apply the moisturizer on your damp skin after a bath or shower to seal in the water.

Here's another tip: Slathering on two thin layers instead of one heavy one can help the moisturizer work longer, suggests Dr. Bark. Just wait a few minutes between applications.

If you notice any stinging, swelling, or redness, discontinue using your moisturizer. And if you find that your dry skin doesn't appear to be healing after a week or two of regular moisturizing, you may need to see a dermatologist for more potent skin medication. *See also* **petroleum jelly**

moleskin. *See* **pads and plasters**

monounsaturated oils Ever since olive oil landed with a splash on America's newspaper pages and palates, monounsaturated oils have been touted as a means of lowering dangerous LDL cholesterol—the kind that's implicated in heart disease—while at the same time preserving levels of protective HDL cholesterol.

This long-standing staple of Mediterranean cuisine also has been linked with beneficial effects on blood pressure and blood glucose levels (potentially helpful for diabetics). In an Italian study involving almost 5,000 people, researchers found that men who were regular olive oil users averaged 2.5 percent lower blood pressure readings and 6.6 percent lower blood sugar levels than nonusers.

But olive oil isn't the only member of the monounsaturated family. A relative newcomer is canola oil, a flavorless oil made from rapeseed. Canola oil contains less monounsaturated fat than olive oil: 58 percent compared to 77 percent. But canola's bright spot is its standing as the oil lowest in saturated fat (just 6 percent). Excess saturated fat in the diet can raise blood cholesterol levels and increase the risk of heart disease. Peanut oil also is considered a monounsaturated oil. (Keep in mind that all oils are a blend of saturated, monounsaturated, and polyunsaturated fats in varying proportions.)

"Monounsaturated fats are proving to be a renewed area of interest in medical research. For many years, we considered them to be neutral in regard to coronary heart disease. But there is evidence now that indicates they can do some good, both for heart disease and cancer, too," says Maurizio Trevisan, M.D., an associate professor at the State University of New York Medical School in Buffalo and an author of the Italian diet study. The cancer work still is in its preliminary stages, he says, but some research has shown that feeding animals a diet high in monounsaturated fat (in the form of olive oil), versus a diet high in saturated fat, may protect against colon cancer.

While olive oil has grabbed much attention, canola oil should not be overlooked. It, too, has been shown to lower LDL cholesterol without reducing HDL cholesterol when substituted for saturated fats in the diet.

SET YOUR PRIORITIES

How can you get more monounsaturated fat in your diet?

First, keep in mind that a low-fat diet should contain no more than 30 percent of calories from fat. "The number one priority is keeping total fat low. Number two is keeping saturated fat low. And number three is seeing that the remaining fat is predominantly monounsaturated followed by polyunsaturated," says Alicia Moag-Stahlberg, a registered dietitian and spokesperson for the American Dietetic Association and a nutritionist at Northwestern University Medical School in Chicago.

The best way of getting monounsaturated fats is by substituting them for other fats in a balanced diet that includes fresh fruits and vegetables, whole grains, lean meats, skinless poultry and fish, and low-fat or nonfat dairy products. Try olive oil on pasta and salads, canola oil for cooking. *See also* **polyunsaturated oils**

motion sickness remedies If you've ever sailed a small boat in a big storm, or spun upside down on too many carnival rides, you know the feeling. You get a little hot . . . a little dizzy . . . a little green. It's time to get off, you tell yourself—before it's too late!

Nearly everyone suffers occasional bouts with motion sickness. Just ask Harrison H. Schmitt, an astronaut and crew member on Apollo 17 who walked on the moon in 1972.

"If you've experienced various levels of seasickness for two or three days, that's what astronauts say it's like," says Schmitt, a former U.S. senator from New Mexico. "Of course, motion sickness may be a little messier in space— the vomitus will just float around the cabin if you don't contain it."

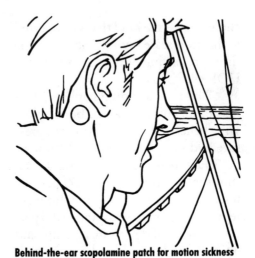

Behind-the-ear scopolamine patch for motion sickness

WELCOME RELIEF

Fortunately for the astronauts— and for Earth dwellers, too—there are many motion sickness remedies to choose from. Perhaps the most powerful is scopolamine, a prescription drug that depresses the central nervous system and the vomiting center inside the brain.

Because scopolamine is short acting, it's commonly affixed to an adhesive patch that people stick behind the ear. The patch releases scopolamine at measured rates for several days.

Unfortunately, scopolamine produces side effects—drowsiness, for example, and an extremely dry mouth— that limit its usefulness. When the Apollo 17 astronauts took scopolamine, it was mixed with the stimulant dex-troamphetamine—a combination called scop-dex—to keep them alert.

"Scopolamine is a very, very powerful drug," says psychophysiologist Robert M. Stern, Ph.D., a professor of psychology at Pennsylvania State University who has performed numerous studies on motion sickness. Had the astronauts taken large amounts of the drug, few would have gotten sick. On the other hand, they wouldn't have been able to function, he adds.

For car trips and sailing expeditions, two over-the-counter products, Dramamine and Bonine, are long-time favorites for combating motion sickness. Slow to go to work, they work best when taken *before* you start feeling sick. Take them half an hour to an hour before your trip begins.

Gingerroot traditionally has been used to beat motion sickness, although there are few studies to prove that it really works. Antinausea wristbands, which press against a specific point on the wrist that acupressurists say controls nausea, also may help. Another suggestion: If you're going to travel, nibble on some nonfatty foods like a cracker or a piece of bread before you leave, Dr. Stern says.

Scientists believe motion sickness occurs when your body and mind receive conflicting signals. In his laboratory, Dr. Stern seats hapless volunteers in an optokinetic drum, a black-and-white striped cylinder. The drum spins while volunteers stay put.

"The brain is receiving signals— 'I'm rotating'—but the vestibular sense in the inner ear is saying, 'Hey, dummy, you're sitting on a stool.' We think it's that discrepancy that makes people feel sick," Dr. Stern says.

TIPS FOR TRAVELERS

When you're traveling—in a boat, car, or plane—you can keep your senses working together by watching the scenery go by, Dr. Stern says.

Stay mentally active. Astronauts aren't likely to get sick during launch because they're too busy, Schmitt says. That's why drivers rarely get sick on long car trips, even when their passengers do. "You need to challenge your central nervous system—namely, the brain," Schmitt says.

Dr. Stern offers these suggestions for beating motion sickness.

Eat a low-fat, starchy meal before leaving. If you're taking a long trip, take additional healthy snacks.

Stay busy. Play a chess game in your head. Memorize license plates. Recite some lines from Shakespeare.

Watch the world go by. Don't try to read in the car. Keep your senses in synch by looking out the window. If kids in the back seat are feeling sick, put them up front where they'll have a better view.

Keep your head still. Vigorous head movements often make nausea worse. *See also* **antiemetics**

Motrin. *See* **ibuprofen**

mouth guards Every night, Dorothy puts on her nightgown, kisses her husband, and slips a plastic apparatus over her teeth that, she says, "makes me look like Rocky Graziano."

Why would anyone want to go to bed looking like a prizefighter? Simple. Because for some people, wearing a mouth guard can shield the teeth from wear and tear and knock out pain in the jaw.

The truth is, Dorothy is a nighttime gnasher. "My tooth grinding used to wake my husband," she says. "I would clench my teeth so tightly during my sleep that I eventually cracked two of them in half. And my jaw and head would ache during the day. This mouth guard may not look glamorous, but it has cured the soreness and headaches."

Technically known as occlusal splints, mouth guards (or night guards) are horseshoe-shaped appliances made of flexible or rigid acrylic that fit over the upper teeth and are typically worn during sleep. Unlike bulky athletic "bite guards," mouth splints are custom-fitted so they conform precisely to your tooth landscape.

The purpose of wearing such a device is not to shield you from a blow to your chops but to protect your teeth if you have the automatic habit of grinding and clenching, a condition known as bruxism.

According to studies, mouth guards eliminate 70 to 80 percent of the symptoms resulting from grinding

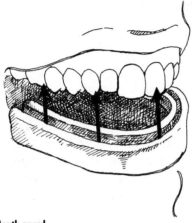

Mouth guard

and clenching. Experts offer several different explanations. One theory is that when your mouth senses this foreign body over your teeth, it sends a message to your brain to refrain from chomping.

TMD RELIEF

Several different types of mouth guards enable doctors to offer a kinder, gentler way to treat temporomandibular joint disorders (called TMD or TMJ). These disorders are an array of painful muscular or joint problems centered around the sturdy hinge linking the lower jaw to the skull. In one study, 80 percent of the patients suffering from TMD improved or were cured when the only form of treatment was

wearing an occlusal splint for at least six months.

"A few years ago, we would have assumed that a TM disorder required either surgery to the jaw joint or adjustment of the teeth," says Jeffrey P. Okeson, D.M.D., director of the Orofacial Pain Center at the University of Kentucky College of Dentistry in Lexington. "The success of mouth guards proves that TM pain is more often the result of bad habits like clenching or grinding teeth than of poor bite. Clearly most TM problems can be successfully treated by wearing one of these temporary appliances at night."

Even if an uneven bite is suspected in your particular pain problem, wearing a specially designed mouth splint that readjusts your jaw slightly forward may bring relief. "The splint works like a crutch," says Dr. Okeson. "It puts the jaw in a better position and keeps the pressure off tender tissues."

What's more, when the force is distributed more evenly, your jaw muscles don't have to work as hard and are less likely to become tired and sore.

Mouth guards can also ease headaches in some cases. In a study conducted at Harvard University, about 80 percent of patients wearing a mouth splint for one to two weeks reported fewer or less severe headaches.

Before any permanent, surgical corrections are made for your TM problem, you should wear a mouth guard for four to six months to see if the symptoms are nonsurgically relieved, suggests Dr. Okeson. If the symptoms *are* relieved, the appliance should be gradually eliminated to see if your problem returns. A return of symptoms may suggest that emotional stress is a factor.

"Mouth guards by themselves do not cure the habit of clenching and grinding," says Dr. Okeson. Studies show that even after long-term use of a splint, bruxism returns when the use of the device is stopped. "To cure bruxism you also need to learn techniques to help you cope with emotional stress and to practice resting and relaxing your jaw," he says.

Good jaw relaxers include applying moist heat to muscles around your jaw for 20 minutes at a time and gently massaging those muscles.

And try to remember not to clench. "Always make sure you leave at least 2 millimeters of space (about the width of a grain of rice) between your upper and lower teeth," suggests John D. Rugh, Ph.D., professor and director of research for the dental school at the University of Texas Health Science Center at San Antonio.

At income tax time or other stressful periods you may notice that your jaw is throbbing again and your face aches. That's likely a sign that you need to step up your relaxation efforts and begin wearing your mouth guard at night again. "If you catch your soreness early on, it may only take a week or so to eliminate it," says Dr. Okeson.

CUSTOM FIT IS BEST

A custom-fitted mouth guard is better than the ready-made kind you may find in an athletic supply store, says Dr. Okeson. In addition to being uncomfortable, a poor fit could cause your teeth to shift. A knowledgeable dentist can take an impression of your teeth and tailor-fit a mouth guard for a few hundred to a few thousand dollars, depending on which kind you get.

The rigid plastic models are more expensive but are generally more durable. The flexible appliances may provide more comfort for some patients. But in some instances, the flexible kind may actually *increase* bruxism, studies show, possibly because the soft material invites chewing.

"Ideally, a mouth guard is neither so bulky that it feels uncomfortable nor so soft that you shred it," says Sheldon Gross, D.D.S., past president of the Amercian Academy of Craniomandibular Disorders.

moxibustion   A pungent odor and a trail of smoke are the distinguishing signs of this decidedly offbeat therapy from the East. Moxibustion uses the smoldering tinder (moxa) of the mugwort herb to stimulate what traditional oriental physicians regard as "energy sites" along the body.

In a typical procedure, an acupuncturist uses a burning moxa stick, which is held above the skin, or a moxa cone, which is burned on a thin disk or platform sitting directly on the skin. It's all quite painless. The patient feels warmth but no burning.

Moxibustion originated in China thousands of years ago and continues to be used there as often as needle acupuncture. The technique is being used more frequently in the West, although it is still not widespread. Interestingly, although a smokeless, electric moxa device does exist, most practitioners prefer burning the traditional herb, because they say it penetrates more deeply than electric moxa.

A BALANCING ACT

Moxibustion is based on the oriental belief that the universe is a balance of yin and yang forces. These forces are said to influence the *chi,* a kind of vital energy that's theorized to flow along 12 lines or meridians beneath the surface of the skin. According to this theory, if energy stagnates in your body or you have an imbalance of yin and yang, bad health can result.

Basically, practitioners say they use moxibustion to stimulate the movement of energy between yin and yang and to bring warmth to offset an excessive coldness. Moxa is placed at certain prescribed points—which correspond to traditional acupuncture sites—in an effort to stimulate the flow of energy, rebalance the yin and yang, and restore good health.

A thorough examination is regarded as the best way to determine whether a patient might benefit from moxibustion. The practitioner looks for signs that supposedly indicate an imbalance of heat and energy, such as a pale tongue, cold or damp skin, flaccid muscles, or a slow pulse. Moxibustion is not used if the person has high blood pressure, inflammation, or other indications of what the practitioner considers to be excess heat in the body.

What's the rule for using moxa versus needles? In the United States, needles are primarily used to treat acute pain conditions such as headaches and neuromuscular problems, while moxibustion is used for conditions that are considered to be caused by low energy or cold, such as anemia, asthma, arthritis, constipation, menstrual irregularities, and gastrointestinal ailments.

Frequently, a practitioner uses both forms. "When I treat arthritis, I use moxa to get the energy flowing and then puncture the meridians for deeper effect," says Haig Ignatius, M.D., a licensed acupuncturist and vice-president of the Traditional Acupuncture Institute in Columbia, Maryland.

Although the procedure has not been studied extensively by Western researchers, practitioners say that, in some cases, moxibustion works just like a hot compress. That is, it increases the blood flow to an area and thus stimulates healing. Also, some acupuncturists claim that the mugwort herb appears to have special healing properties and is able to stimulate the pituitary gland and immune system.

Despite the lack of hard data, there are enough positive patient testimonials to convince a growing number of health professionals that moxibustion can play a part in healing. A typical comment: "I had a severe cold and went to see my acupuncturist. He placed a moxa stick above my head and soon after, I felt alert and invigorated. My cold symptoms didn't immediately disappear, but I felt great."

If you are considering having moxibustion for any reason, look for a practitioner who has been trained properly in this technique. Choose an acupuncturist who is state licensed or licensed by the National Commission for the Certification of Acupuncturists, an accreditation board that requires three to four years of training in all aspects of acupuncture. For help locating such an acupuncturist, contact the American Association of Acupuncture and Oriental Medicine, 1424 16th Street NW, Suite 501, Washington, DC 20036.

music therapy   A crying baby hears its mother sing a lullaby. A dental patient undergoing root canal surgery listens to a Beatles tune on stereo headphones. A woman with arthritis begins taking piano lessons. Amazingly, they feel better: at peace, less apprehensive, more comfortable. They're experiencing the healing power of music.

"Music is pleasing, but it also has tremendous therapeutic value," says Arthur Harvey, a consultant with the program for arts and medicine at the University of Louisville. "When musical sounds reach the brain, they trigger changes in the immune system, the endocrine system, and the central nervous system."

Either alone or teamed with other treatments, music therapy may involve a variety of activities—playing an instrument, singing, composing, or just listening to and discussing music—to improve health.

"Music therapy is an incredibly flexible tool," says Barbara Crowe, a registered music therapist who is director of music therapy at Arizona State University in Tempe. Music can help

learning-disabled children or adults with head injuries develop basic movement, reading, and memory skills. It also can help improve a failing memory. In one study, playing a recorder or handbells helped nursing home patients improve their ability to recall. In mental health programs, music gives troubled individuals a positive, appropriate way to express emotions.

PAIN RELIEF

Many dentists routinely offer their patients music via headphones to help reduce pain and anxiety. But music isn't merely a pleasant distraction. Studies have shown that soothing music lowers pulse rate and blood pressure. And it triggers the release of beta-endorphins, pain-suppressing neurochemicals in the brain. A number of reports show that patients who listen to music before or during surgery are less apprehensive and need less pain medication or anesthetic.

A study at Southern Methodist University found that improvised music, coupled with healing visualizations, reduced pain in a woman recovering from a broken hip. The same report describes how music-mediated imagery helped people with other chronic conditions, including arthritis, diabetes, and lupus.

"As with humor, psychodrama, and other 'expressive art' therapies, more and more health professionals—doctors, nurses, physical therapists—recognize the significant impact of music on health and healing," says Dr. Harvey. At least one medical school has added music therapy instruction to its curriculum.

RECHARGE OR RELAX

You don't have to be musically gifted to take advantage of music's therapeutic potential. "By taking just 3 or 4 minutes out of your day to play selected music or put on some headphones, you can recharge your body," says Dianne Maynard Baker, R.N., a private practitioner in music intervention in Ann Arbor, Michigan. And if you're scheduled for root canal work or surgery, take along some soothing tapes.

For maximum relaxation, slow, quiet, instrumental music is best. Some experts say compositions by Baroque composers like Bach or Vivaldi are ideal. So is music played on a harp, flute, string or wind instrument, or a hammer dulcimer—"a string instrument that seems to be in tune with the body," says Baker. In any case, select music with a beat at or below your heart rate—about 60 beats per minute.

Music therapists use music that, because of its tone, meter, rhythm, pitch, and other elements, can help the healing process. So if you'd like professional guidance, contact the National Association of Music Therapists, 505 11th Street SE, Washington, DC 20003.

mustard plasters Mention mustard and most people think of that spicy yellow stuff they slather on hot dogs. But for centuries, mustard has also been slathered on the body in an attempt to spice up the healing process—specifically, to relieve muscle pain and combat chest congestion.

Instead of applying mustard straight from a jar, however, the technique uses powdered mustard seeds made into a plaster. That's an old term for a pastelike substance spread on some fabric and affixed to the skin.

If you are not fond of mixing up your own medicine in the kitchen, you can purchase plasters containing mustard at a drugstore. These products consist of an adhesive cloth impregnated with dry, powdered mustard, explains Arthur Kibbe, Ph.D., director of scientific affairs for the American Pharmaceutical Association. Liquid is added just prior to application. One type of mustard plaster, for example, is meant to be applied on the back to help relieve muscle aches.

CAN HEAT HEAL?

Is a mustard plaster really such a hot painkiller? Scientists aren't so sure. They do know that when an enzyme in mustard seed mixes with water, it turns it into an oil that feels hot on your skin. "Mustard is a rubifacient, which means it is a local irritant that reddens skin," explains Dr. Kibbe. Supposedly this local warming increases blood flow, produces a soothing feeling, and helps relieve muscle and joint aches.

In a sense, a mustard plaster is like a wireless heating pad. "The mustard plaster makes the skin feel nice and warm. And it may act as a counterirritant. That means the warm sensation blocks out the pain sensation," says James Nordlund, M.D., chairman of the Department of Dermatology at the University of Cincinnati. "Whether a mustard plaster actually heals muscle pain is unproven."

Furthermore, you probably won't find any studies to prove that a mustard plaster effectively combats colds and other respiratory ailments. Yet many natural health practitioners contend that these herbal hot packs do just that. "The warmth generated from a mustard plaster creates bronchodilation [widening of airways] and helps you breathe easier," says Tori Hudson, N.D., medical director of the National College of Naturopathic Medicine in Portland, Oregon.

Mustard plaster fans also claim that it helps stimulate the immune system and speed recovery. As the mustard heats the skin, the blood vessels open wider and flood your chest with germ-fighting white blood cells, Hudson says.

If you would like to try this time-honored remedy next time you have a cold, here's a recipe recommended by the College of Naturopathic Medicine: Mix one part dry mustard powder with three parts flour. Add the white of an egg and enough water to make a paste. Spread the paste between two layers of cloth such as a pillowcase. Put the plaster on your chest for 15 to 20 minutes. Then place a towel wrung out in cold water over your chest and cover with a wool blanket. Leave this on for 30 to 60 minutes. Wait 2 hours and apply the plaster to your back using the same process.

One warning: Never apply mustard directly to the skin—you could burn yourself. If you find that the plaster is too warm, remove it or add more flour to tone down the strength of the mustard. And don't expose the area to direct sunlight during or immediately after application.

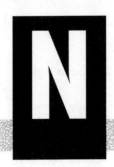

naturopathy (nay-cher-OP-a-thee) A middle-aged Seattle woman suffering from diabetes had difficulty staying on her medication, curbing her appetite for sweets, and controlling her weight. Her condition continued to worsen until her medical doctor referred her to a naturopathic physician. Soon the woman began to improve. She stuck with her medication, changed her diet, and lost weight. Best of all, her blood sugar levels began to reach favorable levels.

Just what miracle cure did the naturopathic doctor offer this woman? None. "I simply administered a number of natural, nontoxic therapies to help her better manage her condition," explains Jane Guiltinan, an N.D. (doctor of naturopathy) in private practice and clinical associate professor at Bastyr College of Naturopathy in Seattle.

By definition, naturopathic physicians are general practitioners trained as specialists in natural medicine. They are not M.D.'s, however. They treat a wide range of ailments and aim to restore health using an array of therapies that can include nutrition, herbal medicine, homeopathy, hydrotherapy, exercise, counseling, physical medicine, and acupuncture.

At the turn of the century, thousands of naturopathic physicians and nearly two dozen naturopathic medical colleges spanned the United States. When pharmaceutical and technical medicine came along and the idea that drugs could eliminate most disease swept the nation, naturopathic doctors and colleges became as rare as two-bit haircuts.

Today, naturopathic physicians are making a comeback. A thousand licensed N.D.'s are located in 25 states. Currently, there are three naturopathic colleges in North America, with a fourth that anticipates opening its doors in the mid-1990s.

ALTERNATIVE FOR SOME

Although many medical doctors regard naturopathy as an unproven approach to healing, some are more tolerant. "Naturopathy can complement conventional medicine," says Jonathan Collin, M.D., a physician in private practice in Seattle, a location where many naturopathic physicians are clustered. "You wouldn't want to go to a naturopathic physician for a pain that mysteriously crops up at age 40 or for an acute condition, such as a broken bone or a heart attack that requires advanced life support," says Dr. Collin. "But naturopathy offers a viable alternative for people who suffer from minor discomforts, chronic pain, or diseases of the respiratory or digestive tract. It's especially good for people who've been diagnosed and treated with conventional medicine with little success."

N.D.'s typically treat people with colds, minor infections, allergies, muscle and joint problems, gynecological disorders, and fatigue and other poorly defined disorders. "Often these patients have gone the medical route and want something more than harsh medications," says Dr. Guiltinan.

Philosophically, the fundamental principles of naturopathic medicine are far removed from those of mainstream medicine. "Instead of aiming to suppress symptoms, naturopaths are more concerned with finding the underlying cause of a condition and applying treaments that work with the body's natural healing mechanism instead of against it," says Dr. Guiltinan. "Naturopathy is based on the belief that, given the right tools, the body can heal itself."

Another difference, the N.D.'s claim, is that they spend more than twice as long with each patient than M.D.'s. "Teaching patients to take responsibility for their own health and how to prevent disease is a basic natur-

opathic principle," says Dr. Guiltinan. "In the case of the woman with diabetes, for example, we helped her keep a food diary and eliminate refined sugar sources from her diet. We prescribed an herbal remedy, blueberry leaf tea, to help stabilize her blood sugar and augment her medicine. We also offered counseling and biofeedback to help her cope with her disease."

To be licensed, practitioners must possess a doctor of naturopathic medicine degree from one of the recognized four-year graduate-level naturopathic medical colleges. According to a spokesman from the American Association of Naturopathic Physicians (AANP), the curriculum of the first two years at Bastyr College in Seattle and the National College of Naturopathic Medicine in Portland, Oregon, focuses on standard medical science and is modeled after traditional medical colleges. The following two years focus on a wide range of natural therapeutics. The accrediting agency for naturopathic medical programs has been recognized by the U.S. Department of Education.

DOUBTS REMAIN

The schooling may be impressive, but critics say naturopathy has a long way to go before N.D.'s will be on an equal footing with M.D.'s.

One major problem: Not everyone calling himself or herself a naturopathic doctor has received proper training. And currently less than a dozen states (mostly in the West) license practitioners. "In most states, anyone who has taken a mail-order course in herbs can hang out an N.D. shingle," says John Weeks, executive director for the AANP. The AANP supports legislation requiring licensing of N.D.'s in all states. To locate a licensed naturopath near you, contact the AANP, 2800 East Madison Street, Seattle, WA 98112.

Another concern is that naturopathic doctors employ some therapies that are scientifically unproven. It may be true that nutrition, exercise, botanical medicine, and stress management—the stock in trade of many N.D.'s—have been scientifically validated as effective treatments for certain conditions. But many other natural therapies lack the kind of scientifically controlled, clinical trials that medical doctors demand.

Currently, the research departments of the naturopathic colleges are investigating ways to carry out controlled research with multiple natural therapies. And they're hoping that efforts such as a collaborative project with Harborview Hospital in Seattle involving chronic fatigue syndrome (CFS) patients will lend scientific credibility to naturopathy. "The study will compare the use of antidepressants with natural methods such as fever/steam treatments," says Dr. Guiltinan. "CFS is possibly caused by a virus. If so, we hope to demonstrate that fever therapy inactivates the virus and supports the immune system."

niacin. *See* **cholesterol-lowering drugs; nutritional therapy**

nicotine gum Pity the suffering soul who's trying to quit smoking. All night, she moans and dreams bad dreams. All day, she grimaces, bites her nails, and obsessively clicks her ballpoint pen. Worse, she grabs junk food instead of cigarettes, gaining 30 pounds on her painful quest to be smoke free.

For many would-be quitters, giving up cigarettes is about as easy as giving up air. But nicotine gum can help you past the worst parts. Here's how.

Each piece of gum contains 2 milligrams of nicotine, which feeds your nicotine craving *without* slowly killing you with the 200 to 600 puffs of cigarette smoke that smokers inhale every day. When you're dying for a smoke, take a chew instead.

"The data are absolutely clear," says Jack E. Henningfield, Ph.D., chief of the clinical pharmacology branch of the National Institute on Drug Abuse. "People who have gotten the gum show an increase in their quitting rate and a decrease in withdrawal symptoms."

Legend has it that Mark Twain once said it was easy to give up tobacco. After all, he'd quit hundreds of times! Smokers, however, know how hard it is to *permanently* stay off cigarettes. Some heroin addicts have said it's harder to stop smoking cigarettes than to quit taking drugs, Dr. Henningfield says.

Nicotine gum eases the excruciatingly uncomfortable physical withdrawal smokers suffer soon after quitting. That means you can tackle the mental and behavioral habit first.

Once that's licked, you can take on the nicotine habit.

Of course, you'll eventually want to quit chewing, too, Dr. Henningfield says. In the meantime, "you're substituting an FDA-approved medicine for a chemical waste dump," he says.

AN AID, NOT A CURE

Nicotine gum isn't a magic cure. In one study, for example, 315 smokers were divided into two groups. One group chewed nicotine gum, while the other group chewed a nontherapeutic placebo gum. After 11 months, 10 percent of the nicotine group had stayed off cigarettes, but so had 7 percent of the placebo group—a statistically insignificant difference.

Nicotine gum seems to work best when it's part of a comprehensive stop-smoking program, with lots of social support and behavioral intervention, says Gary DeNelsky, Ph.D., head of the Department of Psychology at the Cleveland Clinic Foundation and director of the clinic's smoking cessation program.

"If you just hand a heavily addicted person a box of the gum, it isn't likely to do much good at all," Dr. DeNelsky says. The gum can, however, help you "survive" weak moments—when the telephone rings, for example, and your hand automatically dives for the pack.

"In our society, you're probably always within 5 minutes of a cigarette," Dr. Henningfield says. "All you need is one bad traffic jam to get you started again."

When you get your prescription for nicotine gum, ask your doctor how to use it. That's right—you have to learn to chew gum. For example: Chew it slowly. The nicotine in the gum is released each time you chew. To get a steady supply of nicotine, chew the gum until your mouth starts to tingle. Then "park" the gum between your cheek and gum—that's where nicotine enters your body. When the tingling stops, chew until it returns.

Don't drink and chew. Dr. Henningfield says acidic beverages such as coffee and soft drinks inhibit nicotine absorption. In the morning, chew your gum *before* you sip a cup of coffee.

Incidentally, you won't get a sudden nicotine rush if you accidentally swallow your gum. In fact, the gum doesn't produce much of a "blast" at all, Dr. Henningfield says. It's meant to be a stop-smoking aid, not a replacement addiction.

Dr. Henningfield compares nicotine gum to crutches. "Crutches don't heal your broken leg, but they help you hobble around while your body heals."

nitroglycerin   An ingredient in heavy-duty explosives, this mixture of potent chemicals is also a powerful medication for the relief and prevention of angina pain.

Angina pain is what often hits people with partially clogged coronary arteries (atherosclerosis) when they either exercise or fall prey to emotional stress. It's at these times that the heart needs the most blood, which normally comes in abundance with every beat. If, however, deposits of fatty plaque are gumming things up—o-o-o-o-o-w . . . pain.

What can nitroglycerin do? A lot. By relaxing the muscles in blood vessel walls, nitroglycerin acts to dilate both the arteries and veins. That means that more blood can flow into the arteries supplying oxygen to the heart muscle, allowing the heart to work easier and . . . a-a-a-a-h . . . the pain is gone.

An Old Champ

Just how effective is nitroglycerin? "For relieving an acute attack of angina, nothing is better," says Prakash Deedwania, M.D., clinical professor of medicine at the University of California's School of Medicine in San Francisco and chief of cardiology at Veterans Hospital in Fresno. Because of such effectiveness, the frequency of nitroglycerin's use is still on the rise—even after 100 years.

Attacking angina pain *before* it strikes is nitroglycerin's second talent. In this arena, however, nitroglycerin has competition from two modern-era medications, the so-called beta blockers and calcium channel blockers. Neither of the two new kids on the block has proven *more* effective than nitroglycerin, only *as* effective. Doctors may prescribe any one of the three or a combination, depending on the frequency of symptoms and other factors.

Whether you're taking nitroglycerin on a regular basis to prevent attacks

or on an occasional basis to relieve the pain, there's little to worry about. First-timers on nitroglycerin may initially experience headaches; however, these are usually not a problem after the first week. Otherwise, "nitroglycerin is non-addictive and has no serious side effects," says Dr. Deedwania.

Nonetheless, the medication is sold by prescription only. It comes in various forms, including pills, patches, ointments, and nasal sprays. Which one is best for you is something you'll need to discuss with your doctor.

Use It Wisely

Most commonly, nitroglycerin is prescribed as a little pill that you slip under your tongue. It dissolves quickly and, if you're in pain, should provide relief within 5 to 10 minutes. The pills may also be taken before engaging in activities that are known to bring on angina attacks. Nothing could be simpler, but many patients don't use their little pills as they should, says Dr.

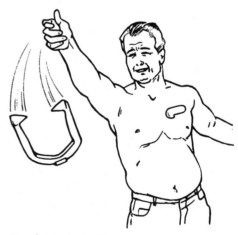

Nitroglycerin chest patch

Deedwania. For them, wearing a transdermal patch that delivers nitroglycerin through the skin continuously for hours at a time may be a handier alternative.

One common mistake is to hoard old pills. "You should renew your prescription at least every three to six months, particularly if the bottle has been opened," says Dr. Deedwania. Beyond six months, the pills tend to lose their effectiveness. To protect nitroglycerin, you should store it in the amber bottle it came in, with the lid tightly closed. Be careful not to keep cotton in the bottle or to mix nitroglycerin with other drugs. It can vaporize or be absorbed into other materials.

If your nitroglycerin is still potent, it should dissolve rapidly with a distinct tingle in your mouth. *See also* **beta blockers; calcium channel blockers**

NSAIDs. *See* **anti-inflammatories**

nuclear medicine. *See* **radiation therapy**

Nuprin. *See* **ibuprofen**

nutritional therapy Everybody and every body needs vitamins and minerals. Ignore your Recommended Dietary Allowance (RDA), and you invite a host of problems, such as anemia, scurvy, and beriberi. But too much of a good thing can be as bad as nothing at all. In large doses, certain vitamins and minerals can be toxic.

There is, however, a middle ground. Below the toxic level, but sometimes above and well beyond the RDA, nutrients may be used to prevent and treat some diseases. But this middle ground is a hazy one, says Sheldon Saul Hendler, M.D., Ph.D., a faculty member at the University of California Medical School in San Diego and author of *The Doctors' Vitamin and Mineral Encyclopedia.* Even the experts are unclear as to whether vitamins and minerals in large quantities should be handled as nutrients or as drugs, he says.

Here's a brief look at just a few of the scientific findings. (Please remember that because nutrients are a double-edged sword—too much can be as dangerous as too little—you should check with your doctor before starting any supplement program.)

VITAMIN A

Let's begin our look at nutrition therapy with a common affliction: wounds. Perhaps you've cut yourself with a kitchen knife or burnt your hand trying to light the candles on your daughter's birthday cake. Studies suggest that vitamin A might be able to speed your recovery. And unlike many of the other vitamin therapies discussed here, the healing effect of vitamin A on wounds may be available *without* a need to turn to supplements, researchers say. A review of numerous studies, published in the *Journal of the American Academy of Dermatology,* concludes that vitamin A is especially important for people with wounds who are taking steroid drugs. Steroids are often prescribed to control inflammation, but they also make skin slower to heal. Steroids or no steroids, this might be the time for you to start eating a diet rich in vitamin A that includes carrots, squash, yams, cantaloupe, and leafy green vegetables.

Further testimony to the power of vitamin A comes in the area of cancer control. A few studies suggest that vitamin A may help heal precancerous sores in the mouth called leukoplakias. In one study, 17 people with leukoplakias took 30 milligrams of extra beta-carotene (a source of vitamin A) each day for three months. Of the 17 people, 2 saw all their sores vanish, and another 12 said goodbye to many. Normally, only 5 percent of such sores disappear on their own. Eating carrots, squash, and other foods high in beta-carotene may offer protection against a number of cancers (including lung cancer), says Shirley Brown, M.D., a co-principal investigator with San Francisco's Preventive Medicine Research Institute and a clinical instructor of medicine at the University of California in San Francisco. "I'd like to see people getting more."

Vitamin A may also have a role to play against a particularly annoying childhood infection. When measles-afflicted kids in South Africa were given large doses (120 milligrams) of vitamin A, they got better faster and spent fewer days in the hospital than did those who were given no supplements. The added vitamin also reduced the incidence of lethal complications.

VITAMIN B₆

If you're a typist, an assembly-line worker, a carpenter, or anyone who does repetitive tasks using the wrists, you may be susceptible to carpal tunnel syndrome, a pinching of the major nerve running through the wrist. Vitamin B_6 might help. Many doctors prescribe it to ease carpal tunnel pain. Patients who respond best are those starting off with some deficiency in the vitamin. If you've had pain and numbness in your hands, you may have carpal tunnel syndrome. See your doctor. And don't be surprised if B_6 is part of your treatment.

Have you ever winced from the pain of passing a kidney stone? If that stone resulted from your body's inability to assimilate oxalic acid (a substance found in many foods), B_6 might have been able to help. Research shows that B_6 reduces the amount of oxalate in the urine and so tends to prevent new stone formation. Sorry, B_6 can't dissolve any stones you may already have formed, and it's not a cure for all kinds of kidney stones. But if your doctor judges you to be a good candidate, B_6 may be prescribed to ward off future stones.

In addition, some studies have suggested that B_6 may help in the control of some forms of diabetes, relieve some of the symptoms of premenstrual tension, help in some forms of infertility, and protect against some forms of cancer, says Dr. Hendler.

FOLATE

This B-complex vitamin comes naturally in citrus fruits, leafy green vegetables, broccoli, whole grains, and liver. One established medical role for folate is as a treatment for two kinds of anemia—the kinds doctors call mega-loblastic and sickle cell anemia. In sickle cell, added folate may help the bone marrow produce more red blood cells. But folate is not a self-treatment for these anemias, cautions Jeanne A. Smith, M.D., anemia specialist at New York City's Harlem Hospital. Some types of megaloblastic anemia are caused by a vitamin B_{12} deficiency. Your doctor has to monitor you to make sure folate supplementation isn't merely masking those symptoms without getting at the cause. Folate supplementation can also mask another kind of anemia, called pernicious anemia.

Folate may help brighten the day for people with clinically diagnosed depression. Scientists have long suspected that some cases of depression, and schizophrenia as well, may be linked to folate deficiency. New evidence suggests that folate supplementation can speed recovery from these mental disorders in some cases.

Of 123 patients diagnosed with either major depression or schizophrenia at an English hospital, 41 (one-third) were found to have some degree of folate deficiency. The researchers gave half of these deficient patients a daily dose of 15 milligrams of methylfolate (the form of folate that most readily crosses into the brain), while they continued to receive standard drug treatment. Over six months, these patients showed significantly more improvement than those folate-deficient patients who did not get the vitamin. The researchers say that "curing" the folate deficiency seems to have enhanced the effect of the drugs rather than hav-

ing a direct therapeutic effect itself. The dose of folate used in this study was far above the RDA.

Research suggests that folate supplementation (again, far above the RDA) may help rescue some people from the harsh side effects of methotrexate, a powerful drug used for rheumatoid arthritis. If you're taking this drug, talk to your doctor about these findings.

NIACIN

Did your last cholesterol test yield a number so high that it sounded like a professional bowling score? Niacin treatment may become part of your doctor's game plan for bringing that number down.

One form of this B vitamin, a form called nicotinic acid, is "abruptly coming to be regarded as one of the substances of choice for lowering blood levels of cholesterol, edging out multi-million dollar drugs that were designed for that purpose but which do the job less well," says Dr. Hendler.

Physicians were first clued in to niacin's potential when they looked at an old study—the Coronary Drug Project, begun in 1966. Among 8,300 men who'd had heart attacks, only those who took niacin to lower cholesterol (out of four drugs tested) had fewer nonfatal heart attacks over five years. And 15 years after the start of the study, the doctors found 11 percent fewer deaths in the niacin takers. Since this study, no other cholesterol-lowering agent has been found to help people live longer.

Niacin is found in enriched or

whole grain breads and cereals, meats, and poultry. But the amount needed to battle cholesterol is well above what you're likely to get in your diet—"unless you consume about 200,000 calories a day!" says Dr. Hendler. In any case, niacin supplements—like all supplements—should only be taken under a doctor's supervision.

VITAMIN C

You're not alone if you take vitamin C—it's the most popular nutritional supplement on the market. And for some very good reasons. Among them is C's apparent ability to, if not prevent, at least calm the common cold. A number of studies suggest that taking vitamin C supplements can cut the time you'll suffer from a cold by more than a third, says Dr. Hendler. Scientific evidence also suggests that your cold will be less severe.

Researchers at the University of Wisconsin studied 16 men who initially had nearly identical vitamin C levels. They gave half of them 500 milligrams of additional vitamin C four times a day and the other half a placebo (a blank pill). Then they put the men in a dormitory for a week with eight other volunteers who had been infected with a cold virus. The 16 men continued their vitamin C or placebo treatment for two weeks afterward.

The cold facts? Seven of the eight men in the placebo group caught colds, while six of those taking vitamin C fell victim. No significant difference here. But there was a big difference between the two groups in the severity of their colds. The men who didn't take C had a much nastier time with their colds than the men who did. Compared to the vitamin C group, there were three times as many aaah-choos, twice as many coughs, and almost twice as many nose-blowing episodes in the placebo group.

Blood pressure also seems to be affected by vitamin C. A study at the Medical College of Georgia, in Augusta, found an association between high levels of vitamin C in the blood and lower blood pressure. Researchers looked at the vitamin C status of 67 men and women (blood levels are a good indication of dietary vitamin C intake) and found that those with high levels of C had lower blood pressure than those with low C levels.

The researchers aren't sure whether a low level of vitamin C actually *causes* a rise in blood pressure. Lower vitamin C intake could simply be a sign of a less healthful diet overall, which can influence blood pressure. "We can't draw any conclusions yet," says Paul F. Jacques, Sc.D., an epidemiologist at Tufts University, where research has yielded similar results. "But the association . . . certainly deserves further investigation."

Surely, vitamin C research will continue on several fronts. This nutrient is recognized as a possible protective agent against various kinds of cancer. Evidence suggests that supplementing with vitamin C can shorten the healing time of tooth extractions and perhaps other kinds of wounds as well. There is also evidence that supplemental vitamin C may help counteract asthma, prevent diabetes, combat gum disease, and help manage certain mental disorders, like manic-depression, says Dr. Hendler. Research has even shown that vitamin C can help the body rid itself of alcohol. And, finally, vitamin C might restore fertility in some men. It's virtually impossible for conception to occur with men whose sperm clump together. In two separate studies, researchers found that vitamin C broke up these clumps, restoring fertility.

Foods high in vitamin C include citrus fruits, strawberries, cantaloupe, broccoli, cabbage, potatoes, peppers, and tomatoes. In contrast to the case with many vitamins, most doctors would probably not object to your taking vitamin C supplements in moderate, but higher-than-RDA, amounts. "I'd say you could go as high as 1 gram (1,000 milligrams) a day, or 2 grams a day when you have a cold, without any danger," says Dr. Hendler.

Vitamin E

Found in vegetable oils, green leafy vegetables, wheat germ, and nuts, vitamin E is currently under study as a possible preventive and therapeutic aid against cancer, heart disease, cataracts, and Parkinson's disease. Final answers are not yet in, but the preliminary data are hard to ignore.

In one study, 14 Parkinson's patients who reported taking vitamin E daily for an average of seven years were compared to a similar group not taking vitamin E. When rated for severity of 41 signs and symptoms, including tremors, rigidity, slowness, and impaired walking and balance, the vita-

min E users were found to have significantly fewer problems than nonusers.

"This evidence does seem to indicate that vitamin E may help prevent Parkinson's and reduce the severity," says researcher Stewart Factor, D.O., of Albany Medical College. "But it's important to keep in mind that the studies were small."

Some women use vitamin E as an aid for symptoms of both premenstrual syndrome (PMS) and menopause. Robert London, M.D., of the Johns Hopkins School of Medicine, says that his research suggests that vitamin E may help relieve a cluster of bothersome PMS symptoms. Relief of hot flashes seems more elusive. Dr. London says women should see a physician before self-prescribing vitamin E for that purpose.

Research also suggests that vitamin E may benefit patients experiencing a powerful side effect from antipsychotic medications. The nutrient may diminish the severity of tardive dyskinesia, an often irreversible condition characterized by abnormal involuntary muscle spasms, usually in the face and fingers.

Calcium

This mineral has a deserved reputation as the nutrient that builds strong bones and teeth—but let's not be guilty of typecasting. Calcium also deserves attention for its effect on blood pressure. Not too long ago, most researchers weren't sure what that effect was. In some studies, calcium helped people lower their blood pressure. In others, it did nothing. In yet others, it *raised* blood pressure!

With a bit more research, it came to light that calcium seems to benefit only those who are sensitive to salt. That is, if your blood pressure rises in response to increased salt intake, calcium may be more likely to lower it. One small study from the New York Hospital–Cornell University Medical Center seems to support this. The results showed calcium had no effect on anyone whose salt intake was low. But when salt intake was high, two things happened: Calcium blunted the blood pressure rise in salt-sensitive patients but slightly increased the blood pressure of patients who were not salt sensitive. If you have high blood pressure, you should be under a doctor's care. If it's determined that you are salt sensitive, calcium therapy might help.

If you're a woman suffering premenstrual woes, you may also wish to discuss calcium with your doctor. Researchers at New York Medical College tested calcium supplementation in 33 premenstrual syndrome sufferers for six months. Seventy-two percent of the women reported significant relief. They had less pain, less water retention, and fewer mood swings during ovulation. And they had less pain during the actual time of their menstruation.

And what's the latest evidence to support calcium's role in maintaining strong bones? In one study, women whose lifetime dietary calcium intake averaged about 1,000 milligrams per day (200 milligrams above the RDA) had 60 to 75 percent fewer hip fractures than women consuming half that amount. Another study showed that both men and women over 60 years old who consumed more than 765 milligrams of calcium daily had a hip fracture rate that was 60 percent lower than people who got less than 470 milligrams.

The best dietary sources of calcium include low-fat and skim milk, buttermilk, low-fat yogurt, and cheese. Broccoli, collards, kale, and turnip greens are also rich in calcium, as are fish such as canned salmon and mackerel when eaten with the bones.

CHROMIUM

The latest look at this mineral suggests you might want to heap the pasta a bit higher and skip that sugary dessert. Such a balancing act at dinnertime may help millions of people with early signs of diabetes, researchers speculate. Their speculation is fueled by a study of the effects of chromium on 17 people, 8 of whom had mild glucose intolerance. This condition, which is characterized by unusually large swings in blood sugar, can progress to diabetes. For five weeks, half the people took chromium supplements (200 micrograms a day, which is officially regarded as the "safe and adequate" intake), and the other half took blank pills. (Americans normally consume an average of just 30 micrograms of chromium a day.) Then they switched pills for five more weeks. In 7 of the 8 glucose-intolerant people, spikes in blood glucose levels after a sugary drink were only half as high while on chromium as when they were unsupplemented.

The researchers believe that adequate chromium could prevent most—

but not all—cases of mild glucose intolerance from progressing to Type II (adult-onset) diabetes. Getting adequate chromium doesn't mean you have to eat more of the mineral or take chromium supplements. You just need to consume fewer chromium depleters (items containing simple sugars, like cookies, pastries, and candy) and more chromium preservers (complex carbohydrates such as found in pasta and potatoes).

MAGNESIUM

"I think the most exciting of all the minerals right now is magnesium. Practically every week there's another paper on its benefits," says Dr. Hendler. These scientific papers touch on some important areas of health, such as heart disease and high blood pressure.

Magnesium is a shocker among nutrients in that up to 90 percent of us may not get our RDA. There's evidence that the 10 percent of us who *do* get our share may be among the healthiest people around. For instance, surveys show that people living in areas where there's lots of magnesium in the drinking water have fewer deposits of fatty plaque in their arteries. Those deposits can lead to heart disease.

Of course, low plaque buildup in areas with high-magnesium water may be due to something other than magnesium. But researchers seem fairly certain that they're on to something. Meanwhile, scientists have raised another possibility: Low magnesium may increase the severity of a heart attack—that is, the number of heart cells that die during the heart attack. Animals

low in magnesium tend to accumulate calcium in heart cells. And during a heart attack, these cells accumulate still more calcium—enough to damage them, studies show.

"If this happens in humans, too, it means low magnesium makes you more likely to die if you have a heart attack," says Sherman Bloom, M.D., of the University of Mississippi, author of some of these studies.

Low magnesium may also be linked to high blood pressure, a major risk factor for heart attack and stroke. At Harvard Medical School and Brigham and Women's Hospital in Boston, researchers looked at diet and blood pressure in more than 58,000 women. Magnesium intake, researchers found, had an inverse association with blood pressure: Women consuming little magnesium developed more high blood pressure than did women getting lots of magnesium. Several other studies have confirmed this.

In Germany, researchers who looked at long-distance runners and bodybuilders advised that dietary supplementation with magnesium may help prevent muscle spasms. German researchers also gave supplements of magnesium to over 500 expectant mothers and noted a decrease in premature labor, heftier babies, and a drop in the number of birth-related problems.

Adequate intake of magnesium may also help prevent certain kinds of kidney stones, reduce the pain of menstrual cramps, assist in the treatment of some cases of arrhythmia (irregular heartbeat), and possibly ward off migraine headaches. Magnesium-rich foods include whole grain cereals, legumes, and many fruits and vegetables.

POTASSIUM

A banana at breakfast may help give high cholesterol the slip. And a baked potato at dinner may help take the steam out of high blood pressure. That's the suggestion of a study on the effects of the mineral potassium, which is abundant in these foods.

The researchers discovered this possible potassium bonus when they divided 37 men and women with mild high blood pressure into three groups. One group took 2,340 milligrams of potassium daily (slightly more than the estimated minimum requirement) in supplements. Another group took that amount plus magnesium, while another took a non-therapeutic placebo. After eight weeks, the two potassium groups' blood pressure plunged, compared to the placebo group's. Their cholesterol also took a nosedive compared to the placebo group. Those taking both potassium and magnesium, however, didn't do any better than those taking potassium alone.

"Strong evidence from a number of studies suggests that a diet low in potassium may lead to high blood pressure," says George Webb, Ph.D., associate professor of physiology and biophysics at the University of Vermont College of Medicine. And some studies have suggested that taking extra potassium may help lower blood pressure. But this is the first study in humans that seems to suggest that getting enough potassium may also help cut cholesterol—another heart disease risk factor.

Potassium may also reduce the risk of death from strokes. In one 12-year study of 850 Californians, a 400-milligram increase in daily potassium intake—that's about one additional banana or glass of orange juice a day—was associated with a 40 percent reduction in the risk of stroke-related deaths. At least three studies have confirmed these results.

Other foods high in potassium include tomatoes, broccoli, watermelon, and dried apricots.

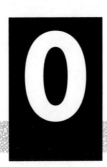

oatmeal, colloidal Sink your spoon into a bowl of oatmeal and you'll be giving your insides a health boost. But sink into a bathtub filled with finely ground powdered oatmeal—called colloidal oatmeal—and you might help soothe your itchy skin.

"An oatmeal bath is a cheap, handy home remedy for many dermatological irritations," says Paul Lazar, M.D., clinical professor of dermatology at Northwestern University in Chicago and author of *The Look You Like.* "For conditions such as poison ivy, for example, oatmeal can calm itchiness with the same effectiveness as calamine lotion."

It's not that there is some special chemical or enzyme in oatmeal that makes it such a great grain for relieving irritated skin, says Dr. Lazar. "Oatmeal's therapeutic value simply lies in its ability to hold water," he explains. When oatmeal comes in contact with water, it puffs up and forms a slimy gel that holds the moisture next to your skin. The water is absorbed by the skin's top layer, soothing any burning and itchiness. Oats also contain a small amount of oil, which helps seal in the water, making your skin more supple. "The effect is the same as a mild moisturizer," says Dr. Lazar.

Just don't try dumping your favorite oat cereal into your tub—you'll wind up with a clumpy, gummy mess. "In order to be therapeutic in the bath, oats must be ground into fine, colloidal oatmeal powder, which will disperse throughout the water and form a thin water-holding coating on your skin," says Thomas Gossel, Ph.D., chairman of the Department of Clinical Pharmacy at Ohio Northern University in Ada.

Fortunately, you don't have to grind the grain yourself. The well-known commercial colloidal oatmeal bath product, Aveeno, is a readily dispersible powder consisting of finely ground whole oats. Aveeno also makes an oilated bath treatment (containing mineral oil as well as colloidal oatmeal) that provides a better protective barrier on the skin. In addition, Aveeno cleansing bars are sometimes recommended as a soap substitute for sensitive or extremely dry skin conditions.

How well do these oatmeal products work? More than 25 years ago, researchers found that colloidal oatmeal baths taken twice daily helped relieve contact dermatitis, prickly heat, eczema, and other itchy, dry skin conditions. Despite the lack of updated studies, doctors continue to recommend colloidal oatmeal preparations for skin problems.

Chickenpox heads the list. "Twice-daily colloidal baths are helpful for patients with chickenpox because they are nonirritating and soothing. In addition there is a slight anti-inflammatory effect," says Lawrence Charles Parish, M.D., clinical professor of dermatology at Jefferson Medical College in Philadelphia.

If an itchy, red rash is driving you to distraction, make a beeline for your bathtub, suggests Fredric Haberman, M.D., medical director of the Affiliated Dermatology and Plastic Surgery Center in Saddle Brook, New Jersey, and New York City and author of *The Doctor's Beauty Hotline*. Here is Dr. Haberman's recommendation for itchy rashes: First run warm water into the bathtub. As the tub is filling, add a colloidal oatmeal product. (For even dispersion, use a flour sifter). Then get into the tub and soak. After about 20 minutes, get out and pat your skin dry with a clean, soft towel. Afterward, apply an over-the-counter 0.5 percent hydrocortisone cream to affected areas. The cream can be reapplied every 4 hours if necessary.

Remember not to oversoak. "Frequent bathing may further dry out and irritate your skin no matter what you add to the bathwater," notes Joseph Bark, M.D., chairman of dermatology at St. Joseph's Hospital in Lexington, Kentucky.

Ask your doctor for more advice on taking colloidal oatmeal baths for your specific skin condition. If you get the go-ahead, just be sure to take it easy getting in and out of the bathtub—oatmeal mixed with water can create a slippery coating on tub surfaces.

oil of wintergreen What do many throat sprays and liniment rubs and some toothpastes have in common? They feel tingly—either in your mouth or on your skin. That's because these products often contain an oil distilled from the wintergreen bush.

Oil of wintergreen gets its zippy odor and taste from methyl salicylate, its main ingredient. "This substance has the unique ability to make your skin feel hot and cold at the same time," says Thomas Gossel, Ph.D., chairman of the Department of Clinical Pharmacy at Ohio Northern University in Ada. That's why it's often the active ingredient in those "deep-penetrating" rubs used for temporary relief of arthritis and minor aches and pains.

If you have sore muscles and don't mind the strong medicinal smell, a massage that includes wintergreen's active ingredient might be worthwhile.

"Some patients tell me these massages produce significant relief from backache and neck pain," reports Brian

Bowyer, M.D., assistant professor of physical medicine at Ohio State University. "The methyl salicylate dilates [widens] blood vessels, which increases blood flow and produces a sensation of warmth, which helps promote relaxation," says Dr. Bowyer.

Still another theory—which might explain oil of wintergreen's soothing effect on swollen, sore joints—comes from James Nordlund, M.D., chairman of the Department of Dermatology at the University of Cincinnati. "Methyl salicylate is absorbed into the tissues in very low levels. And since it has aspirin-like properties [aspirin is acetylsalicylic acid], these rubs may act as a painkiller and anti-inflammatory at the site of pain," says Dr. Nordlund.

More than likely, however, methyl salicylate's benefits may simply stem from the fact that it acts as a counterirritant. "The pleasant cool and warm sensations crowd out the pain sensation," says Dr. Nordland.

USE WITH CARE

If you are aching to try one of these products containing oil of wintergreen or its main ingredient, you should follow some precautions. Methyl salicylate can be absorbed rapidly through the skin, says Dr. Nordland, so apply the rubs in thin layers. With each layer of application, the effect becomes more pronounced. Three layers, for example, would probably give you a very strong effect.

Never cover a rubbed area with a heating pad or anything except your normal clothing. You could increase the absorption of methyl salicylate and severely burn and blister your skin. And stay out of direct sunshine.

If you do have to bandage or wrap an area, it's recommended that you wash the area after the rub has penetrated to avoid excessive skin irritation. (Washing will not take away the effectiveness of the rub, but it will take away the strong odor.) And don't use these products at all if you are allergic to aspirin.

A final reminder: Never use pure oil of wintergreen directly on your skin. And never drink the stuff. Manufacturers use minute amounts of this minty-tasting oil to flavor food, drinks, and breath products. "But swallowing what seems like a small amount, less than 1 teaspoon, could be toxic or even fatal," says Dr. Gossel. Keep the kids away from oil of wintergreen products.

olive oil.   *See* **monounsaturated oils**

onions   This vegetable was once the breakfast of Olympians? Considered a symbol of the universe? So revered that its very presence prompted the people of central Asia to build temples wherever it bloomed?

Yes, such is the charmed history of the onion. As a member of the allium plant family, its closest relatives are garlic, scallions, and leeks. But the onion alone can make you cry.

Here's news that could dry those tears: Sulfur compounds in onions similar to those that make your eyes water may also bestow some important health benefits. Recently, the onion has attracted attention for its cancer-fighting potential. Some researchers suspect this vegetable may also be capable of keeping your arteries clear, and there are even hints it can fend off asthma attacks.

"I think the results are encouraging in all these areas," says Eric Block, Ph.D., chairman of the chemistry department at the State University of New York at Albany and an expert on the chemistry of onions and garlic. He says the National Cancer Institute has even targeted a nationwide study to see what the effects are when onions are made a regular part of the diet.

Who knows? The glory days may return for this humble denizen of your pantry.

LESS STOMACH CANCER

The clearest link between the onion and human health comes from Chinese researchers, who compared a group of 564 stomach cancer sufferers to a group of 1,131 healthy people. They found that people who reported eating the greatest amount of onions, garlic, scallions, and Chinese chives were the least likely to have stomach cancer. The people who indulged the most in those vegetables had only 40 percent of the risk for stomach cancer as people who rarely ate them.

Laboratory studies show that those sulfur compounds in onions slow the rate at which selected tumors grow and multiply. Onion oil was found to be even more potent than garlic oil against a specific tumor-producing chemical that New York University

Medical School researchers dabbed on the skin of mice.

Scientists don't know exactly how the onion compounds fight tumors, says Sidney Belman, Ph.D., author of that study. But the principal mechanism appears to be the same whether the onion is battling tumors, artery disease, or asthma attacks, according to Dr. Block. In short, the sulfur compounds block extra oxygen from being introduced to the cells. And this affects the manufacture of prostaglandins, naturally occurring substances that govern processes like inflammation and blood clotting.

Certain cancer-causing substances elevate prostaglandin levels in the body. In the New York University Medical School study on mice, the onion chemicals countered this effect.

HEART BENEFITS?

Because the onion has anticlotting properties, it may also turn out to be an ally in the fight against heart disease. In scientific studies, onions have consistently enhanced fibrinolytic activity, the blood's ability to break up dangerous clots that lead to heart attacks.

Pound for pound, garlic is actually five times more potent than onions when it comes to inhibiting blood platelets from forming clots. But that difference may not count for much when you consider people's eating habits, says Amar Makeja, Ph.D., a professor of biochemistry and molecular biology at George Washington University Medical School who has studied these effects. "Every salad bar, for example, has onions. But you don't see garlic offered. Obviously, people eat more onions than garlic."

Onions may boost HDL cholesterol levels, too. HDLs (high-density lipoproteins) are the "good guys" that cart off excess cholesterol to the liver, where it's reprocessed or removed from the body. In a Boston study, 50 cardiovascular patients who consumed onion oil equivalent to one medium onion a day for a year showed higher levels of HDL and enhanced fibrinolytic activity, says Isabella Lipinska, Ph.D., a researcher with the Institute for the Prevention of Cardiovascular Disease of New England Deaconess Hospital.

Up until now, we've been talking largely about properties shared by both onions and garlic. But onions stand on their own as a potential anti-asthma agent. Researchers in Germany have identified several substances in onions that they believe interfere with prostaglandins in a way that heads off an asthma attack. In a study of laboratory animals who were challenged with an asthma-aggravating substance, the protective effects of this chemical lasted 12 hours.

Unfortunately, you'd have to eat about 15 pounds of onions to get enough of the chemical to produce this effect, Dr. Block calculates. The findings are still very preliminary. But an onion-based asthma drug is conceivable in the future.

Given all of the available evidence, might boiled onions, onion soup, and onion-rich salads be healthful additions to your diet?

Absolutely, agree Dr. Belman, Dr. Lipinska, and Dr. Makeja.

Cooked onions will be kinder to your stomach than raw. "You'll still get the HDL and anticlotting benefits, although you'll lose the antibacterial effects," Dr. Lipinska says.

You might do best of all by eating onions with your favorite fatty foods. Try onion soup as an appetizer for a meal featuring a roast, for example. Studies in India suggest that when you eat onions with fats like butter, you won't get as much of a rise in blood fat levels as you would had you eaten the butter alone, Dr. Makeja says.

If you want to cut those onions without irritating your eyes, put the cutting board in your sink and run water on the onion as you slice it. The chemical that causes the tears is soluble in water. *See also* **garlic**

orthoses   Move over, corrective shoes. Orthoses are taking over.

These custom-fit, prescription inserts for shoes are designed to improve your walk. Podiatrists say they can alleviate foot, knee, and lower back pain.

Don't confuse orthoses (sometimes called orthotics) with ordinary insoles. Insoles can provide extra cushioning, a plus for people whose feet are too rigid to wear an orthosis or for those who, as a result of the aging process, don't have much of a fat pad left to protect the underside of their feet, says Ellen Cohen-Sobel, D.P.M., Ph.D., assistant professor of orthopedics at the New York College of Podiatric Medicine in Manhattan. But off-the-rack insoles don't offer support specific to your type of foot.

Orthoses do. They're created from a cast impression of your feet. They incorporate the corrections a podiatrist finds necessary after analyzing the way you walk. Most are made from thermal plastics.

They offer two big advantages over corrective shoes: One is that you can switch them from shoe to shoe, provided they fit. (Women may need separate orthoses for their high heels and flats.) This means you get custom-fit support without sacrificing fashion. But the fundamental difference is this: Podiatrists say that orthoses enhance movement; most corrective shoes work by limiting movement.

"Corrective shoes do stop the pain, but it's like putting a cast on the foot," says Howard Dananberg, D.P.M., co-founder of The Walking Clinic in Bedford, New Hampshire. "Because the foot no longer moves, muscles

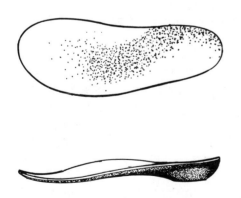

Orthosis (top and side view)

become weak. So people who wear corrective footwear long enough can become addicted to it. They can't do without it.

"The point of an orthosis is to position the foot so it can support itself," he says. "If you help the foot move correctly, it will use the weight of the body to strengthen itself."

HEEL PAIN EASED

Experts say orthoses are great for relieving heel pain, thanks to their cushioning and shock absorption action. Dr. Cohen-Sobel says they also prevent aggravation of existing corns, calluses, and bunions.

They also correct a common condition, functional hallux limitus (FHL), which Dr. Dananberg feels may be at the root of many ailments. Here's what happens: The ball of the foot temporarily locks instead of flexing, preventing the normal dissipation of the power of the stride. According to Dr. Dananberg, this faulty release of power forces the body to adjust through the skeleton. The gradually resulting poor posture, he says, can lead to pain in the knees, back, and even the jaw.

Are orthoses forever? Sometimes yes, sometimes no. Some people wear them for six months to two years, then take them out and never have pain again, Dr. Dananberg says. This is often the case when an injury has aggravated feet that were already vulnerable because the individual wasn't walking right. By correcting the original problem, orthoses can speed healing of the injury and prevent a recurrence.

A drawback with orthoses is that their cost is not covered by some medical insurers. It can cost you anywhere from $250 to $600 for a diagnosis and creation of your orthoses. *See also* **shoes, therapeutic**

osteopathy (os-tee-OP-ah-thee) In many ways, you'd be hard-pressed to spot the differences between an osteopath (D.O.) and a medical doctor (M.D.). Their training is similar. So is the amount of time they spend in school and the number of classes they take. D.O.'s, like M.D.'s, are physicians who are licensed to practice medicine and surgery in all 50 states. In fact, they often specialize in the same areas—such as internal medicine, neurosurgery, and urology. So when you step inside an osteopath's examination room, you can expect him or her to do the same things an M.D. might—whether it's prescribing medication, ordering a scan, or simply whacking your knee with a rubber hammer.

What the osteopath also may do— and here is where they begin to differ from medical doctors—is take a close look at your body *structure*—at the relationship between your posture, bones, and muscles and the way those interact to affect your overall health.

"We feel that any human body that is structurally in normal alignment is better able to combat disease than one that is not," says Joseph W. Stella, D.O., past president of the American Osteopathic Association and vice president for medical education at the Allentown (Pennsylvania) Osteopathic Medical Center. "We don't say proper alignment cures disease," Dr. Stella adds. "We say it helps."

TWO SPECIAL TOOLS

To help keep people healthy and in alignment, osteopaths often use two hands-on techniques: palpation along with manipulation. Here's how they work.

Palpation. Plan on getting touched—maybe a little, maybe a whole lot—when you visit an osteopath. Osteopaths call this touching and probing palpation; *you* might call it looking for trouble spots. Osteopaths are trained to feel for external signs—damp skin, tight muscles, a restricted range of motion—that indicate internal or external problems, says Richard Bachrach, D.O., an adjunct professor at the New York College of Osteopathy in New York City.

Where you hurt isn't necessarily where the problems are, Dr. Stella says. For example, your gallbladder is under the liver and to the front of your body, but gallbladder *pain* may appear under the right shoulder blade, he explains.

Researchers have found that some conditions—for example, an acute or impending myocardial infarction (heart attack)—consistently may be discovered by palpation. (The infarction causes a tightening of the upper back muscles.) It's very unlikely, of course, that an osteopath would diagnose a heart attack only by palpation. "We would diagnose it by a cardiogram, lab work, and so on," Dr. Stella says. "The palpation may only be of *assistance* in making the diagnosis."

Manipulation. Used to restore functional alignment, this osteopathic option helps improve the movement of blood, lymph, and nerve impulses throughout your body, Dr. Bachrach says. If tight muscles in your back compress nerve fibers, for example, signals may be blocked from reaching their destinations. By relieving the tightness, osteopathic manipulation can help reduce the pressure on the nerve, which allows your body's signals to get where they need to go.

There are many types of manipulation. The doctor may relax the muscles around your spine to help give vertebrae a normal range of motion. Or he may press rhythmically against your chest, to stimulate the flow of lymphatic fluids throughout your body.

Osteopathic treatment doesn't necessarily stop there, of course. You may still need surgery, a prescription, or a week in bed, Dr. Stella says. But a pair of sensitive, well-trained hands can help. "Any condition other than an out-and-out fracture will benefit from osteopathic manipulation," he claims.

oxygen therapy Imagine trying to breathe through a flattened straw and you'll have an idea of how difficult it is to take in air if you have emphysema or some other type of chronic obstructive pulmonary disease (COPD). Constantly being short of breath can make you move as slow as a turtle and leave your limbs numb, your head muddled, and your spirits low. Your heart strains as even a stroll to the end of the driveway feels as though you are hiking up Mount McKinley.

Studies have shown that supplemental oxygen given on a continuous basis eases the strain on the heart and helps get the needed oxygen to the brain and body so COPD patients can think better, move better, and sleep better. Moreover, full-time oxygen therapy prolongs life.

Until recently, COPD sufferers had no choice but to stick close to their oxygen tanks—big clunky cylinders filled with compressed oxygen. These tanks look like the cylinders used to fill helium balloons and weigh as much as a full-grown man.

If they needed to venture outside, they could use a smaller, baby-sized "transfer" tank, filled with oxygen from the bigger tank. On the downside, these 10-pound take-along tanks only carry enough oxygen to last 2 hours. As for the bigger cylinder, it only holds about 24 hours' worth of oxygen, which means refills must be delivered daily.

But newer oxygen "concentrator" devices eliminate the need for daily refills. These electronic plug-in devices, which are about the size of a TV console, use filters to sieve nitrogen from the air, leaving behind relatively pure oxygen. Because these models continually manufacture a fresh oxygen supply, they are a lot cheaper than buying compressed oxygen. The concentrators also can be equipped with long oxygen tubing so patients can move around the house. A smaller version can be taken along in the car or plane to be plugged in at a hotel.

PORTABILITY BREAKTHROUGH

The biggest boon for the breathing impaired, though, has been portable liquid oxygen tanks. These Thermos-type units and their refills contain up to a seven-day supply of cooled oxygen.

Smaller devices fitted with shoulder straps are called "strollers" or "liberators." These strollers are filled from the larger reservoirs and may last a few hours to all day, depending on how much oxgyen you use. Control knobs adjust the flow rate of oxgyen as needed.

As with all supplemental oxygen tanks, oxygen is delivered through the nose by a set of double clear plastic tubes called cannulae that rest in front of the nostrils. The oxygen supplements the breath you take in naturally.

Studies comparing portable liquid oxygen devices to stationary tanks showed that the former improved both the length and quality of life. "A major reason for this was probably that patients could receive their oxygen while away from home, something not possible with stationary oxygen," says Thomas Petty, M.D., director of academic and research affairs at Presbyterian and St. Luke's Hospital in Denver. The studies also showed less heart strain and better brain function and exercise capacity with ambulatory oxgyen compared with stationary oxygen.

As Dr. Petty puts it, "The 'oxygen-packing patient' is a member of a grow-

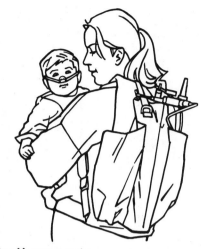

Portable oxygen carrier

ing fraternity of people—400,000 in the United States—whose lives and happiness are enhanced by the availability of portable oxygen." The strollers allow them to garden, golf, tinker with the car, even take trips from coast to coast. They simply take their portable stroller and their reservoir, which can be refilled en route and at their final destination.

But as we'll see, COPD patients aren't the only ones to benefit from oxygen therapy.

HEADACHE STOPPER

Sam Jones has one in his office, his car, and his den at home. A telephone? No, an oxygen tank. Sam has a tank handy so he can inhale oxgyen at the first hint of a headache.

This is not just an occasionally throbbing temple we're talking about. Sam gets cluster headaches—head-mashing pain that repeatedly strikes sufferers, typically males, in clusters of short attacks lasting from 6 to 12 weeks. The pain is so severe that cluster headaches have been dubbed "suicide headaches."

Fortunately, Sam's doctor knew about research showing that inhaling 100 percent oxygen for 15 minutes is as effective in aborting cluster headache as ergotamine, the standard headache medication.

"If you suffer from cluster headaches, you have a 75 percent chance of oxygen halting them," says George H. Sands, M.D., headache specialist at Long Island Jewish Medical Center, New Hyde Park, New York.

Cluster headaches are believed to be caused by an expansion of blood vessels triggered by the release of serotonin, a chemical found in the brain. Possibly, says Dr. Sands, oxygen has an effect on the pain pathways of the brain.

It's safe to use as often as four times a day, says Dr. Sands. But because you are inhaling 100 percent pure oxgyen through a mask (not the supplemental oxygen used by COPD patients), you should not use it for more than a half hour at a time. If you suffer from cluster headaches, ask your doctor for more details about the oxygen treatment. *See also* **hyperbaric oxygen**

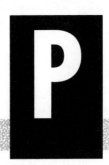

pacemaker If you're an active individual who has an irregular heartbeat, today's pacemakers may be just the ticket to a steadier ticker.

Of course, nothing responds like the heart's own natural pacemaker as you race across the court to meet that serve or cool down after your aerobics class. But the performance gap is narrowing. The one-speed pacemaker of the past has given way to a generation of instruments capable of adjusting your heart rate as needed. That means you can continue to golf or master your racquetball game, provided your doctor says it's okay.

These battery-operated devices are small enough to be implanted in a large vein and are directed toward a chamber of the heart—typically the right chamber. They pulse with electricity, stimulating contractions of the heart muscle in people whose own biological contraction mechanism is faulty.

The actual beat is produced biologically in the heart's sinoatrial node, which is located near the top of the right atrium. From the node, the signal for contraction flows throughout

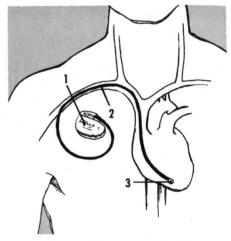

Pacemaker (1) with lead wire (2) and electrode (3)

the heart's pumping chambers, providing a rhythmic and coordinated pulse. The pulse rises and falls with changes in emotional states and activity levels.

Most people who need pacemakers have trouble with transmission of that signal throughout the system.

Today's pacemakers more closely mimic the natural rhythms of the heart by stimulating both the large and small chambers (the atrium and the ventricle) in sequence, instead of just one chamber, as the older models did. One current model responds to the number of breaths you take per minute. Another "reads" the electrical signals of the cardiac tissue to determine how fast your heart needs to beat.

But pacemakers aren't for everyone with heartbeat irregularities. Before you agree to one, make sure you get a second opinion. A *New England Journal of Medicine* study of 382 pacemaker patients suggests that 20 percent of pacemakers aren't needed. Many abnormal rhythms simply don't warrant the costly ($12,000) devices.

Even when they are necessary, pacemakers can cause problems. They can cause infections, they occasionally stop doing what they are designed to do, and they can cause irregular heartbeats. They also need to be replaced after a certain period of time, depending on the particular model, because the battery does not last forever. On the plus side, they offer effective protection against the threat of sudden fainting or death due to heart failure.

pads and plasters   Pity your poor skin. Something is always rubbing it the wrong way. First it was the handle of the garden hoe (it gave you a pea-sized blister on your palm). Then it was those pointy, high-heeled shoes you wore on your vacation. They gave you corns and calluses as souvenirs.

When your skin is under this kind of pressure, you may need to invest in some protective padding.

Moleskin is a handy padding that has been used to protect sensitive areas of the body for years. Despite its odd name, this feltlike material has nothing to do with moles; it's actually made from sheep's wool. Moleskin comes in self-adhesive sheets that can be cut to fit over sensitive areas on fingers, toes, heels, and other areas that are prone to friction.

Moleskin or other padding can't really help a blister that's already formed, says Emily Omura, M.D., director of dermatopathology at the University of Alabama in Birmingham. But if you have a blister that's already burst and is raw and oozy, you might want to purchase one of the newer blister pad kits. They include an antibiotic dressing and a spongy material that absorbs pressure and reduces friction while the site heals. The kits also come with thicker pads that you can use later to prevent more blisters from forming.

CUSHIONS FOR CORNS

Your feet are the most friction-prone part of your body. Those poor soles may be crammed into fashionable but narrow footwear that jams your toes together like packed sardines. Or, they may be stuck in ill-fitting athletic shoes. During a workout, your shoe may move one way while your foot moves the other way. And there's the rub.

Corns, calluses, and bunions are your foot's natural defense against all that rubbing and pressure. Unfortunately, as these thickened skin areas get thicker, they press on nerve endings. Then, these natural "protection" pads become a pain in the foot.

If moist, whitish, soft corns between the toes are your problem, hobble to the store for some lamb's wool. A wad of wool stuffed between your toes could give them the space they need, suggests Jerome Litt, M.D., assistant clinical professor of dermatology at Case Western Reserve University School of Medicine in Cleveland, Ohio, and author of *Your Skin from Acne to Zits.* "By reducing the pressure that was responsible for the corn in the first place, these growths usually disappear by themselves," Dr. Litt says.

Need a quick way to cushion hard corns on the top surface of your toes? For instant relief, you can't beat those small, self-adhesive foam rubber foot pads, says Dr. Omura.

Hard corns frequently form over the top of the fifth toe (or on the tip of the third or second toe if your shoes are very pointed). Just the pressure of the top of the shoe riding on these cone-shaped masses can feel like you're walking with a sharp pebble in your shoe.

"A doughnut-shaped pad encircling the corn lifts your shoe away from the corn and also relieves pressure from neighboring toes," says Dr. Omura. Doughnut-shaped pads work well for bunions, too. You can also fashion these from moleskin sheets, she adds.

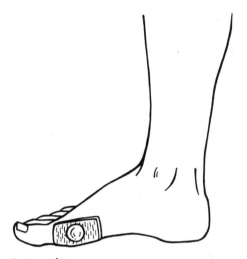

Bunion pad

GETTING PLASTERED

For a really bothersome corn or callus, you might want to take the next step and apply a *medicated* foot pad, sometimes called a plaster.

These medicated pads are less messy than old-fashioned plasters. In Grandma's day, a plaster consisted of a pastelike mixture containing some type of strong—often hot—medicinal herb. The plaster was spread over the skin and adhered as it cooled to body temperature.

Today's medicated corn and callus plasters are self-adhesive cushion pads with disks of salicylic acid. This strong substance chemically pares down the upper layers of skin. If you're not careful, though, salicylic acid can eat into healthy skin, as well. Therefore, some precautions are in order.

For starters, don't use acid plasters at all if you have diabetes or circulatory problems, advises Dr. Omura.

To remove corns, use only the nonwaterproof plasters that contain 20 percent salicylic acid. The waterproof corn plasters—and *all* callus plasters—contain double that amount of acid. "Never use the strong acid plasters on the tops of your toes. Your skin is thin

P

there and the risk is greater that the acid could burn into healthy skin," says Dr. Omura. "Save the strong plasters for very thick, painful calluses on the soles of your feet."

"Take care to protect the neighboring skin when using acid plasters," says Nelson Lee Novick, M.D., associate clinical professor of dermatology at Mount Sinai School of Medicine in New York City and author of *Super Skin: A Leading Dermatologist's Guide to the Latest Breakthroughs in Skin Care.* Before working on your foot, cut a cardboard template to the exact size of your corn or callus. Then, use it to cut out the exact fit from the adhesive plaster. But don't apply the plaster yet.

First soak your foot in lukewarm water and pat dry. Gently file the rough skin from your corn or callus with a pumice stone. "Don't use sharp instruments such as scissors, razors, or callus parers to shrink thickened skin," says Dr. Novick.

Next apply the plaster and leave it on for five days. (A thin film of petroleum jelly applied to the skin surrounding the plaster will help prevent irritation to that area.) Then remove the plaster, leave it off overnight, and file the dead skin in the morning. Apply another plaster for five more days. If your corn or callus hasn't budged in ten days, see your doctor. *See also* **mustard plasters**

painkillers   The annoying aches of bumps and bruises . . . unrelenting toothaches . . . the agony of a migraine. It's unfortunate, but pain, in varying degrees and endless varieties, is fre-

quently a fact of life. And it's not always short-lived: Some 80 million Americans suffer long-term, chronic pain.

The good news is, we have nearly as many painkilling medications (or analgesics) as we have pains. That's important because different pains respond to different remedies. Aspirin, for instance, is often great for headaches, but it won't help much if you've just had major surgery. Morphine, on the other hand, knocks out the worst pains, but you wouldn't want to use it against the mild aches and pains you get every day.

Here's a brief overview of the options.

Aspirin. You might think this humble pill, a fixture in nearly every purse and medicine cabinet, must have outlived its usefulness by now. There are many newer analgesics on the market. Why bother with this old warhorse?

Despite its age, aspirin isn't heading for pasture just yet. Physicians still choose aspirin as a frontline defense against all kinds of pain. Aspirin may not relieve headaches and backaches *better* than ibuprofen or indomethacin, but for most people it appears to work just as well. It's cheaper, too.

Aspirin blocks your body's production of prostaglandins, chemicals that initiate pain and inflammation when you're hurt. Since aspirin relieves pain *and* swelling, it's often the drug of choice for arthritis and other joint disorders.

However, aspirin isn't always the best choice. Some people don't respond to its painkilling power. It has also been linked with Reye syndrome, a children's brain and liver disorder that sometimes is fatal. More commonly, aspirin is hard on the stomach. Regular users may experience pain, cramping, or ulcers.

Acetaminophen. Also available over the counter, acetaminophen has been billed as one of the safest analgesics on the market. In fact, pediatricians often recommend it for their young patients. Although acetaminophen relieves pain about as well as aspirin, it won't do much to relieve swelling.

NSAIDs. Nonsteroidal anti-inflammatory drugs, called NSAIDs, are designed to offer as much pain relief as aspirin, with fewer unpleasant side effects. In fact, some of the NSAIDs have been found to relieve pain as well as codeine.

Ibuprofen, an over-the-counter NSAID that appears to reduce intrauterine pressure and the frequency of uterine contractions, now is the drug of choice for women who suffer painful menstrual periods. Ibuprofen also works as well as aspirin for relieving headaches and other mild-to-moderate aches and pains.

There are many prescription NSAIDs: Voltaren, Indocin, Naprosyn, and Feldene are some well-known brands. The NSAIDs are quite selective; you may have to try several before you find the one that's right for you.

Unlike narcotics, the NSAIDs don't impair mental or physical functions, nor are they likely to be addictive. However, NSAIDs do have a "ceiling effect"—higher doses don't necessar-ily give extra pain relief. If you're in a lot of pain, you may require something stronger.

Narcotics. These analgesic heavyweights are prescribed for the worst kinds of pain—after surgery, say, or for a really bad toothache. Narcotics such as codeine, morphine, and meperidine are extremely effective. They also may cause nausea, constipation, and respiratory depression.

Unlike aspirin and the NSAIDs, which inhibit prostaglandin production, narcotics go right to work in your brain where pain is received. Because they don't have the "ceiling effect" of the NSAIDs, higher doses of narcotics are sometimes used to relieve severe pain.

This doesn't mean that people who take morphine after surgery will continue to crave it when they go home. Narcotics, taken to relieve pain, don't appear to produce feelings of euphoria. So when people stop hurting, they stop taking the drugs. *See also* **acetaminophen; aspirin; ibuprofen**

papaverine   (pah-PAV-er-in) There are some things men never talk about. A dropped pass in the homecoming game always is a conversational no-no, as are the details of business deals, earlier marriages, and so on. As for impotence, well, that gets *buried.*

Men, it's time to speak up—to your doctor, at least. For many of the estimated ten million impotent (and extremely quiet) men in the United States, treatment may be an injection away. Enter papaverine, a smooth muscle relaxant that expands blood vessels and increases blood flow to the penis (just what's needed to get—and maintain—an erection).

Doctors may inject papaverine diagnostically to determine if a man actually is capable of developing an erection, says John Morley, M.D., director of the Geriatric Medicine Education and Clinical Center at the Veterans Administration Medical Center in St. Louis and director of geriatric medicine at St. Louis University Medical Center.

If a man *is* capable of getting an erection, then he might inject papaverine into his penis at home to give nature a little help.

"The majority of men are taught to inject the drug themselves," Dr. Morley says. "They take a small needle and push it all the way in—about half an inch. Whenever they want to have intercourse, they inject the papaverine, and they have an erection."

AN EASY PROCEDURE

The injections aren't as bad as they sound, Dr. Morley says. The 27- to 30-gauge needles slip in easily. There's a moment of burning, but little pain. "Most people have very little trouble getting used to it," Dr. Morley says. "Once they've done it, they find the injections very easy to do."

Erections typically occur in 5 to 15 minutes, and last for about an hour, he says.

For men who haven't been able to have sex for a long time—in some cases, for many years—taking a shot is easy indeed, says psychologist Alvin Baraff, Ph.D., director of MenCenter in

Washington, D.C. However, Dr. Baraff says he's heard of men for whom papaverine was too much of a good thing.

"I know one man who took an injection and then walked around for about 5 hours, waiting for his erection to go down," Dr. Baraff remembers.

Stories about papaverine and priapism—a painfully persistent erection that occurs independently of sexual desire—aren't uncommon. Doctors agree, however, that priapism is dose-dependent: The less papaverine injected, the less likely that an out-of-control erection will occur.

Dr. Morley says doctors aren't yet sure what side effects may follow the long-term administration of papaverine injections. Fibrous growth in the penis has been reported, as have bruising and general aches and pains. Liver damage is also a potential problem.

Even though papaverine injections appear relatively safe, few men *want* to keep taking them. There's something about penile punctures, for even the slightly squeamish, that's somewhat unpleasant.

A TEMPORARY ASSIST

Many men start out with papaverine, then move on to less invasive erection aids—vacuum devices, for example, which use suction to draw blood into the penis. Other men opt for penile implants, which are painless *and* permanent.

For some men, however, one shot of papaverine is enough, Dr. Morley says.

"For those who have psychogenic [originating in the mind] impotence,"

Dr. Morley says, "just injecting papaverine and showing them they *can* get an erection will sometimes produce an instant cure." Even men whose impotence stems from physical problems may need only temporary help. Papaverine "improves the blood flow to the penis, and they may have a spontaneous cure after about four injections," Dr. Morley says.

Papaverine injections seem to work best for young men, Dr. Morley says; older men are more likely to bruise. Of course, people with unsteady hands or poor eyesight may have good reason for staying away from needles. *See also* **penile implants**

pectin When you bite into that big, juicy apple, you're munching it. When you gnaw carrots or beets, you're getting loads of it. Grapefruit are packed with it. So are oranges, okra, and potatoes. Home canners wouldn't be without a good supply of it in their kitchen. So what is it?

Pectin, a type of fiber found only in fruits, vegetables, and nuts.

Although not as powerful as the fiber found in wheat bran, pectin does help keep things flowing smoothly through the digestive tract. But pectin's real job seems to be its ability to help lower cholesterol. In a study at the College of Medicine at the University of Florida, volunteers who took 15 grams of pectin a day—about what you'd get in 2½ cups of grapefruit—lowered their cholesterol 7.6 percent. What's more, they did it without changing their usual diets.

Most of us don't like grapefruit *that* much. But pectin isn't hard to find. Other citrus fruits are also rich in pectin. A tomato salad delivers a hefty pectin punch, as do broccoli and carrots. If you have a juicer, you even may get a taste for pectin pop—warm or on the rocks! Just make sure you scrape the sides of the juicer—that debris is where the pectin is.

Pectin also helps people take the pounds off. Like other foods rich in soluble fibers, pectin appears to slow gastric emptying. That means people eating lots of pectin tend to feel full longer.

In a California study, volunteers were given egg sandwiches, first alone, then with 15 grams (about ½ ounce) of supplemental pectin added. Not surprisingly, they felt fuller after eating the pectin-laced sandwiches. That's good news if you want to lose weight. After all, the longer you feel satisfied, the less often you'll be tempted to raid the refrigerator.

Like other fibers, pectin increases the time it takes your food to digest. That helps your body maintain a steady supply of glucose, reducing the giddiness you could feel when your blood-sugar goes on its daily roller-coaster ride.

Pectin is beginning to show up on food labels and in health food stores. But you don't have to rely on pectin powder to get your share. A grapefruit does just as well. *See also* **apple**

penicillin For thousands of years, bacteria with long, mysterious names—*Staphylococcus aureus, Streptococcus pneumoniae, Escherichia coli*—spread disease and pestilence throughout the world. Human victims, unable to combat these aggressive germs, simply suffered and died.

Then, in 1928, a stray bit of mold contaminated some staph cultures growing in Alexander Fleming's laboratory. The staph quickly died, and antibiotics were born.

The penicillins—named for the mold, which belongs to the genus *Penicillium*—are powerful weapons in the fight against infectious diseases. Drugs such as ampicillin, amoxicillin, and penicillin V, now made from synthetic materials, are the drugs of choice for treating many bacterial infections, including cystitis, gonorrhea, and strep throat. While the penicillins most commonly are prescribed for minor infections, they also help combat life-threatening diseases such as pneumonia and meningitis.

There are more than a dozen penicillins, each of which targets specific types of bacteria, says Sacramento internist Joshua Hoffman, M.D. Amoxicillin and ampicillin, for example, kill bacteria in the ear, nose, and throat. Cloxacillin, on the other hand, goes after infections of the skin, soft tissues, and respiratory tract.

While some antibiotics simply stop bacteria from reproducing, the penicillins are bactericidal—they actually destroy bacteria. They do this by weakening the bacteria's cell walls. Then, when the germs expand, they disintegrate and die.

STOPS STREP THROAT

Doctors see a lot of strep throat, a painful throat infection. Caused by B-hemolytic streptococci, a strep throat is a very red, sore, and angry throat. Left untreated, it may even lead to scarlet fever or heart problems. Penicillin, the primary antibiotic used for strep, can destroy most of the invaders within a few days.

Some recalcitrant germs often survive this initial assault, however. To make sure *all* the bacteria are killed, doctors generally prescribe one or two weeks' worth of penicillin. That reduces the risk that the infection will return, Dr. Hoffman says.

Over time, bacteria, like people, adapt to their environment. And because bacteria reproduce in a matter of hours, they adapt much more quickly than people do. So it's not surprising that in the 50 years since penicillin was introduced, many bacteria have become immune to one or more antibiotics. Scientists always are looking for new drugs to fight these resistant germs. If ampicillin, amoxicillin, or penicillin V doesn't eliminate an infection, some other antibiotic probably will.

A FEW DRAWBACKS

In some ways, the penicillins are almost *too* effective—they often kill good bacteria along with the bad. For example, antibiotics may kill the bacteria that limit the amount of yeast (candida) in the body, resulting in an infectious overgrowth of yeast in the mouth, vagina, or bowel.

"If you alter the population of bacteria in your colon, certain bacteria can become prevalent and cause very serious infections," says Dr. Hoffman.

"There's a significant incidence of bacterial colitis induced by antibiotics."

Penicillin allergies are quite common, and in rare instances, people experience severe reactions. In fact, some 300 people every year are thought to die from penicillin-induced anaphylaxis. When doctors suspect a penicillin allergy, they generally use another antibiotic. When penicillin must be used, skin tests help determine how serious the reaction might be. *See also* **antibiotics; tetracycline**

penile implants Most men would sooner admit to armed robbery than confess they can't get an erection.

There's a big problem with all this square-jawed silence about impotence: Many of these men—it's estimated there are ten million chronically impotent men in America—might be candidates for penile implant surgery, says Bruce MacKenzie, founder of the Tennessee-based Impotence World Services and Impotents Anonymous.

Penile implants, primarily made from silicone rubber, are surgically inserted in the shaft of the penis to make it sufficiently rigid for vaginal intercourse. Penile implant operations were first performed in the 1960s. Now, some 30,000 men have the surgery each year.

MacKenzie says he got *his* penile implant in 1981. The difficult part for most men, he says, is getting past the embarrassment and into the doctor's office.

"Impotent men thrive on denial," he says. "We get calls from men saying,

'I'm not impotent; I just can't get an erection.' Some people say they've had the problem 15 years, and they didn't do anything about it because they didn't know anything could be done."

Penile implants are relatively simple surgeries, says John Morley, M.D., director of the Geriatric Medicine Education and Clinical Center at the Veterans Administration Medical Center in St. Louis and director of geriatric medicine at St. Louis University Medical Center. There's little pain, and complications are rare.

Implants don't reduce the sensations you feel during intercourse, Dr. Morley says. If you had orgasms in the past, you'll probably have them after the surgery, as well.

OPTIONS TO CONSIDER

Penile implants, like cars, come in different styles and sizes. (Even if you dream of Cadillacs, however, your doctor may insist you get a Fiat.) Here's how the two basic types work.

Malleable implants. Also called semirigid, the malleable implants consist of two flexible rods or cylinders that are surgically inserted into both sides of the penis. The rods may then be bent in different directions, like pipe cleaners.

When you're ready for intercourse, for example, simply bend your penis outward. Time to get dressed? Bend it back toward your body for concealment.

Malleable implants have several disadvantages. They don't get as hard as natural erections. Nor does the penis change size: Men with malleable implants have permanent enlargement.

On the other hand, the malleable implants have few moving parts, so malfunctions are rare. The surgery also is quite simple, Dr. Morley says, requiring only 20 to 30 minutes and a local anesthetic.

What does it feel like to have a malleable implant? Men who aren't impotent normally have "one or two small erections as they go through the day," Dr. Morley says. "The semirigid implant feels exactly the same as those."

Inflatable implants. Unlike the malleable implants, which never change size, inflatable implants mimic the penis's natural behavior. Erections rise and fall—on command, of course. You don't have to wait for nature.

Inflatable implants consist of twin cylinders connected to a pump and fluid-filled reservoir. The cylinders are inserted in the penis; the pump may be concealed in the scrotum; the reservoir goes in the abdominal cavity.

When you squeeze the pump, you get an erection. Squeeze again, the erection goes away.

MacKenzie swears by his inflatable implant, which has worked without problems for a decade. For one thing, the erections look like the real thing. And while he appreciates *getting* an erection, there are times when it's also nice to be able to get *rid* of it—in the locker room, for example.

WHICH IS BEST?

Dr. Morley says he generally recommends the rugged malleable implants. Inflatable implants tend to break down after five years, he says, which means additional surgery. Cost also is a factor. Inflatable implants cost about four times more than the malleable implants.

"When we compared the inflatable type with the malleable type, we found patient satisfaction was identical," Dr. Morley says.

Of course, not every man is a candidate for penile implantation. Urologists rarely recommend the implants for men whose impotence stems from psychological rather than physical causes. And men who want intercourse very infrequently may look into less invasive remedies.

Whichever alternative you choose, let your embarrassment go, MacKenzie says. "People should accept chronic impotence for what it is—a treatable condition, just like heart disease or a broken leg." *See also* **papaverine**

peppermint   When a waiter brings some red-and-white-striped candy mints along with the dinner check, it's not so you'll leave him a bigger tip.

The refreshing, icy-cool-tasting peppermint has a long tradition as a stomach soother that can relieve the gassy, bloated feeling that sometimes occurs after eating (even in the finest restaurants).

Because of its pungent taste and pleasing aroma, peppermint has been one of the best-loved herbs ever since this hybrid was found sprouting among the spearmint bushes in England in the late 17th century. Since then, the herb has flavored everything from candy to alcoholic drinks.

But peppermint has a serious, therapeutic side to it, as well. The oil it contains stimulates the flow of bile to the stomach, promoting digestion. But it's the oil's antispasmodic (muscle relaxant) properties that give peppermint the power to free turbulent gas trapped in your belly. Specifically, peppermint oil relaxes the muscular closure between the stomach and the esophagus, allowing gas to escape. In other words, ingesting peppermint gives you a good burp.

If you are prone to heartburn, however, stay away from peppermint. "If the muscle closure is *too* relaxed, stomach acid could escape back up into your esophagus and cause the typical burning sensation," says Arthur I. Jacknowitz, Pharm.D., professor and chairman of the Department of Clinical Pharmacy at West Virginia University.

Although controversial, some studies suggest that this muscle relaxant feature—as it affects the intestines—might make peppermint an effective aid for relieving irritable bowel syndrome, a condition characterized by constipation, diarrhea, bloating, and stomach cramping.

"Theoretically, peppermint interferes with the mobilization of calcium ions, the substances responsible for the contractibility of the intestinal muscles," says Dr. Jacknowitz.

TEA FOR THE TUMMY

If a grouchy tummy is your bane, you may want to try sipping peppermint tea. The tea is better than mint candies, says Varro E. Tyler, Ph.D., professor of pharmacognosy at Purdue University. "Many mints are made with artificial flavoring and not the real McCoy," he says.

The recommended healing technique: Steep 1 or 2 teaspoons of peppermint leaf in hot water for several minutes. Then sip the tea slowly.

But don't give the tea to infants or children, says Dr. Tyler. "Young children may experience a choking sensation from the menthol found in peppermint oil."

Some people have taken peppermint to quell hunger pangs, because it can calm a growling stomach. But this could backfire. Peppermint may actually trigger the appetite, says Dr. Tyler. The muscles are only calmed temporarily. Then you may have hunger pangs stronger than they were before.

COOLING AND SOOTHING

Peppermint's benefits are not limited to soothing stomach and intestinal troubles. Peppermint's menthol acts as a counterirritant on your skin. That means it causes a cooling sensation that counters the sensation of pain. This is why menthol is included in many topical pain-relieving substances such as cough drops and muscle rubs.

Additionally its cooling and soothing properties probably account for peppermint's prominence in formulas for relaxing baths and also in recipes for teas to help you sleep. There is little scientific evidence to support these uses, however.

One Italian study conducted on lab animals suggested that peppermint extract has a sedative action on the central nervous system. But ironically, some U.S. researchers have found that a sniff of peppermint may actually help maintain concentration and alertness.

This much is known for sure: If sipping or dipping in peppermint makes you feel good, go ahead and indulge in moderation, says Dr. Jacknowitz.

But if you're purchasing a peppermint product—whether it be a tea or a bath soak—make sure the label specifies peppermint and not just "mint." The mint family includes the flavorful spearmint, as well as lavender and rosemary. Only peppermint contains menthol, however. *See also* **menthol**

peppers, hot Many of our favorite culinary combustibles—steaming tacos, blistering burritos, and atomic enchiladas—call for peppers: fresh peppers and dried peppers, large and small peppers, peppers of all shades of red, green, and yellow. Peppers with one ingredient in common: capsaicin.

Capsaicin is the stuff that makes hot chili hot—or, sometimes, *H-O-T!* Capsaicin is so hot, in fact, it can be detected by the tongue even when it's diluted to 1 part in 11 million. This scorching stuff isn't merely a shortcut to heartburn, however. A diet of capsaicin-rich foods can break up sinus and chest congestion, and may help ward off infections too. And mixed in a cream and applied to the skin, capsaicin is making a reputation as a potent painkiller.

A HEALING TORRENT

What happens when you take a bite of something really, really hot?

"Basically, it stimulates glands in your nose, which then starts running," says Gordon Raphael, M.D., associate clinical professor of medicine at George Washington University in Washington, D.C. "Your eyes tear and you sweat. You salivate to get what's hot out of your mouth."

Essentially, all that wheezing, gasping, and blowing can help reduce cold and flu congestion almost instantly. In fact, the pepper principle does some of the same things for your stuffy head that a hot bowl of chicken soup—or an over-the-counter expectorant—might do, Dr. Raphael says.

There's another benefit to courting the chili burn, according to Dr. Raphael. The resulting nasal Niagara Falls contains the antibacterial compounds lactophenin and lysozyme. "These things being secreted are fairly potent, anti-infectant chemicals that serve as a first-line defense," he says. "So eating some of those spicy foods may help you get over colds, and they can certainly help keep your nose clear," Dr. Raphael concludes.

SHINGLES PAIN SOOTHED

It is a happy coincidence when foods for our insides also contain medicines for our outsides. Capsaicin ointment, doctors believe, can help relieve many types of pain, including the pain of shingles, a rash caused by the herpes virus.

In one study, 32 elderly people with painful shingles received either a tube of capsaicin cream or a placebo, a similar-looking cream with no special properties. Both groups were told to

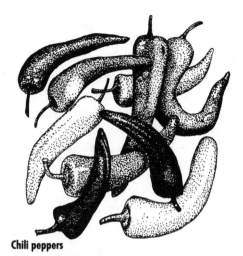

Chili peppers

apply the creams several times a day. After six weeks, 80 percent of the capsaicin group reported a decrease in their pain levels, compared to just 31 percent of the placebo group.

Capsaicin is thought to inhibit the skin's supply of substance P, a chemical messenger responsible for carrying pain sensations from your skin to your brain. As you might expect, capsaicin produces its own burn, but doctors say that generally goes away after a few days.

The painkilling power of capsaicin isn't limited to herpes sores. In one study, Canadian researchers asked 18 women to apply capsaicin cream for postmastectomy pain. Of the 14 women who completed the study, 12 reported some improvement, and 8 of those showed "good or excellent responses."

Capsaicin also has been found to relieve diabetic neuropathy, a condition that causes burning pain on the bottoms of the feet.

Capsaicin also may block some types of inflammation. How? Inflammation is your body's response to inju-

ries and pain. Take away the pain (by depleting substance P), and your brain may not sound the inflammation alarm.

On the other hand, capsaicin actually may speed the healing times of some injuries. Since it dilates (widens) blood vessels, it helps increase the supply of white blood cells, and that's good for healing.

Apart from scientific studies, there's an abundance of anecdotal evidence that capsaicin relieves all sorts of pain. In *The New England Journal of Medicine,* a doctor tells of two men who successfully used capsaicin cream to relieve leg and foot pain. In the *Lancet,* a British medical journal, another doctor reports that one woman, a double amputee, "completely relieved" her pain with regular applications of the cream.

Doctors agree more tests are needed before they render a verdict on capsaicin. However, conducting those tests in a fully objective manner might be a little tricky, since most people easily spot the difference between placebo creams and the real thing—capsaicin burns!

Pepto-Bismol. *See* **bismuth**

petroleum jelly This nontoxic, odorless, gel-like ointment—which actually *is* distilled from petroleum—has been called a "first-aid kit in a jar." For over 100 years, petroleum jelly (or petrolatum) has been used as a lubricant, a protectant against friction, and as an effective home remedy for soothing dry skin and minor skin irritations, from dishpan hands to diaper rash.

The secret to petroleum jelly's effectiveness, experts say, is its ability to provide a superthick barrier on the skin and to seal in moisture. "Your skin thrives on water," says Paul Lazar, M.D., clinical professor of dermatology at Northwestern University in Chicago. "When water is lost from your skin, due to harsh weather or overcleansing, for example, it becomes dry, itchy, rough, and prone to cracking. Coating your skin with petroleum jelly traps water in the skin cells, and allows the skin surface to become soft and smooth, minimizing cracks and roughness."

In fact, when it comes to rehydrating skin, petroleum jelly has been proven the very best barrier there is. In tests measuring its effectiveness, petroleum jelly was found to be nearly 100 percent occlusive, meaning that it almost totally prevented any water from escaping from the skin's surface during a specified period of time. As a result, petroleum jelly has become the gold standard against which all newly developed dry skin products and moisturizers are measured.

The drawback is that pure petroleum jelly is greasy and doesn't spread easily over large areas, says Dr. Lazar. However, petrolatum is often a key ingredient in the more spreadable creams because it's so effective in relieving the symptoms of dry skin.

If you have sensitive skin, though, you may find that a thin coating of pure petroleum jelly is less irritating than slathering on a dry skin product loaded with extra ingredients. "Petrolatum has no fragrances or other additives, and very few people are allergic to it," says Nelson Lee Novick, M.D., associate clinical professor of dermatology at Mount Sinai School of Medicine in New York City and author of *Super Skin: A Leading Dermatologist's Guide to the Latest Breakthroughs in Skin Care.*

A DAB FOR WHAT AILS YOU

Applying a dab of petroleum jelly straight from the jar is often the most effective way to treat minor skin irritations. If, for example, your nasal passages are so dry they sting each time you inhale, a dab of petroleum jelly might help you breathe easier.

Petroleum jelly is also helpful for soothing painful anal fissures. "If you are taking Accutane an unpleasant side effect can be dried tissues in the anal area," says Dr. Bark. "Applying a little petroleum jelly can help to rehydrate the tissues and provide soothing lubrication as well."

Runners and walkers are often advised not to leave home without taking along petroleum jelly as a protection against friction and winter winds. If your thighs are on the generous side, for example, smearing them with petroleum jelly can help prevent chafing. Slathering some on your feet could keep you a step ahead of painful blisters. And here's a tip for facing the great outdoors: "If you run regularly and harsh winds are battering your face, first try a layer of moisturizer, seal it in with petroleum jelly, and then wear a soft cotton face mask," suggests Dr. Bark. "It may not be elegant, but it works."

Petroleum jelly will also lick chapped lips, according to Fredric Haberman, M.D., medical director of the Affiliated Dermatology and Plastic Surgery Center in Saddle Brook, New Jersey, and New York City and author of *The Doctor's Beauty Hotline*. "First smear your lips with a thick coating of petroleum jelly. Next hold a warm, wet washcloth against them for several minutes. Then, with a fresh cloth wrung out of very warm water, gently massage more petroleum jelly into your lips. Continue massaging until most of the petroleum jelly has been absorbed. Blot your mouth immediately and apply a lip lubricant or conditioner."

With all this dipping into the petroleum jelly jar, you may think that contamination would be a problem, especially since the pure product contains no preservatives. But here's the good news. "Petroleum jelly doesn't support bacteria growth," says Thomas Gossel, Ph.D., chairman of the Department of Clinical Pharmacy at Ohio Northern University in Ada. "A 4-ounce jar could last 20 years."

pet therapy   At last count, Americans owned about 58 million dogs, 49 million cats, 8 million birds, 43 million fish, and untold millions of guinea pigs, iguanas, and assorted other swimmers, creepers, and crawlers.

Clearly, we love our pets. A study of 500 pet owners, for example, found more than half of them shared beds with their pets; 54 percent said they celebrated their pets' birthdays.

Now for the really good news. Pets aren't merely fun to play with; they're good for your health, too. Here's how.

In a landmark study, researchers interviewed 96 people, all with serious heart problems, who had been admitted to a large university hospital. People were asked about their incomes, their social ties—and their pets.

One year later, 78 people were still alive. Of the 39 people who *did not* own pets, 11 (28 percent) had died. Of the 53 people who *did* own pets, only 3 (6 percent) had died. Having a pet to care for, the study suggests, may actually be a predictor of survival.

Many researchers have suggested that dogs and other pets have a calming influence on people of all ages. In one study, for example, simply being near a dog reduced blood pressure in children. It's also been noted that stroking an animal may lower your pulse and blood pressure. Not surprisingly, it relaxes the pet, too.

Doctors don't know exactly what it is about pets that makes us feel so good. One theory: The emotional bonding that often occurs between people and pets may ward off some of the loneliness, depression, and other psychological distress that prevent us from feeling our best.

FEWER DOCTOR VISITS

A study conducted by the School of Public Health at the University of

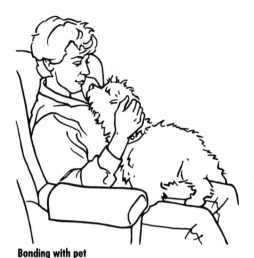

Bonding with pet

California at Los Angeles found pet ownership may reduce the demand for physician services among the elderly.

Over the course of a year, researchers kept tabs on nearly 1,000 Medicare enrollees, more than one-third of whom owned pets. It was found that pet owners saw their doctors less often than nonowners—a measure of continued physical well-being. In times of stress, moreover, nonpet owners were more likely to visit their doctors than were the pet owners.

Doctors long have noted that the positive emotions people share with pets may be as strong as the love between parents and children. That's why pet therapy now is a fixture in many nursing homes, retirement centers, and even prisons. Pets make people feel good about themselves *and* the animals.

"Forces that connect people and animals are especially strong and enduring," explains Leo Bustad, professor emeritus at the College of Veterinary Medicine at Washington State University in Pullman.

Dr. Bustad describes a woman in a nursing home who, following a stroke, spent her days on a couch, curled up in the fetal position, unresponsive to people. After she was moved into a "pet-therapy room" with a Persian cat named Handsome, the woman started inviting people to watch her new friend.

Pets bring good will, it seems, wherever their paws take them. For example, animals in one program were brought to a hospital for the criminally insane. Morale went up, and violence and destructive behavior went down.

Pets aren't for everyone, of course. If you don't like animals, stroking a 150-pound German shepherd probably will make your blood pressure go *up,* not down.

But if you do like animals, a pet in your home is bound to let loose a lot of good feelings. A powerful tonic when you're blue, a friendly dog, cat, or goldfish may be just what the doctor ordered.

phenobarbital   One of the wonder drugs of recent decades, phenobarbital has been used as an anesthetic, a sleeping pill, and an antianxiety drug. Today, it's primarily used to control—and prevent—the violent, grand mal convulsions that accompany some types of epilepsy and head injuries.

"To prevent seizures, phenobarbital is often used following neurosurgery, or when there's been trauma to the brain," says E. Don Nelson, Pharm.D., professor of clinical pharmacology at the University of Cincinnati.

Phenobarbital inhibits seizures by

depressing the entire central nervous system. It's fast-acting and inexpensive, it works at relatively low doses, and it generally produces few side effects. However, people sometimes complain of unwanted sedation.

Phenobarbital has been used to treat asthma, high blood pressure, and, in combination with other drugs, pain, but it probably isn't very effective for these conditions, Dr. Nelson says. In fact, phenobarbital may actually *increase* people's sensitivity to pain.

"Historically, it was given to people with asthma just to calm them down, but there are other, safer drugs," Dr. Nelson says. "It shouldn't be given to someone with hypertension because there are other, specific drugs that lower blood pressure."

DANGEROUS EFFECTS

Apart from treating convulsions, phenobarbital rarely is used these days. "It's a dangerous drug," Dr. Nelson says. "The biggest problem with phenobarbital—with all the barbiturates—is that if you combine them with alcohol, you're going to have a serious overdose on your hands."

Because of its effects on the central nervous system, phenobarbital may increase depression in people who already are depressed. It also has a narrow margin of safety: Breathing difficulties, or death, may occur when people take more than the prescribed amounts.

In children, the long-term use of phenobarbital may have serious consequences. In a study published in *The New England Journal of Medicine*, re-searchers concluded that the mean IQ of children treated with phenobarbital was 8.4 points lower than that of children who didn't receive the drug.

Phenobarbital also disrupts rapid-eye-movement (REM) sleep, the sleep stage during which dreams occur. People who take phenobarbital often wake up feeling tired.

Phenobarbital largely has been supplanted by newer, safer drugs, but it still has defenders. "It's so old and well established, I think it will always have a place in the treatment of grand mal epilepsy," Dr. Nelson says. "The older physicians, the ones who have a lifetime of experience using this drug, use it skillfully. The younger physician, on the other hand, will just select something that's safer to begin with." *See also* **anticonvulsants; barbiturates; sedatives**

phototherapy. *See* **light therapy**

physiatry (fih-ZYE-a-tree) A twist of fate—and physiatry—spared Joe from surgery for a pinched nerve. Every medical professional he consulted agreed he needed the operation. But the top surgeon for the job was out of town for two weeks. And that was just enough time for the more conservative methods of physiatry to come to Joe's rescue and make surgery unnecessary.

A stroke at age 25 left Beth almost completely paralyzed on one side—and wondering if she'd ever manage on her own again. But she was back to work in six months and living independently, thanks in part to her physiatrist, who saw to it she had every kind of therapy she needed to regain her independence.

Such is the strength of physiatry. Physicians in this small but growing medical subspecialty have broad training in both physical medicine and rehabilitation. Following graduation from medical school, physiatrists spend five years undergoing specialty training and gaining experience before becoming certified, says physiatrist Leon Reinstein, M.D., of Sinai Hospital in Baltimore. Their knowledge of physical medicine equips them to treat structural complaints such as back pain, arthritis, and work-related disorders caused by repetitive motion. As rehabilitation experts, they typically work in tandem with other health professionals to help people with disabling injuries return to as productive a life as possible.

Can a physiatrist help you? To find out, here's a closer look at the profession and its contributions to patient care.

Top Diagnosticians

There are three things you ought to know right off the bat about these practitioners of physical medicine. First, they emphasize nonsurgical remedies. "We're like orthopedists who don't operate," says Randy Braddom, M.D., physiatrist and vice-president of medical affairs for Moss Rehabilitation Hospital in Philadelphia. "If people do need surgery, we refer them to surgeons."

Second, physiatry is the only medical specialty that requires training in electrodiagnosis. So if you have a

pinched nerve like Joe had, the physiatrist may supplement your physical exam with an electromyography study, a diagnostic procedure that records the electric potentials developed in muscles. "What we do is put a small wire in a few muscles and take measurements," Dr. Braddom says. "I can tell in the case of a pinched nerve, for example, which one is affected, how badly, and how long the problem has been there. Also, we can make a diagnosis with almost 100 percent accuracy for carpal tunnel syndrome [a painful disorder involving nerve compression at the wrist], and with 90 percent accuracy or more for low back and neck pain."

And that leads to our third point. Dr. Braddom claims that physiatrists are "probably the best diagnosticians in the musculoskeletal area.

"If someone has neck or back pain, or really, any musculoskeletal problem from a herniated disk to tennis elbow, it's worth seeing a physiatrist first," Dr. Braddom says. "We can provide accurate diagnosis and treatment for acute and chronic pain." Once physiatrists find the source of pain, they use physical means like stretching, heat, cold, and exercise to bring relief. In Joe's case, anti-inflammatory drugs, traction, and exercise sufficed to overcome the pinched nerve.

Rehab Specialists

Some conditions, of course, can't be fixed. For example: stroke, spinal cord injury, amputation, and neurological problems like multiple sclerosis. Here, the physiatrist's aim is rehabilitation rather than cure—to help the patient regain as much of his ability to function as possible. Does the patient need physical therapy? Braces or artificial limbs? Psychological, social, or vocational support? Practical guidance in accomplishing day-to-day duties? All of these questions are addressed by the physiatrist.

It's up to the physiatrist to plan the treatment, provide follow-up, and coordinate the activities of the other members of the rehab team. (These might include a rehabilitation nurse, occupational and physical therapist, brace maker, pharmacist, dietitian, psychologist, and speech pathologist.)

"We're not just managers," says Dr. Braddom, correcting a common misperception about physiatrists. "Like an architect, we draw a blueprint of the treatment and oversee it to make sure it is built correctly. Since a patient's needs may change from day to day, the rehab plan must be changed on a daily basis. During rehabilitation the physiatrist is also the patient's regular physician, the one who takes care of his or her medical problems."

Someone suffering from crippling rheumatoid arthritis, for instance, would receive help on a number of fronts. The plan might call for local heat and massage treatments to relax the muscles, self-relaxation training and posture therapy, and suggestions to adapt eating, dressing, walking, and personal hygiene routines, says Mayo Clinic physiatrist Joachim Opitz, M.D. Anything that can help restore a person's self-reliance—whether simplified clothing, special cutlery, even labor-saving ways of or-ganizing the kitchen—is incorporated into the therapy.

physical therapy   If all you know about physical therapy is what you've seen in the movies, you probably think it's all about teaching heroic accident victims or war veterans to walk again. Physical therapy *can* bring about some pretty spectacular recoveries.

But if you think that's all there is to it, you could be missing out on some of the things physical therapy can do for you. The garden-variety muscle aches that accumulate as you move through a typical day are the province of physical therapy, too.

Maybe you've had a really stressful week at the office and find your lower back pain flaring up. You could get a massage. But if you ask your doctor to refer you to a physical therapist, you'll get comparable relief for those cramped muscles—plus lessons in how to prevent the pain from coming back. With home exercise and regular treatments, you may be able to beat the problem entirely in four to six weeks, with the physical therapist's help.

The state-licensed members of this health care profession are trained to use physical treatments—including heat packs, ultrasound (sound wave) therapy, manipulation of joints, and exercise—to help you restore movement and eliminate pain. They do an individual evaluation of your problem, then create a treatment plan to fix you up.

"We have the advantage of being part of the standard medical system," says Patricia King, a licensed physical therapist and assistant professor of the program in physical therapy at the University of Tennessee at Memphis. "We work closely with doctors and are trained to refer patients with untreated medical problems to physicians."

MANY WAYS TO HELP

Here are just a few examples of ways physical therapy can help.

If you've been badly burned, physical therapy can help prevent the loss of motion that usually occurs when the healing skin creates scarring over joints.

If you've got pneumonia, bronchitis, or emphysema, physical therapy can help clear your congested lungs. Your therapist will position you so that gravity can assist in the clearing and tap specific places in your chest to dislodge phlegm.

If you've just had a stroke, physical therapy may be able to help you recover some—if not all—of the capacity for movement you had before the stroke disabled you. "We won't be able to change the fact that you've had a stroke," says Ken Davis, licensed physical therapist and former director of practice for the American Physical Therapy Association. "But we can teach you how to adapt your life to make the most of the capacity you do have."

Nor can physical therapy change the course of rheumatoid arthritis. But you can learn postures that will prevent arthritic limbs from becoming deformed, Davis says.

Physical therapists can also help you move more freely if you've just had surgery for scoliosis (spine curvature), or shoulder, knee, or hip injuries.

As you can see, this is a *diverse* profession. The 71,000 licensed physical therapists in the United States today have found a home in all kinds of settings: sports medicine clinics, industry, schools, academic research departments, hospitals, hospices, home health agencies, nursing homes—even private practice. In the hospital alone, you'll find physical therapists working alongside pediatricians, obstetricians, cardiopulmonary specialists, neurologists, orthopedic surgeons, and physiatrists.

Physical therapists take a four- to six-year college degree program before they are eligible for a license. Their training equips them to diagnose routine muscle and joint complaints without a doctor's intervention.

More often than not, your doctor will refer you to a physical therapist if your condition warrants. However, 24 states have laws allowing people to contact physical therapists directly, without a physician's referral, Davis says.

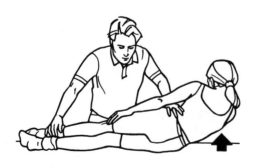

Physical therapy for scoliosis

pillows Not all pillows are created equal. Some can actually be therapeutic tools for good health and proper posture. Others ought to be sued for nonsupport.

Ideally, a pillow should function as a means of support for the head and neck and help your body form a healthy line when you sleep, says Louis Sportelli, D.C., a Palmerton, Pennsylvania, chiropractor and former chairman of the board of the American Chiropractic Association.

In many cases, the right pillow can actually help people with neck and shoulder pain, says Dr. Sportelli. Conversely, the wrong pillow could not only aggravate an existing condition, it might even be the cause of pain, he says.

Even if you don't suffer from neck or shoulder pain, you shouldn't take your pillow for granted, says Dr. Sportelli. After all, you're going to be spending 5 to 8 hours a night—or more—with it.

What matters is that you choose a pillow that makes your neck feel good— whether that pillow be flat or thick, soft or hard, or maybe no pillow at all, says Valery Lanyi, M.D., a New York City physiatrist and associate professor of rehabilitation medicine at New York University. It also helps to experiment with placement of the pillow to see what's most comfortable, she adds.

"All people are built differently," says Dr. Lanyi. "Some people report discomfort with certain kinds of pillows, while others may not.

"There are many conditions in which positioning the body—rightly or wrongly—can make a difference," Dr. Lanyi says. "I usually make a detailed examination before deciding whether to make a recommendation about pillows."

Sometimes a strategically placed pillow relieves leg and knee pain, says Dr. Lanyi. In other cases people with neck and back pain may benefit from creative placement of pillows.

People with lower back pain caused by disk problems should sleep in one of two positions, says Dr. Sportelli. "They should either sleep on their back with one pillow beneath their knees and one cradling their head, or they should sleep on their side with a pillow between their knees," he says.

The reason for the pillow between the legs is "that you don't want the upper leg to strain by having to angle to meet your other leg," says Dr. Sportelli. He says that many people with disk problems are most comfortable curled into the fetal position.

SPECIALIZED SUPPORT

Some people who don't sleep well with ordinary store-bought pillows report that they make better headway at night with specially constructed pillows, says Dr. Lanyi. For example, "there are pillows that can be heated and cold-pack pillows that can be cooled with ice. These can sometimes be helpful in controlling headaches and preventing muscle spasms around the neck," she says.

Therapeutic pillows come in var-

P

ious shapes and sizes. There are pillows designed to supplement your regular pillow. Cylindrical in shape, they slip right inside the regular pillowcase to give an extra lift to people who prefer an unusually high pillow. Others are stand-alone pillows shaped like hourglasses that give soft support for the sides of the head while cradling the neck in their center indentation. If you prefer sleeping on your back, you'll probably love the hourglass pillows.

Another pillow option is the firm variety filled with buckwheat hulls. These pillows conform to the shape of each sleeper's neck and head. But like anchovies and olives, these pillows are an acquired taste; many people need a week or two to adjust to the feel of the hulls.

There also are pillows with built-in, battery-run vibrators. People who like neck massages swear by them. Light sleepers who are turned off by the characteristic buzzing noise are likely to swear *at* them.

People with circulatory problems or leg swelling after arthoscopic knee surgery may want to purchase a special, wedge-shaped pillow that slips under the legs. "Available at medical supply stores, it's a must for people who have had knee joint replacements," Dr. Sportelli says.

PILLOWS TO GO

People who travel might find that their comfort is well worth the slight inconvenience of taking their special pillow with them, says Dr. Lanyi. Another alternative for travelers is to take one of the many available crescent-shaped, blow-up pillows along with them on trips.

"People tend to fall asleep on airplanes and then their head lolls around," says Dr. Lanyi. "Even inexpensive blow-up pillows will prevent this. I travel with one."

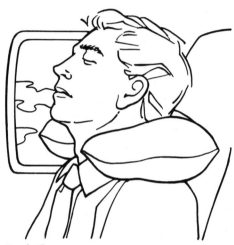

Travel pillow

Taking your own pillow to the hospital for an overnight stay or longer is also a good idea, suggests Dr. Lanyi. "Hospital pillows are notorious," she says. "People who have something wrong with their neck get a better night's rest if they take their own pillows with them. When my husband went to the hospital, I took him his neck pillow because he couldn't fall asleep."

But don't get *too* attached to your favorite pillow. While children can keep their security blankets for year after year without ill effects, adults should promptly replace their old pillows when they begin to deteriorate, says Dr. Lanyi.

"Pillows have their own life expectancy," she says. After that, they're liable to let you down. *See also* **mattresses and beds**

placebo (plah-SEE-bo) In the days when magic and medicine went hand in hand, it wasn't unusual for potions to contain exotic, but medically questionable, ingredients:

> Eye of newt, and toe of frog,
> Wool of bat, and tongue of dog,
> Adder's fork, and blind-worm's sting,
> Lizard's leg, and howlet's wing.

These days, of course, you would have to be pretty sick before you'd imbibe this unappetizing brew from *Macbeth*. But modern placebos, which may have no active ingredients whatsoever, have been found to relieve conditions as varied as depression, chronic headaches, and chest pains.

Latin for "I will please," placebos are pharmacologically inert substances that sometimes have beneficial effects. Researchers commonly use placebos in drug studies so they can differentiate physical from psychological improvements. People who take active drugs more often will show improvement than those taking placebos.

But it doesn't always work that way. Even in so-called blind studies (when volunteers don't know which type of pill they're getting), as many as 30 to 50 percent of the people receiving placebos report at least some improvement in their condition. This is called the placebo effect.

"In one study, patients got better even when they *knew* they were taking placebos," says Howard Brody, M.D., professor of family practice at Michigan State University and the author of *Placebos and the Philosophy of Medicine: Clinical, Conceptual, and Ethical Issues.* "One lady said, 'Every time I took the pill, it was like a reminder that the doctor was concerned about me.' "

When a known drug improves some condition it's not *supposed* to improve, it's called an impure placebo. Aspirin, for example, is known to relieve headaches. Taken to improve weak vision, on the other hand, it's a placebo.

Placebos aren't always drugs. Many diagnostic procedures also elicit the placebo effect. For example, your doctor may order an x-ray even when he's relatively sure you don't have a fractured bone. But the test may relieve anxiety, which in turn helps relieve the pain. Of course, it also gives the doctor a chance to confirm the diagnosis.

HOW PLACEBOS WORK

If you improve after taking a placebo, does that mean the problem was all in your head? Not necessarily, Dr. Brody says. (Some research suggests that the body releases endorphins, opiate-like painkillers, into the blood of placebo responders.)

Besides, when placebos are dispensed from the hands of a caring physician, it's really only natural that people feel a little bit better. Indeed, placebos draw their power from the caring relationship people form with their doctors, says Howard M. Spiro, M.D., professor of medicine at the Yale

School of Medicine and editor of the *Journal of Clinical Gastroenterology.*

In his book, *Doctors, Patients, and Placebos,* Dr. Spiro says as many as half of the volunteers in some ulcer studies improve after taking placebos. "They're being watched in the study, and they're getting an enormous amount of attention," Dr. Spiro says. "The attention, the care, the coming back to report—all of this is helpful."

Generally, placebos are thought to work best for illnesses without detectable physical causes: ulcers, for example, and premenstrual tension. Placebos are thought to be least effective for treating serious diseases such as cancer and heart disease.

All placebos are not created equal. "People assume that if it stings, it must be more powerful," Dr. Brody says. That's why people injected with sterile water have a greater placebo response than those injected with a milder saline solution. Large pills give more relief than small ones, and capsules work better than pills. Not surprisingly, surgery often stimulates a very potent placebo response.

Positive words also are helpful. In one study, taped messages ("You will not feel sick, you will not have any pain . . .") were played while people had surgery under general anesthesia. Compared to other surgical patients, they had fewer postoperative fevers and gastrointestinal problems, and they spent less time in the hospital, as well.

Still, placebos—and more conventional medicines—sometimes get more thanks than they deserve, Dr. Spiro says. Most people go to the doctor only when they've been sick for several days or weeks. By that time, of course, the illness probably was ready to depart on its own. People credit the pills, he says, but the real medicine was time. *See also* **affirmations; imagery; TLC**

plantain (PLAN-tayn) If you're one of those people who hates cultivating a blue-ribbon lawn, take heed. You just may have an excuse to quit getting your grass in gear.

You see, if you declare war on weeds in your lawn, you could be wiping out plantain, a broad-leafed herb of the plantago family with about 200 different species worldwide. In fact, plantain thrives so well in cultivated areas that some American Indian tribes referred to it as "white man's footsteps."

But what your green-thumbed neighbors consider to be an infiltrating menace that's about as welcome in their yards as a congregation of fire ants could actually be a blessing in disguise, says Varro E. Tyler, Ph.D., a professor of pharmacognosy at Purdue University.

"Plantain has a long-standing reputation around the world as a topically applied remedy for all kinds of bruises, cuts, and abrasions," says Dr. Tyler. It's also used by nursing mothers to treat cracked nipples, as well as by people whose skin cracks easily in cold weather, he says.

CRUSH TO ACTIVATE

To apply plantain, take a fresh leaf and pulverize it by using a hammer or a mortar and pestle "to break

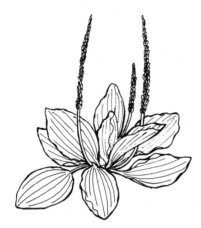

Plantain

up the cells," Dr. Tyler says. Don't expect a thick liquid to ooze out the way gel flows from a pulverized aloe plant, he warns. "When you take a fresh plantain leaf and crumble it up, it's moist like a damp cloth—not saturated with moisture."

You can apply the crushed plantain directly to the affected part of the body, says Dr. Tyler. "Just use something to hold it in place—like a bandage or tape and gauze," he says.

Some people simply bruise the leaf and apply it directly to the skin. Others mix pulverized leaf into petrolatum and use it in a salve or ointment, he says.

The plantain leaf contains a substance that has an antibiotic effect when applied locally, says Dr. Tyler, "so it kills microorganisms on the skin."

But contrary to what physicians from Shakespeare until the recent past thought, plantain is not a cure for poison ivy, says Dr. Tyler. Nor does eating the leaf have any therapeutic effect. Besides, plantain contains a lot of tannin "and is not very tasty," he says.

Plantain is best used simply as a folk remedy for external injuries, says Dr. Tyler. When he was collecting such remedies years ago for one of his books, a woman from Lafayette, Indiana, wrote him to praise plantain. "She had roller-skated a lot as a kid," says Dr. Tyler. "And her mother put so many plantain leaves on her scraped knees that classmates dubbed her 'the girl with green knees.'"

plant therapy   No, we're not talking about giving your lilies stem-straightening exercises or a bulb bypass along with their next helping of fertilizer. Plant therapy isn't for plants. It's for people. Advocates of plant therapy (also called horticultural therapy) say that people who spend time growing and nurturing plants get much more out of it than dirt under the fingernails.

The power of plants to calm the nerves, hoist the spirits, and turn a blue day into a rosy-red one may date back to the origin of man. "I believe there's a primal association, locked somewhere in our genes, that makes us feel comfortable, safe, and happy around plants," says Richard H. Mattson, Ph.D., director of the horticultural therapy program at Kansas State University. "We need our daily quotient of green," he says.

GREEN MAGIC

Although anyone can benefit from working with or just being around greenery, horticultural therapy is often used by professionals to treat those with mental or physical disabilities. At Friends Hospital in Philadelphia, for example, Martha Straus, who has a bachelor's degree in horticultural therapy, directs a program that dates back to 1879. How therapeutic can plants be in such a setting? Straus tells one story of a young woman who entered the hospital following an attempt to kill herself.

As part of her treatment, the woman was taken to one of the hospital's two greenhouses and given a jade plant to care for. "She told me that when she took this little plant in her hands, she wanted to live. She was looking forward to the future—to seeing how her plant was going to grow," says Straus. When the young woman left the hospital six weeks later, she took many plants with her—and a *much* healthier state of mind.

Magic? Maybe. "It's very hard to put into words. Unlike most other therapies, horticultural therapy deals with a living thing. Something green, and growing, which responds to your care, or lack of care," says Straus. Caring for and cultivating another living thing can do wonders for a person's confidence and self-esteem, she says.

Much of the success of plant therapy has been reported by word of mouth (through the grapevine, so to speak). However, a number of formal studies have sprouted in scientific journals, confirming the power of plants. They tell us that green therapy really flowers when it comes to beating stress.

In one Kansas State study, 20 adults were taken in shifts into a greenhouse to get down and dirty with the pots and plants. According to several common measures of stress—blood pressure, heart rate, and skin temperature—the experience appeared to be a calming, stress-reducing one for all. Other studies have shown similar results. "Relaxation occurs very quickly, usually within 15 minutes," says Dr. Mattson.

BEGINNING IS EASY

Plant therapy under professional supervision is used in nearly 300 hospitals across the country, according to the American Horticultural Therapy Association in Gaithersburg, Maryland. But you can apply plant therapy right in your home, office, or backyard. Millions do.

Douglas Lundsgaard spends at least several hours every week unwinding with his apple, cherry, and pear trees, strawberry vines, raspberries, currants, grapes, and assorted vegetables. "It's a nice respite from an orthopedic practice," says the 48-year-old-surgeon, speaking by cordless phone directly from his garden in Eugene, Oregon. "Plants take my mind off my problems and allow me to be expressive. I like the feeling of nurturing and the calming effect," he says.

Tending plants offers benefits to the body as well as the mind. "Some guys go down to the health club and work out. Me, I go home to my garden and turn over some soil—and I probably get as much exercise as they do!" says Dr. Lundsgaard.

If you think that caring for plants may be good medicine for you, pick up a watering can and get started. "All you need is a few seeds, a little bit of soil, and motivation," says Dr. Mattson.

He recommends starting off on a small scale, "perhaps with only one plant." You don't even have to buy your plant. "You can get started with what's in your garbage!" says Dr. Mattson. That is, the top of a pineapple, a seed from an orange, or a bud from a potato can all produce healthy plants. (If you're not sure how, check some basic gardening books.)

The ongoing care of a plant or several plants shouldn't require much time or energy—unless you want it to. "Unlike pets, plants won't leave a mess on the floor, and they won't drag fleas into the house," says Dr. Mattson. Nor do plants need to be brushed, fed daily, or taken for walks on cold, wet mornings.

plasters.   *See* **pads and plasters**

poetry therapy   "Poetry," said romantic poet William Wordsworth, "is the spontaneous overflow of powerful feelings." The same thing might occasionally be said of therapy, which is why some experts—called poetry therapists—believe that the reading and writing of verse can help people discover, and perhaps resolve, some of the vexing problems in their lives.

All poetry, ranging from classic couplets by Tennyson to popular songs by Melissa Manchester, can be a therapeutic icebreaker, says Nicholas Mazza, Ph.D., associate professor of social work at Florida State University and editor of the *Journal of Poetry Therapy.*

"When people come for counseling, they are sometimes reluctant to talk about certain aspects of themselves," says Dr. Mazza, who is also a clinical social worker. "It's sometimes easier for them if they can talk about a poem or a song. They can say, 'It's not me; I'm just talking about the poem.' The poem provides an entry point to therapy."

People who find it difficult to make decisions, for example, might be asked to read Robert Frost's *The Road Not Taken:*

Two roads diverged in a wood, and I—
I took the one less traveled by,
And that has made all the difference.

"When people read this poem, they're able to see that all decisions involve loss, and they begin to see where they're stuck in their own lives," Dr. Mazza says.

Poetry therapy works especially well for children, Dr. Mazza says, who often can't articulate what they're feeling inside. A poem such as *Tree House* ("a tree house, a free house/a secret you and me house") can help them talk about themselves, he says.

Of course, poetry therapy can involve more than simply reading verse. Some people begin to resolve their problems by writing their own poetry. One adolescent boy, for example, who was sexually abused by his father, describes himself in a poem as "falling apart." After several verses, however—

The hope was barely in sight,
But giving up was not my style,
So I decided to go on and fight,
To make my life a longer mile.

"If you write something down, you begin to have control over it. When you have control over your problems, you can begin to solve them," Dr. Mazza says.

SAYING IT HELPS

Alice Walker, a Sacramento speech and language pathologist, says she sometimes uses simple rhymes to help people with apraxia — a neurological disorder that hinders speech — learn to speak more clearly. During practice sessions, "people might start out simply saying certain combinations of letters over and over, but that gets pretty boring," Walker says. "Poetry helps keep their interest up. Also, when they come to a rhyme they can guess what the next word will be, and that helps their progress."

Gloria Frym is a San Francisco poet who once taught creative writing to prisoners in the county jails. Poetry — and healthy doses of encouragement — helped open some unlikely doors, she says. "One student wrote autobiographical poetry about her experiences as an inmate — she's now a second-year law student," Frym says.

Of course, you don't have to have serious problems before you can benefit from poetry therapy, Dr. Mazza says. "I believe that if there were more poetry in people's lives, there would be less need for therapy. Poetry can be very healing," he says.

Beginning poets shouldn't worry about the *quality* of their verse, Dr. Mazza warns. "Sometimes good writing does take place, but that's not the goal. After all, when you start thinking in terms of literary merit, you might get depressed if rejection notices come in."

polyunsaturated oils You're seated at the breakfast table with a steamy muffin and a tub of some kind of self-proclaimed heart-healthy spread. You slowly pull the knife across the spread and ease it near the container lip, wishing wistfully for the good ol' days when coffee was coffee, eggs were eggs, and butter was butter.

But you're a smarter person for dipping into that polyunsaturated tub margarine rather than slicing into a stick of butter, nutritionists and doctors agree. That's because butter is high in both saturated fat and cholesterol, which can make your blood cholesterol level rise and put you at risk for heart disease. Polyunsaturated oil, on the other hand, can actually help lower cholesterol.

To get our bearings, let's look at the total fat picture for a moment. The three types of fats in the diet are saturated, monounsaturated, and polyunsaturated. Most fats contain some of each form, but saturated fats, which are hard at room temperature, are more abundant in meat and dairy products, lard, butter, and coconut and palm oils. A greater portion of monounsaturated fats are found in canola, olive, and peanut oils. Polyunsaturated fats come from vegetable sources (called omega-6's) and from deep-water fish and some plants (called omega-3's). Highly polyunsaturated oils include soybean, corn, safflower, and sunflower.

GOOD-FOR-YOU FATS

Polyunsaturated and monounsaturated fats are part of the "good fats" you'll want in your diet because they have been proven to lower blood cholesterol when substituted for saturated fats. In addition, polyunsaturates contain essential fatty acids, nutrients your body needs just like vitamins or amino acids, says Jacqueline Dupont, Ph.D., national program leader for human nutrition at the U.S. Department of Agriculture.

"All food fats provide energy and some other useful functions, but it's absolutely necessary to get the polys," says Dr. Dupont. "They do lower LDL cholesterol [the harmful kind] without question, and you've got to have them for other nutritional reasons, as well."

Researchers are debating polyunsaturated fats' effect on HDLs, the desirable high-density lipoprotein cholesterol. High levels of HDLs are associated with a lower risk of heart disease. Some evidence suggested that polyunsaturated fats lowered HDLs as well as LDLs, an effect that would lessen their benefits. But studies are showing that polyunsaturated fats don't depress HDL levels over the long term.

Polyunsaturated fats have been overlooked somewhat with all the excitement about monounsaturated fats like olive oil, Dr. Dupont says. However, polyunsaturates should not be replaced by monounsaturates. "It's absolutely necessary to get the polyunsaturated fatty acids," she explains, because they are important for healthy skin, fertility, and many other vital functions.

Even the "good fat" polyunsaturates should make up only 10 percent of the calories in your diet, according to American Dietetic Association and American Heart Association guidelines. Another 10 percent should come from saturated fats and another 10 percent from monounsaturated fats. This may take some work, since the average American consumes 37 percent of total calories from fat, including about 14 percent saturated.

The best ways to include polyunsaturates in your diet is to substitute soybean, corn, safflower, and sunflower oils for saturated fats in cooking. You also may select light and diet tub margarines for use as spreads. These are a better on-the-table choice than butter or stick margarines, which become more saturated during the solidifying, hydrogenation process.

It is possible to get too much of the polyunsaturated fatty acids, Dr. Dupont says, reminding that 10 percent of calories from this type of fat is tops. "It's enough," she says, "but not too much." *See also* **monounsaturated oils**

positive attitude.   *See* **affirmations**

posture therapy   We'd all like to have better posture. But the big difference between most of us and those rare individuals who actively make changes in the way they stand or sit can be summed up in a word: Pain. They've got it, and so they're willing to work with a posture expert to get rid of it.

Posture therapy is more than snapping into position the moment someone barks "straighten up." A lot of bodies can't even do that—or hold themselves that way for very long without strain. That's because years of slouching, slumping, and sedentary living—or repeating the same movements over and over at work—have shortened key muscles and overstretched others. Fortunately, posture therapy can provide specific aid to the neediest muscles, and the rewards can be great.

NECK PAIN RELIEVED

Consider the case of Deena, a 30-year-old schoolteacher whose round-shouldered, head-forward stance contributed to years of intermittent neck and shoulder aches. The pain finally became bad enough for her to consult physical therapist Patricia King, on her doctor's advice.

King, assistant professor of the physical therapy program at the University of Tennessee, Memphis, began with a diagnosis: Deena's back and neck muscles were weak, the muscles and joints around her shoulders and midback were tight, and her favorite sleeping pose didn't help matters. Plus, she was constantly on the go and never found time to relax.

The prescription? Hot packs, ultrasound, and electrotherapy to relax the tight muscles. King also worked with the joints to loosen them. And she gave Deena home exercises to strengthen the appropriate frame-supporting muscles and to stretch the tight muscles and joints.

"One of the problems with a lot of self-stretching programs is that people tend to skip over the stiffest areas," says King. "That's why some people go to an exercise class and get worse.

Evaluation by a physical therapist and hands-on therapy to improve muscle and joint mobility in the right areas is so important."

Deena felt some relief after two treatments, although therapy lasted three months overall. The improvements in her head and neck posture even eliminated a problem her dentist had found with her bite, King says.

Another postural success story: Westfield, New Jersey, physical therapist Brian Miller helped a nearly bedridden woman, who had had back pain for 20 years, progress in just two months to the point where she could go shopping and cook with relative ease. "She's in much less pain than when she started with posture therapy," says Miller.

All of Miller's clients get "homework," too. "They have to work a lot on paying constant attention to their posture," he says. "I teach them to adopt different cues. For instance, if they work in an office, I tell them that every time they catch themselves looking at the clock, they should stop for a moment and scan their posture. If anything's off, that's the time to realign."

Who else can posture therapy help? When King studied women with pelvic pain, she found that posture therapy brought complete relief to 12 of 59 women and significant relief to 39 others. Treatment took six weeks to four months.

ON-THE-JOB RELIEF

Physiatrist Richard Bonfiglio, M.D., chairman of rehabilitative medicine at Mount Sinai Hospital in Chicago, is among the specialists who focus on work-related posture disorders. Educating people about good posture practices on the job can help them recover faster from lifting injuries and prevent re-injury, he says. Even more common today in some industries than on-the-job back injuries, however, are the neck, shoulder, and arm problems of computer operators. Sometimes, something as simple as adjusting the height of the chair or keyboard can make a big difference, Dr. Bonfiglio says. Other job injuries may require special exercises to strengthen muscles that are constantly being used to capacity. "If you can strengthen the muscle enough so that you are doing the job using less than 50 percent of that muscle's strength, you'll cause less trauma," he says.

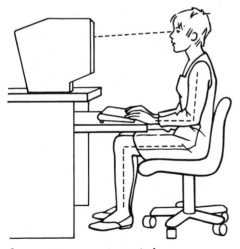

Correct posture at computer terminal

Here are some additional on-the-job posture tips from Dr. Bonfiglio.

At your desk, use a lumbar roll pillow that fits in the small of the back to improve your sitting posture.

Don't cradle the telephone between your ear and shoulder. That can cause nerve irritation. Instead, use a cradle attachment or get a speaker phone.

Arrange your desk so that items you use frequently are close enough that you don't have to stretch and reach.

If you must stand in one position for long periods, put first one foot and than the other up on a low stool. Continue to alternate. By taking weight off muscles, this can cut down on fatigue.

Don't use your back to lift. Bend your knees instead. Keep the object close to your body. And if you turn, turn the entire body. Don't twist.

Aside from physical therapists and physiatrists, who else offers posture therapy? Osteopaths and chiropractors work with body alignment, but they don't emphasize posture education, according to Miller. But there are various bodywork systems that aim to teach better posture. Miller incorporates three of these into his practice: the Alexander Technique, the Feldenkrais Method, and Trager Psychophysical Integration. *See also* **Alexander Technique; Feldenkrais Method**

potassium. *See* **nutritional therapy**

poultices When natural substances—usually herbs—are mashed and placed on the skin to promote healing, the concoction is called a poultice. Often the material is heated, then spread on gauze. The gauze is laid directly on the part of the body that needs treatment, then covered with a piece of wool to hold in the heat.

Herbalists and other natural healers claim that poultices can soothe sore areas, speed healing, and purify the area by drawing out foreign matter and pus. "They're particularly good for boils, bee stings, and other skin inflammations," says Wade Boyle, N.D., a naturopathic doctor who maintains a practice with a medical doctor in Evans City, Pennsylvania. They are not always appropriate for open wounds, however.

Onion poultices are probably the most well known, says Paul Bergner, editor of *Medical Herbalism: A Clinical Newsletter for the Herbal Practitioner.* He says they were especially popular among medical doctors in the 1800s.

"Poultices were not that uncommon even 50 years ago," adds Dr. Boyle, who also wrote the book *Herb Doctors: Pioneers in Nineteenth Century American Botanical Medicine.* Even though herbalists continue to use them, as do some naturopathic doctors, their popularity has waned. "Poultices are neglected because they're messy and a little bit labor-intensive," he says.

What other ingredients might you find in a poultice?

Everything from aloe vera to pine tar. Herbs are probably the most common, but garlic and red potatoes are often used, too, says Boyle. Debra Nuzzi, a Boulder, Colorado, herbalist, also lists clay and charcoal.

Are poultices safe?

In general, yes, says Kentucky dermatologist Joseph Bark, M.D., chairman of dermatology at St. Joseph's Hospital in Lexington: "In my 14 years in practice, I've seen very few problems associated with them." On occasion, though, people may put parsley, limes, or celery on the skin and then develop a rash when they go outdoors. That's because those substances can make skin oversensitive to sunlight, he says.

"Personally, I think foods are better eaten," Dr. Bark says. "When applied as a poultice, some natural materials can add moisture to the upper, dead layers of the skin, but most don't penetrate it. Aloe, however, in the concentrations you find in the fresh plant, has been found to promote healing. But many allergies are caused by its use, and I do not recommend this or naturopathic poultices of any kind."

Herbalists claim that poultices work in several different ways, depending on the material used.

"I think some work on the basis of osmosis," Dr. Boyle says. "They draw fluids and other impurities out of the inflamed area. Others have a direct medicinal effect. Others have an absorbent quality—they glom on to any noxious material and neutralize it."

Comfrey as a poultice is "so potent that it can help regenerate tissue," Nuzzi claims. It contains a substance called allantoin, which she says is a "cell proliferant." But never use a comfrey poultice on an open wound, because it contains toxic substances that would be harmful if absorbed.

POULTICE POINTERS

To make a poultice from a fresh herb, crush the material with a mortar and pestle or place it in a blender with enough water to allow for easy blending, Nuzzi says. (Use distilled water to ensure purity.) Spoon the mixture onto the skin and wrap with gauze, or protect the skin with a thin, clean, colorless cloth before putting the material on it.

John Bastyr, N.D., D.C., a Seattle naturopathic doctor who has been in practice for 59 years, says he favors cold poultices over warm ones. He advises leaving the poultice on for 30 minutes at a time, or until the skin warms it. Repeat with a fresh application every few hours.

Here are a few other suggestions from poultice enthusiasts. (Note: Because these measures are not scientifically proven, they should not be used as a substitute for appropriate medical care.)

For arthritic joints. Make a solution with Epsom salts (2 cups Epsom salts in 1 gallon of warm water). Dip a towel into the solution and place it on the affected area. Hold it in place until the skin gets good and warm (about 15 to 20 minutes), remove the towel, and massage in castor oil. "This is old-fashioned, but it still works," claims Bastyr. "I use it all the time."

For a mild sore throat. Grate up a carrot very fine and sandwich it between two layers of cloth. Cover it with a cold compress and a piece of wool. "Leave the carrot poultice on your throat for 30 to 45 minutes," says Bastyr. You can reuse it as long as there is color left in the carrots, he says.

For boils. Use slippery elm or echinacea powder, moistened into a paste, says Nuzzi. Apply to the skin and wrap with gauze.

For bee stings and drawing out splinters. Use a fresh plantain leaf, Nuzzi says. Its astringent nature is recommended for drawing foreign matter out of tissue. Pine resin is also very good for removing splinters, she says.

power of suggestion. *See* **placebo**

prayer Few remedies are as ancient — or as universal — as prayer. Long before there were doctors, people prayed for health. Witness, for instance, the Old Testament prophet Jeremiah, who prayed, "Heal me, O Lord, and I shall be healed." People today still pray, and "Dear Lord, make me better soon!" rises from innumerable sickbeds and waiting rooms.

Today, of course, we heal with surgery and adhesive strips, antibiotics and electron microscopes. Is there still room in our medicine cabinets for prayer?

Many people think so.

When researchers from Duke University surveyed 106 elderly people about their beliefs, 72 percent said they prayed every day. What's more, nearly two-thirds said their relationship with God helped them cope with loneliness — a condition that in the elderly often is linked with depression and suicide.

"There's no question that mental attitude affects the way we react to disease," says the Rev. Glenn Asquith, Jr., Ph.D., a former hospital chaplain and now an associate professor of pastoral theology at the Moravian Theological Seminary in Bethlehem, Pennsylvania.

In his book *Healing Yourself,* Martin L. Rossman, M.D., tells of a patient who steadfastly refused medical treatment for a precancerous cervical condition. However, she did agree to pray; six weeks later, her problem was gone.

Of course, prayer isn't an adequate substitute for a thorough medical checkup and treatment, Dr. Rossman warns. Prayer isn't likely to mend a broken arm or instantly eliminate a nasty case of the flu. Prayer might, however, *help* your body heal—if you think it will.

"We know now that as the mind becomes more at peace, the body is better able to fight disease," says Robert Cartwright, a healing minister at New Life Clinic and visiting pastor at Hiss United Methodist Church in Baltimore. "How does prayer work? Even in the healing ministry, we don't know."

THE POWER OF BELIEF

Technique seems to be secondary. Some prayers are highly structured, says Dr. Asquith, while others are improvisational. Style matters less than belief, he says.

Indeed, if your belief is strong enough, you may be able to share your healing powers with other people, Paster Cartwright says. "Intercessory prayer is tremendously effective," he claims.

In a study at San Francisco General Medical Center, people outside the hospital were asked to pray, during a ten-month period, for 192 patients in the coronary care unit. However, they *didn't* pray for an additional 200 patients in a second group. The prayer group

"had less congestive heart failure, required less diuretic and antibiotic therapy, had fewer episodes of pneumonia, had fewer cardiac arrests, and were less frequently intubated and ventilated," the study concluded.

If prayer heals, you might expect people who pray (or get prayed for) most frequently will be healthier than people who pray less often. Members of the clergy do, in fact, have lower mortality rates than their lay brethren. Some religious groups, including the Mormons, have some of the nation's lowest cancer mortality rates.

Of course, other factors besides prayer may be responsible. Many religions encourage healthy diets and eschew dangerous substances such as tobacco and alcohol. In addition, religious groups typically offer their members encouragement and emotional support—always important for mental and physical health.

WHEN DISASTER STRIKES

In the event of a catastrophe—an earthquake or airplane crash, for example—prayer may be one of several useful coping mechanisms, says Carol North, M.D., an assistant professor of psychiatry at Washington University in St. Louis who has interviewed people after disasters.

People who weren't religious before an accident weren't likely to turn to prayer, she says. However, prayerful people consistently said prayer got them through the worst times.

"The people who had religion, in general, found it to be a great strength during crises," Dr. North says.

Pastor Cartwright says prayer, regularly practiced, works best. People who pray only in a pinch may not get the same results.

"A lot of people, when anything goes wrong, pull out the fire extinguisher they call prayer," he says. "Generally, though, the prayer that is most effective is the one that lets you become more aware of where you are in life; it's important to pray and meditate to change your lifestyle and to gain personal understanding." *See also* **Relaxation Response**

prednisone (PRED-nih-sone) When rheumatoid arthritis makes your joints swell, this prescription steroid drug goes right to work. If you've twisted your ankle, bent your back, or knocked your knee around, prednisone almost immediately can help reduce the inflammation.

Prednisone reduces swelling by inhibiting your body's production of prostaglandins, compounds that help get inflammation started. Injected into an injured joint, prednisone seals the lining; inflammation-causing cells can't get in. What's more, it depresses the activity of white blood cells, cells responsible for much of the swelling that accompanies injuries.

In one study, 74 people with inflamed tendon sheaths (a condition known as "trigger finger") received injections of triamcinolone, a prednisone derivative, right into their joints. Seventy of the people reported immediate relief.

Prednisone doesn't have to be injected to produce benefits. If you have asthma, for example, a prednisone-charged inhaler can help prevent airway inflammation. Taken rectally, prednisone even reduces the swelling of ulcerative colitis.

In one study, prednisone was credited with restoring some neurological functioning to people with acute spinal cord injuries. Doctors participating in The National Acute Spinal Cord Injury Study treated 316 patients with methylprednisolone (a form of prednisone), a nontherapeutic placebo, or naloxone hydrochloride (an opiate-receptor blocker). People who received prednisone within 8 hours of their injuries showed significant improvement over people in the other groups.

Prednisone, in short, is a versatile drug — versatile in its benefits *and* in its dangers. Relatively safe for short-term use, it gets more dangerous the longer you take it. Side effects can include osteoporosis, runaway infections, and prolonged healing times. That's why doctors generally ask people to begin their treatment with aspirin or other non-steroidal anti-inflammatory drugs before resorting to prednisone. *See also* **anti-inflammatories; cortisone; hydrocortisone; steroids**

proctosigmoidoscopy (prok-to-sig-moi-DOS-ko-pee) Few things in our anatomy seem so mysterious as the snaky curves of our lower intestine — that dark, winding Amazon of rectum, sigmoid colon, and descending colon. Not so long ago, doctors could only "see" inside as far as they could feel with their index fingers. Then along came proctosigmoidoscopy. Using lights, flexible fiberoptics, lenses, and cameras, it lets doctors visually explore the length of the bowel.

In proctosigmoidoscopy—it's also called sigmoidoscopy, or simply lower endoscopy—doctors slide a hollow scope inside the rectum. The scope, with fiberoptics and lenses, lets the doctor see what it sees. In addition, surgery may be performed simultaneously by slipping in an electrocautery (a cutting device) or laser along with the scope. Thus, a polyp may be removed the moment it's discovered.

Proctosigmoidoscopy doesn't require anesthesia, although sedatives sometimes are given.

SCREEN FOR CANCER

The procedure generally is used to screen for cancer. Every year, more than 53,000 people in the United States die from colon cancer, and doctors would like to lower that figure by detecting more tumors at an earlier, more operable stage. The American Cancer Society recommends that people aged 50 years and older undergo proctosigmoidoscopy every three to five years.

Naturally, most people don't look forward to having their bottom tampered with. "First, there's the preparation. You drink a gallon of special liquid, which goes in one end and out the other," says William Ruderman, M.D., chairman of the Department of Gastroenterology at the Cleveland Clinic in Florida. Two enemas follow. Then comes the actual procedure.

Gastroenterologists use different scopes to look at different parts of your lower intestine, says Dr. Ruderman. And depending on the procedure, there may be varying degrees of discomfort. Proctosigmoidoscopy isn't especially pleasant, but it shouldn't be painful. "It's an undignified experience, but that's about it," he says.

In rigid sigmoidoscopy, a 7- to 8-inch scope that looks like a periscope pokes into the rectum. The least costly of the lower endoscopy procedures, it's also the least comfortable, according to Dr. Ruderman.

Flexible sigmoidoscopy is used more often, he says. The flexible sigmoidoscope, ranging in length from 14 inches to nearly 24 inches, searches for cancers and ulcers as far as the sigmoid colon.

15-MINUTE PROCEDURE

"I tell people in advance that they'll feel a sensation of fullness," Dr. Ruderman says. "If it hurts, it means the scope is twisting the colon, or bending it or stretching it. That can be avoided with modern endoscopic techniques."

Like the flexible sigmoidoscope, the colonoscope also searches the intestine for polyps. However, it's about 4½ feet long and sedation usually is required.

Dr. Ruderman says most proctosigmoidoscopies done today take less than 10 or 15 minutes from insertion to completion. However, they will take longer if polyps are biopsied or removed. *See also* **endoscopy**

progressive relaxation Yes, even if you're practically conservative, you can still use this technique. The "progressive" in progressive relaxation doesn't refer to a position on tax legislation or civil rights, but rather to the manner in which you progress from one body part to another during a typical session.

Lauded by many experts for its ability to knock out stress, the purpose of this technique is to teach you to recognize the difference between physical tension and relaxation so that you can consciously choose to relax. You do this by alternately tensing and relaxing various body parts. With practice, you should be able to deeply relax within a few minutes.

Since its introduction about 70 years ago, a number of studies have shown the effectiveness of progressive relaxation at beating stress. And as doctors have turned their attention to the powerful link between stress and disease, progressive relaxation has been recognized as a bona fide health-giver. For instance, one study published in the medical journal *Behavioral Medicine* found that regular practice of progressive relaxation may help to lower cholesterol levels. Other therapists have reported success using progressive relaxation to treat stress-related problems such as headaches, ulcers, high blood pressure, and colitis.

READY...SET...SQUEEEEZE

Want to give progressive relaxation a try? Find a comfortable spot, either sitting or lying down. Gently close your eyes. Inhale and clench your right hand into a hard fist. Hold it for 5 to 7 seconds. Exhale and relax. Feel the tension drain from your hand and forearm. Note the difference between how your arm feels relaxed and how it feels tensed. Rest for about 45 seconds. Repeat the exercise again.

Next do the same with your left hand. Tense. Relax. Repeat a second time. Now move your attention throughout the major muscles of your body. From the hands, move to the bicep muscles in your upper arms. Make a muscle. Squeeze. Hold it. Relax. Repeat. Do the same with your facial muscles (make a frown), neck, upper back (try to pull your shoulders back as though you were trying to touch them together behind you), chest (pull your shoulders in front of you), stomach, thighs, and calves. Tense and relax each muscle area in order.

There are many variations of progressive relaxation, and most stress therapists are familiar with at least one. There are also many tapes on the market to guide you through a session.

Mohammad R. Sadigh, Ph.D., director of psychology and psychophysiological services at The Gateway Institute, a center for pain and stress management in Bethlehem, Pennsylvania, likens progressive relaxation to a bicycle with training wheels. "It's often used as an introduction to relaxation techniques because it's simple. On the other hand, it can be cumbersome," he says.

Quite unlike other relaxation techniques in which the body plays a passive role (such as meditation or autogenic training), "you'll look strange doing progressive relaxation in the waiting room of your dentist," says Dr. Sadigh. Progressive relaxation is also not ideal for those whose stress is accompanied by muscular pain. All that tensing could make matters worse. *See also* **autogenic training; biofeedback; meditation; stress management**

Prozac. *See* **antidepressants**

prunes Like many high-fiber foods, prunes are a time-honored recipe for promoting gentle, regular bowel movements. What's more, they're rich in pectin, a type of fiber known to help lower cholesterol.

Prunes—they're simply dried plums—are about 6.6 percent fiber. That means they add bulk and moisture to your stool.

However, prunes aren't rectal dynamite, despite their fearsome reputation. Like all fiber-rich foods, prunes promote regularity, not explosions.

Many prune lovers take their favorite fruit first thing in the morning. Some start the day with prune juice. Others prefer prune slices sprinkled on their cereal. On epecially hot afternoons, you might sample prune spritzers—a tall glass of prune juice laced with sparkling water.

However, don't eat prunes by the pound when you're not used to them, doctors warn. Give your body time to adjust to all that fiber.

psychoanalysis In turn-of-the-century Vienna, a white-bearded doctor with a penchant for cigars would ask his emotionally troubled patients to lie down on a couch and talk about themselves. His name was Sigmund Freud, and he called his treatment psychoanalysis. It was the first "talk" therapy. Today, there are dozens more—but the original is still preferred by some.

Freud theorized that psychological problems, such as depression, anxiety, and phobias, stem from childhood experiences, often very unpleasant ones. Most of these experiences, he believed, lie buried in a realm of the mind that he called the unconscious. Psychoanalysis digs up and examines this unconscious. How? Freud used a number of tools, including dream analysis and free association, a process in which patients utter any thought that pops into their minds.

Beware—psychoanalysis is *not* for those in a hurry. Or those on a budget. The unconscious does not reveal itself willingly. Many psychoanalysts insist on a minimum of several sessions a week, although some require less. The sessions may continue for years, even decades.

Psychoanalysts argue that short-term therapies, such as cognitive therapy and behavior therapy, don't get to the underlying causes of psychological problems. Not like psychoanalysis can. "Psychoanalysis is not a quick cure for what's bothering you—it's an educational process," says Martin Fisher, Ph.D., professor and director of training at Adelphi University's Institute of Advanced Psychological Studies and a psychoanalyst in private practice in Manhattan. "Where does education end? For some," he says, "it's a lifetime thing."

HARD TO MEASURE

Psychoanalysis gets modest reviews from some psychology experts. Richard L. Wessler, Ph.D., chair of the psychology department at Pace University in Westchester, New York, says that several short-term therapies, such as cognitive, behavioral, and interpersonal therapy, have been proven effective in a large number of studies for many psychological problems, from panic attacks to winter doldrums. But "there's little evidence that psychoanalysis can treat these conditions," he says.

Psychoanalysts argue that these other therapies grew up in an era of laboratories and experimentation; psychoanalysis did not. Instead of clinical studies, they point to thousands of individual case histories. People who have felt depressed, lonely, anxious, or alienated have had their lives revamped through psychoanalysis, says Bertram P. Karon, Ph.D., a professor of psychology at Michigan State University and president of the Division of Psychoanalysis of the American Psychological Association. Even people with more serious psychological problems, like schizophrenia, have been helped, he adds.

Nevertheless, Dr. Karon admits that success in psychoanalysis is often hard to measure. Good psychotherapy, he says, can provide several important—yet intangible—benefits: It may give you greater insight, bring you closer to your feelings, enhance your self-control, give you greater freedom, and make you a more effective human being. "As psychoanalysts, we do not treat a symptom, but a person," says Dr. Karon.

WHAT'S ON YOUR MIND?

Some psychotherapists today cling tightly to Freud's teachings. Others have veered off a bit. But all psychoanalysts seek to tap the unconscious, and Freud's free association is still among the most popular methods.

How does free association work? You may be asked to lie down on a couch, with the therapist sitting behind you. He'll ask you to say whatever comes to mind. You start . . . "I don't feel like being here today . . . I'm tired . . . I noticed the carpeting is dirty . . . I see a new picture up on the wall . . ." While you talk, the therapist seeks patterns. "Eventually, I'll hear the 'music.' It may be anger, neediness, or fright," says Dr. Fisher. "When I can bring the music and the source of the music together, we're making progress," he says.

One 25-year-old man had been seeing Dr. Fisher for about a year, plagued with feelings of anger and anxiety. One day he came in, sat down, and joked about how his chair was not as large and soft as Dr. Fisher's chair. Anger seeped through the humor. After some investigation, it turned out that the man's present torment was related to his father mistreating him as a child. After unlocking this chunk of his unconscious, "a whole new avenue for exploration opened up . . . with months of further analysis, the young man's life began to improve significantly," says Dr. Fisher.

In looking for a psychoanalyst, check credentials. Most will have an M.D. or Ph.D. degree, although some qualified practitioners may have an M.S.W. (master's of social work) or a masters-level degree in psychology. Just as important as a therapist's credentials, says Dr. Karon, he or she "should display kindness and compassion." *See also* **behavior therapy; cognitive therapy; dream therapy; interpersonal psychotherapy**

psyllium   (SIL-ee-um) Do you have flea-wort around the house? No, don't run out and get the dog dipped. Fleawort has nothing to do with pests. It's simply the name of the plant that produces psyllium seeds, a key ingredient in many laxatives.

Psyllium, rich in soluble fiber, soaks up water in your bowel, which makes stools larger, softer, and easier to pass. All natural, it's less aggressive than many over-the-counter laxatives.

Doctors also are recommending psyllium for lowering cholesterol. When volunteers at the University of Minnesota took 3 teaspoons a day of psyllium extract, their total cholesterol

levels dropped an average of 4.8 percent. What's more, they lowered their LDL cholesterol (the artery-blocking type of cholesterol) 8.2 percent.

You won't find psyllium seeds in corner grocery stores or produce markets. Not yet, anyway. But many health food stores stock whole-seed psyllium, which you can grind yourself.

Psyllium also is added to some breakfast cereals and, of course, many natural laxatives.

Some people take a few spoonfuls of psyllium every day to help lower their cholesterol *and* soften their stools, says Larry Bell, M.D., author of the Minnesota psyllium study.

If you already eat a lot of bran, fruits, and vegetables, you may not need psyllium supplements, Dr. Bell says. However, psyllium is a fast, easy way to fill your fiber tank. If you frequently forget to pack fruit for lunch, or you don't much care for grains or vegetables, keep a bottle of psyllium as a backup, he suggests.

Psyllium's stool-softening talents make it a natural choice when constipation comes around, Dr. Bell says. Unlike many laxatives, it doesn't flush you out; it does bulk your stool and promote easier, more regular bowel movements.

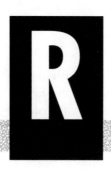

radiation therapy   Perhaps more than any other disease, cancer stirs our deepest fears—fears of pain, prolonged illness, and early death. But 40 to 50 percent of all cancers, if detected at an early stage, are potentially curable. Radiation therapy often plays a crucial part in stopping this dreaded disease.

Tumors are bombarded with high doses of radiation that disrupt the genetic material in each cancer cell, preventing it from dividing. As cancer cells die, tumors shrink and, in many cases, disappear entirely.

Radiation therapy has been around since the late 1800s, when it first was used to irradiate breast cancer. Today, doctors use computers, surgical implants, and high-energy x-ray machines to aim cancer-killing radiation right where it can do the most good—and cause the least harm.

The faster a cell divides, the more vulnerable it is to radiation, says William Hendee, Ph.D., the senior associate dean and vice-president of the Medical College of Wisconsin. Radiation therapy works because cancer cells divide much more quickly than do healthy cells—in some cases doubling in number in just a few hours.

Two types of radiation therapy, internal and external, are discussed here. A third type, used to irradiate tumors during surgery, is rarely used because few operating rooms can afford—or have space for—the bulky x-ray machines used for the procedure.

PLANTING "SEEDS"

"With internal radiation therapy you actually put radioactive materials inside the body," Dr. Hendee explains. Tiny rods, needles, or "seeds," implanted in or near a tumor, deliver large amounts of radiation right where it's needed.

Internal radiation commonly is used for organ cancers—those of the uterus, cervix, bladder, and prostate—which may be difficult to treat in other ways. "Quite often, prostate cancer is treated by implanting small radioactive seeds of iodine-125 right into the prostate," Dr. Hendee says. "You get high doses of radiation to the cancerous tissue, but beyond the prostate the dose falls off rapidly, sparing most of the surrounding tissue."

Some radioactive implants are removed after a few days, while others—usually those that quickly become inert— may be permanently left in the body. The radiation emitted by these implants isn't likely to be harmful to people nearby. Hospitals may put people in private rooms, however, until the radiation "cools" to safer levels.

AIMING THE BEAM

With external radiation therapy, doctors irradiate tumors by shooting x-rays, gamma rays, or electron beams right through the body. X-rays and gamma rays most frequently are used for cancers deep inside the body, while the less penetrating electron beams generally are used for cancers near the surface.

As with diagnostic x-rays, radiation treatments are painless. However, huge amounts of energy are needed to destroy cancer cells. The goal, Dr. Hendee says, is to blast cancer cells while sparing surrounding cells. It isn't always easy.

"We can precisely aim the beam, but it's hard to know where the cancer is at any given time," Dr. Hendee says. "How do we know it hasn't gotten a little bigger or a little smaller? We also have to recognize that the patient is alive and breathing and moving—it's a big challenge."

Most people who receive radiation therapy come to the hospital five days a week for about a month, Dr. Hendee says. "If you give radiation every day, you can get ahead of the rate at which the cells are dividing, and, in time, destroy the cancer," he says.

In some cases—a tumor on the brain stem, for example—cancers may be treated only with radiation, or with radiation and chemotherapy. In some cases, radiation is used to shrink a tumor before surgery, or used after surgery to destroy residual cancer cells.

About half of all radiation treatments are palliative—used simply to relieve pain when there's little hope for a cure, Dr. Hendee says. By shrinking terminal cancers, palliative radiation can help make the illness less uncomfortable.

FEELING THE EFFECTS

Most people, in an average year, receive 0.2 rad (a standard unit of measurement) of background radiation. By contrast, they may receive *4,000* rads in just a few treatments of radiation therapy. Not surprisingly, the body doesn't appreciate this sudden change.

Many people feel fatigued and nauseated while undergoing radiation therapy. Gastrointestinal discomfort, bleeding gums, and heightened sensitivity to pain are sometimes reported. Fortunately, these side effects usually end with the therapy.

More worrisome is the possibility that radiation therapy increases the risk for additional cancers. "There's no question that people who have radiation therapy have a higher incidence of second tumors," Dr. Hendee says. "But you have to wonder if some people are *intrinsically* more likely to get those."

What's in store for the future? A fourth type of radiation therapy, still experimental, uses artificial cells to attack cancers inside the body. Modeled after the body's natural attack cells, these monoclonal antibodies are designed to "bomb" cancer cells with radiation. Unfortunately, Dr. Hendee says, they have sorry aim, landing as often in normal tissue as on cancers. However, if the wrinkles can be removed from this technique, it may be the most efficient way yet to irradiate, and kill, cancers in many parts of the body. *See also* **chemotherapy**

reflexology   To poets, the eye mirrors the soul. To reflexologists, the sole mirrors the soul.

Reflexology is based on the theory that the feet and hands contain specific points that correspond to different parts and organs of the body. Careful manipulation of those points, practitioners believe, may offer relief for anything from arthritis and bedwetting to whiplash and wrist sprains. Angina, epilepsy, flatulence, jaundice, phlebitis, sore throats, strokes—all can be eased or relieved, reflexologists claim, by their "heeling" art.

FEET OF STRENGTH

The map of the foot used by reflexologists mirrors the anatomy of the head and torso, according to Nancy Byers of the International Institute of Reflexology in St. Petersburg, Florida.

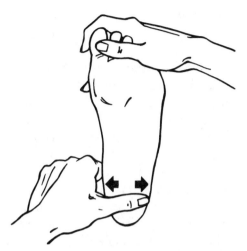

Reflexology treatment for sciatic pain

Stimuli for the brain, head, and sinuses are in the toes; eyes and ears are where toes meet the rest of the foot; the ball of the foot contains lungs and heart; colon, kidneys, and other organs are in the arch.

Current practice, Byers says, is derived from what's called the zone theory, which divides the body into ten straight vertical lines from the top of the head to the tip of the toes.

Specific organs in each zone can be stimulated, reflexologists claim, by stimulating (reflexing) the corresponding spot on the feet—the left foot representing the left half of the body, the right foot the right half. Any twinge or sensitivity in a certain spot of the foot, they say, can indicate a possible problem with an organ in the corresponding zone.

Reflexologists are quick to point out that none of the thousands of nerve endings in the feet go directly to organs elsewhere. Instead, they talk of reflexes and electrical impulses surging from spots on the foot to other areas in the zones.

No scientific studies, Byers concedes, back up the claims that reflexology has healing power. She also admits her art is controversial. "Medical professionals are not going to recognize something out in left field."

The evidence of reflexology's effectiveness, she claims, is in the many reported case studies—the man hopelessly paralyzed from the waist down who read about reflexology, worked his own feet, and began to walk again; the woman who lay restlessly awake each night until she received one treatment and slept like a baby; the person who spent weeks in physical therapy trying to cure neck pain, then was worked on for an hour and arose from bed the next day with not even a slight crimp.

"There's no proof," Byers says, "except that it works."

TOES AND CONS

Most physicians and scientists aren't so ready to toe the reflexology line. Some dismiss it completely; others acknowledge that it "seems to work" but still want to see clinical tests to verify its effectiveness.

"I personally haven't heard of any scientific evidence to support most of the claims" of reflexology, says Glenn Gastwirth, D.P.M., director of scientific affairs for the American Podiatric Medical Association. The association itself has no official comment on or view of the practice, he says.

Turning the theory on its head,

Dr. Gastwirth wonders why—if positive manipulation of the feet really does affect body organs—damage to the feet doesn't have a corresponding negative impact.

"If a [surgeon's] blade cuts across areas that are worked on by a reflexologist, wouldn't there logically be an effect on some of the organs or systems?" he asks. "Or if there's trauma to the foot—a broken toe, a laceration, a burn, the foot's crushed or amputated—what happens to the other organs?"

Thomas DeLauro, D.P.M., executive vice-president for academic and clinical affairs at the New York College of Podiatric Medicine, also points to the lack of clinical research on the claims of reflexology. "Based on our knowledge of neural anatomy," he says, "we're confused at the connection" between the feet and the organs in the body. "Obviously, people get better from it" for whatever reason. "We can't dispute it; we just can't explain it."

GAINING A FOOTHOLD?

Whether or not reflexology does relieve everything from appendicitis and eczema to cirrhosis and scoliosis, it, like any other massage, does feel good. The intense thumb pressure improves circulation and reduces tension, Byers says. "It relieves stress and lets the body heal itself," and for the person who has gone the traditional route to solve a medical problem but has found no cure, it can be "an effective alternative."

Suzanne Levine, D.P.M., diplomate of the American Board of Ambulatory Foot Surgery and clinical assistant podiatrist at the New York College of Podiatric Medicine, also believes it's a good alternative treatment. Some of her patients have benefited from reflexology, and she would "never dismiss it totally." It's "like acupuncture and acupressure," she says. "It's massage taken one step further."

While she agrees with her colleagues that there is no medical proof of the healing claims, she also agrees reflexology eases tension, increases circulation, and balances the flow of energy in the body. "There's something to be said for relaxation and removing stress," she says.

Relaxation Response In this special but natural state, mind and body quiet down. Thoughts drift past, stripped of their power to agitate you. Your brain produces more of the slow brain waves, which signal deep relaxation. You take fewer breaths per minute, using up to 20 percent less oxygen. Even your heart rate decreases by about 3 beats per minute. This is the body's Relaxation Response, a term coined by cardiologist Herbert Benson, M.D., chief of the Division of Behavioral Medicine at New England Deaconess Hospital in Boston.

Regular practice in attaining this state can help you alleviate back pain, headaches, insomnia, depression, and other harmful effects of stress, says Dr. Benson, who is also an associate professor of medicine at Harvard Medical School. It can aid in the prevention and treatment of high blood pressure and related conditions such as heart attacks and strokes, according to Dr.

Benson. It can also relieve chronic muscle tension. One patient of Dr. Benson's found that her persistent neck pain disappeared whenever she elicited the state, and soon it was gone for good.

Dr. Benson is quick to point out that the Relaxation Response is not a cure-all: "It will help you only to the extent that your disease is caused by stress, or made worse by it." Your doctor can help you determine how useful it can be.

GETTING THERE

You can elicit the Relaxation Response through the practice of meditation, yoga, autogenic training, progressive muscle relaxation, the presuggestion phase of hypnosis, repetitive prayer, t'ai chi exercises, or a related discipline. Or you can simply use the following bare bones approach that Dr. Benson says is a distillation of all these disciplines. His studies at Harvard Medical School have shown that the following technique is as effective as any.

First, pick a personally meaningful word or phrase that you can focus on. Sit comfortably and close your eyes. Consciously relax your muscles. Allow yourself to become aware of your breathing. Each time you inhale, repeat your word or phrase to yourself silently. Thoughts will intrude, but let them drift past. Continue to repeat your word or phrase in a relaxed, passive way for 10 to 20 minutes, without trying to make anything happen. If you can, practice this twice a day.

"We find a great many people

choose prayer to focus on," says Dr. Benson, author of *Your Maximum Mind*. "As such, the Relaxation Response becomes a bridge between medicine and religion." And while adding the power of your faith can make this healing state even more effective, the Relaxation Response will work whether you believe in it or not, he adds.

STRESS BUSTER

Mentally focusing on something meaningful or engaging in a physical activity such as t'ai chi or yoga interrupts the flow of anxious or fearful thoughts that normally occupy part of your mind. Such thoughts increase the activity of your sympathetic nervous system, which normally becomes more active during emergencies or stress, releasing hormones that affect heart rate and blood pressure. Increasing the activity of the sympathetic nervous system aggravates the effects of stress, Dr. Benson says.

No matter what discipline you choose to achieve the Relaxation Response, Dr. Benson says the two essential steps to interrupt stress are these: repeating your chosen word, sound, phrase, prayer, or muscle activity, and passively disregarding other thoughts that come to mind.

To get even more mileage out of the Relaxation Response, Dr. Benson suggests using the period immediately after your practice session to "feed" yourself something positive. Read an affirming book, focus on your goals for personal growth, or visualize yourself as healthy. During the Relaxation Response, he says, apparently there is

more harmonious communication between the two hemispheres of your brain, and that can set the stage for enhanced creativity and openness to change. *See also* **autogenic training; hypnosis; imagery; meditation; prayer; yoga**

retinoids   They may sound like creatures from a bad science fiction movie — *Invasion of the Retinoids from Planet X* — but scientists are actually discovering powerful uses for this group of natural and synthetic vitamin A–like drugs, ranging from acne treatment to cancer prevention.

"I think retinoids have an important and optimistic future," says Thomas Moon, Ph.D., a professor of epidemiology at the University of Arizona in Tucson. "They've gone through a roller coaster of ups and downs. At one point, some thought that they were going to be wonder drugs. Then it was thought that they had no effect at all. But now they're coming back."

Retinoids have been used for several years to treat skin diseases. One of the most common of these drugs, isotretinoin, also called Accutane, has successfully been used to battle acne.

Another vitamin A offshoot, tretinoin, may help erase stretch marks. Fifteen of 16 patients who applied a 0.1 percent tretinoin cream to their stretch marks daily for 12 weeks saw the scars fade and in some cases disappear entirely. The drug is the first successful treatment for stretch marks, and researchers believe that it may be useful in treating other types of scars. It works by encouraging the movement of cells that make collagen (a connective-tissue protein) and elastic fibers to the scar site.

But the beauty of retinoids is more than cosmetic. Researchers are uncovering evidence that the drugs may be useful weapons in our war against certain types of cancer.

Skin Cancers Reduced

Accutane, for example, may prevent skin tumors from recurring in the same area of the head and neck where a cancer has been surgically removed. In a study of 103 patients who took oral daily doses of the drug for a year following successful skin cancer surgery, researchers found that only 4 percent had tumors recur. In comparison, new tumors arose in 24 percent of a group of patients who took a nontherapeutic, look-alike drug.

Retinoids also are being studied as a possible treatment for leukemia. Researchers in China and France report that transretinoic acid may be effective against acute promyelocytic leukemia, says Peter H. Wiernik, M.D., associate director of the Albert Einstein Cancer Research Center at Montefiore Medical Center in New York City.

Dr. Wiernik has used the drug to treat four patients, and all have gone into remission. He is planning a large-scale study of the drug involving patients in the United States, Canada, and Australia.

"We're finding that it works. It puts patients with acute promyelocytic leukemia into complete remission," Dr. Wiernik says. "The questions that remain are how long will the remission last and what can be done to enhance the duration of that remission and the survivability of the patient."

There is also evidence that retinoids heal leukoplakias, precancerous sores inside the mouth that are common among people who chew tobacco. More than half of the 21 people suffering from the sores who participated in a British Columbia Cancer Research Center study had no detectable disease after treatment. Experts estimate that only 5 percent of such sores disappear naturally.

Meanwhile, researchers continue to explore other uses for the drugs. Dr. Moon, for example, is involved in several ongoing retinoid studies at the University of Arizona. One of them involves 301 women who are at high risk for developing cervical cancer. The women's physicians are applying a transretinoic acid cream to the cervix that researchers believe may prevent cancer.

"The idea is to stop the progression of a precancerous condition into cervical cancer," Dr. Moon says. "There are indications that the treatment is safe."

Chemotherapy Alternative

Other researchers have investigated Fenretinide, another retinoid, as a chemotherapy. While the drug didn't cause remission in the 31 people with breast cancer and melanoma who participated in a study, researchers still believe it is worth further investigation because of its relatively mild toxicity.

In fact, one of the attractive aspects of retinoids as a cancer treatment is that they appear to be effective but have milder effects than traditional chemotherapy, Dr. Moon says. Dry skin and flulike symptoms are the most common side effects of retinoid therapy.

"Because of the nature of the disease, cancer patients traditionally have had to tolerate some very severe side effects, some of them life-threatening. The retinoids are much milder than that," Dr. Moon says. "Clearly, it would be best if they didn't produce those flulike symptoms, but hopefully the next generation of retinoids will be just as effective but have fewer side effects." *See also* **acne remedies**

RICE This neat little acronym stands for Rest, Ice, Compression, and Elevation—the perfect first-aid combination for minor muscle strains and sprains. You can use it on ankles, elbows, hands—almost any sprained joint. Skip the compression part and it can ease sprained back muscles, too.

The first thing you need to know about RICE is that the faster you apply it, the better. Quick action can limit the pain, swelling, and disability that follow in the wake of an injury, says Edward Haughn, D.O., cofounder of Northwestern Michigan Sportsmedicine in Traverse City, Michigan.

Those symptoms have a purpose, but only up to a point. "The body has a way of protecting itself. Back when our ancestors were running through the woods with clubs, they didn't have a doctor waiting with a cast in case

they got hurt," Dr. Haughn says. That's why nature, unless it's stopped with appropriate treatment such as RICE, does everything it can to immobilize an injured joint. And to keep it immobilized longer than you may care to wait. Luckily RICE may help bypass all that.

HOW TO USE IT

To use RICE, just remember these four steps.

1. Rest. If you've injured your ankle or shin, take the weight off of it immediately. Whatever you've injured, take care not to move it.

2. Ice. Apply an ice pack to the injured area for 15 to 30 minutes.

3. Compression. Wrap the area with a compression bandage to help restrict further swelling.

4. Elevation. Raise the injury above the level of your heart. If you're treating a sprained ankle with RICE, for instance, propping the ankle on a stool won't do much. Lying down and using pillows to raise it above your heart is better. Doing this slows the flow of fluids to the injury site, minimizing swelling.

You can reapply the technique as needed, during the first 24 to 48 hours. You'll only need to keep the ice on for 15 minutes at a stretch with these subsequent applications. At night, remove bandages to avoid circulation problems. If you don't, the swelling could intensify.

After the first 48 hours are up,

you can minimize any remaining pain with an ice massage. An easy way to do this is to freeze water in a large paper cup. Peel away the top of the cup, and rub the injured area for 10 to 15 minutes until it turns bright red.

If you suspect a fracture, consult a doctor after you've given yourself the initial RICE first-aid treatment. Signs of a fracture include sudden and severe swelling, pain at the ends of the bones, any noticeable deformity, and loss of function in the injured area. *See also* **cold therapy**

Rogaine.   *See* **minoxidil**

R

S

salt When Roman statesman Cicero warned, "Trust no one until you have eaten much salt with him," he clearly knew zilch about the dangers of consuming too much sodium chloride. To the ancients, salt was manna from the heavens. They preserved food with it. They used it to make chewy snacks. (One of their favorites was beef jerky.) They even soaked aching muscles in it.

Of course, now we've heard it's best to go easy on the salt. Studies of its potential harmful effects on our health keep popping up like dirty dishes in the sink. Most notably, excess dietary salt may be linked to high blood pressure, water retention, and problems with calcium levels in the body.

GERM KILLER

But the ancients were right in their belief that salt, under the right conditions, can heal. For one thing, it can help kill certain germs such as those that cause sore throat or inflamed gums, according to microbiologist David Marshall, director of the University of Miami Wound Care Information Institute.

For swollen gums or a sore throat, stir 1 teaspoon of salt into an 8-ounce glass of warm water, recommends Daniel Mowrey, Ph.D., director of the American Phytotherapy Research Laboratory in Salt Lake City. Swish the mouthwash around in your mouth for a minute, and spit it out.

POPPING PILLS

In the not-too-distant past, salt tablets were often recommended for athletes and others who toiled physically in hot weather. The thinking was that because sweat contains a lot of salt, if you sweated too much, you would lose too much salt and create an imbalance in your body.

We are primarily made up of saltwater, explains Ross D. Feldman, M.D., professor of medicine and pharmacology at the University of Western Ontario School of Medicine. In fact we have about ½ pound of salt in our body, so if we don't have enough salt, our blood pressure drops.

But Dr. Feldman says when this happens, all you need to do is drink a simple cup of beef bouillon or chicken soup. It's rare that people need to take salt tablets.

Possibly the only people who may need to take salt tablets are those with low blood pressure, and that condition is rare, he says.

SALTWATER SOAKS

One notion that *has* proved to be true is that soaking in saltwater can be beneficial. A study by the Soroka Medical Center in Israel found that patients with rheumatoid arthritis improved dramatically after daily immersions in Dead Sea bath salts. (The Dead Sea is ten times saltier than the Mediterranean.) Scientists say the patients could move their hands and walk better after soaking. Dead Sea bath salts are available at some drugstores.

Saltwater soaks have also been used as an effective home remedy to cure sweaty feet, says podiatrist Suzanne Levine, D.P.M., diplomate of the American Board of Ambulatory Foot Surgery and clinical assistant podiatrist at the New York College of Podiatric Medicine. Why? Because when saltwater comes in contact with skin cells, it tends to suck the water out of them. The cells tend to shrivel and dry up.

sclerotherapy   Varicose veins not only make you feel blue—they can make you *look* blue from hip to toe. But fortunately, an injection technique called sclerotherapy may be able to help. "Sclerotherapy results in obliteration and removal of varicose veins," says D. Brian McDonagh, M.D., a phlebologist (vein specialist) in Schaumburg,

Illinois, and founder of the Vein Clinics of America.

Varicose veins aren't all alike. "There are the large, ropelike varicose veins that both men and women get when their surface veins become flooded with blood," Dr. McDonagh says. "And there are very small, burgundy-colored spider veins which come off a vein located deeper in the legs. The latter are exclusively a problem for women."

Large varicose veins form when a valve malfuntions in a perforating leg vein (one that connects the surface veins and the deep veins). Blood backs up in the vein, distending it. Smaller varicose or spider veins, found mostly in women, are caused by female hormones, especially during pregnancy.

Women with small vein disease are particularly good candidates for sclerotherapy, says Dr. McDonagh. Unlike surgery, which would require too many incisions to be a practical solution, sclerotherapy can be an effective treatment to eradicate this problem, he says. Proper physician training and experience are critical.

VEINS FADE AWAY

With this method, which was developed in Europe, the doctor injects a special solution (such as sodium tetradecyl sulfate) into the offending vein. "The goal is to eradicate existing vein disease without damaging the surrounding tissue," Dr. McDonagh says.

The term *sclerotherapy*—which comes from the Greek word for "to harden"—is actually a poor choice of words. After the vein is injected, it only temporarily hardens, says Dr. McDonagh. The real good of the procedure comes when the inflammation and hardening subside, leaving a minuscule band of scar tissue in its place, he says. In effect, the useless vein dries up and withers away to nothing.

Voilà! Your legs no longer resemble a topographical map of Minnesota's 1,001 lakes—and because there is no surgery, there is absolutely no scarring, says Dr. McDonagh.

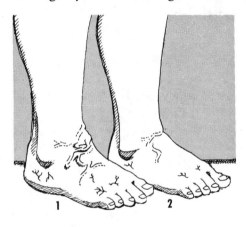

Before (1) and after (2) sclerotherapy

However, he cautions that people seeking sclerotherapy should determine that they are consulting a competent physician who has considerable experience with the procedure. He says that people should only choose doctors to do the procedure "who are very fastidious and take great care prior to and during the treatment." Lists of qualified doctors may be obtained from your local medical society or by sending a self-addressed, stamped envelope to the North American Society of Phlebology, 511 Encinitas Boulevard, Suite 111, Encinitas, CA 92024.

One thing to consider about sclerotherapy is that although the procedure has a greater than 80 percent five-year cure rate, there's no guarantee that other veins won't break down in the future. "That's because you have 214 perforator veins per leg—we're talking 428 for both," says Dr. McDonagh. "If you had 428 teeth in your head you'd never get out of that dental chair. So I can fix it when one of these veins breaks down and floods your system, but neither surgery nor injections can cure varicose veins." One bad vein almost inevitably is followed by others.

Another drawback is that many insurance companies don't reimburse for the procedure, a practice that annoys Dr. McDonagh. "Companies should stop dismissing varicose veins as merely a cosmetic problem," he argues. "Not only can such veins cause aching, pain, leg ulcers, dermatitis, and heaviness, but they can destroy the psyche of some people who have them."

He tells the story of one woman with longtime varicose veins who told him after her sclerotherapy that she'd have to inform her husband that she could swim after all. "Can you imagine? She denied that she could swim just to avoid exposing her legs at the beach," he marvels.

sedatives Sleep charges our batteries, gives us our much-needed rest, and prepares us for tomorrow's challenges. As one poet says:

O Sleep, the certain knot of peace,
The baiting-place of wit, the balm of woe,
The poor man's wealth, the prisoner's release,
The indifferent judge between the high and low.

Of course, people who stay awake all night, anxious and full of stress, may not appreciate Sir Philip Sidney's paean to sleep. They *will* appreciate a doctor's prescription for sedatives, which can help people cope with temporary anxiety and insomnia.

Actually, sedatives go by many names, depending on what they're used for. If you take a sedative to relieve anxiety, for example, it may be called an anxiolytic, or a minor tranquilizer. Taken to help you sleep, sedatives are called hypnotics. In other cases, they are muscle relaxants, pre-anesthetics, and anticonvulsants.

POPULAR PRESCRIPTIONS

Regardless of the name, sedatives are among the most widely prescribed drugs in the world. In fact, approximately two billion doses of diazepam (Valium), one of the most popular sedatives in the United States, are prescribed every year.

In the past, the sedatives of choice were the barbiturates. Today, most doctors prefer the benzodiazepines—drugs such as diazepam, flurazepam (Dalmane), lorazepam (Ativan), and oxazepam (Serax). Of every 20 prescriptions written in the United States, 1 is for a benzodiazepine.

"From a pharmaceutical point of view, the benzodiazepines are just about a perfect drug," says E. Don Nelson, Pharm.D., a professor of clinical pharmacology at the University of Cincinnati. "They relieve anxiety without causing a great deal of sedation."

A nervous father with a child in the hospital might take sedatives to calm his anxiety. People who lie awake all night because of recent traumas—a divorce, for example—might take sedatives to help them get to sleep.

All sedatives work by depressing the central nervous system. So even though the benzodiazepines produce less sedation than some other drugs, they do cause some drowsiness. In addition, they tend to disturb normal sleep, so some people wake up feeling tired.

The primary difference between many of the benzodiazepines is the speed with which they work. Some of the fast-acting benzodiazepines may be used for the emergency treatment of convulsions or severe panic attacks. Slower-acting drugs may be used for the long-term (more than a few weeks) relief of anxiety.

LINGERING EFFECTS

While some sedatives are quickly eliminated from the body, most remain for days, Dr. Nelson says. That may be especially serious for elderly people, whose systems naturally work more slowly. To prevent dangerous accumulations of drugs in the body, doctors often prescribe sedatives for only a few days or weeks at a time.

Mixed with other substances, sedatives may be extremely dangerous. "When the benzodiazepines are combined with alcohol, they can be deadly," Dr. Nelson warns. However, the benzodiazepines are much safer than the barbiturates, and fatalities are rare.

Sedatives really aren't meant for long-term use, Dr. Nelson says. People with persistent anxiety, insomnia, or panic attacks need to resolve—not medicate—their problems. But when things get tough, sedatives can help, he says: "Most people who take sedatives take them for two weeks or less." *See also* **antianxiety drugs; barbiturates; phenobarbital; tranquilizers**

Seldane. *See* **antihistamines**

self-help audiotapes   Virtually unheard of 15 years ago, self-help audiotapes now seem right at home in cassette decks everywhere. Americans spend millions of dollars a year on taped therapy. Listeners say the tapes help them relax, kick bad habits, and learn new skills—all while commuting to work, washing the dishes, or running in the park. (Try that with 10 pounds of textbooks.)

There are many types of self-help tapes. As you might expect, weight-loss tapes abound. They exhort listeners to lose weight and feel good about themselves, too. Other tapes encourage people to exercise, to improve their work habits, to positively change their lives. Some tapes simply help people learn new things—playing the har-

monica, for instance, or mastering a foreign language. *Es muy bueno!*

A WAY TO UNWIND

Stress-reduction tapes are especially popular. Tapes filled with soothing voices and gentle music can help anyone unwind, says Naida Colby, a registered nurse and consultant with the Minnesota Center for Health and Rehabilitation who makes her own relaxation tapes.

The music on her tapes is recorded in largo—a stately tempo which Colby says slows your brain activity and gives you a healthy, relaxed sleep. The words on relaxation tapes aren't as important as the tempo, she says.

"I can put someone into an alpha-theta rhythm [the brain waves characteristic of light sleep] just by saying rest . . . rest . . . rest," she says. "It's almost like hypnosis."

Many tapes do help people relax, and relaxation always is helpful for healing, says Claire Etheridge, Ph.D., a clinical psychologist in Laguna Beach, California.

Although Dr. Etheridge frequently prescribes relaxation tapes for her clients, she says people need to be careful about what they listen to—and where they do their listening.

"People should not listen to relaxation tapes while they're driving," she says. "You get some nice music in the background, with a voice talking, and that can be very dangerous because you may fall asleep."

However, a relaxation tape may be very soothing (and safe) at the end of the day, *after* you finish your commute, Dr. Etheridge adds.

"When we go into an alpha state, we put our critical mind—that part that jabbers at us—to rest," she says. "You automatically begin to get in touch with your spirit, more in touch with your soul."

PORTABLE PERSUASION

Once the listener is in a relaxed and receptive state, many tapes go on to deliver a motivational or instructional message. However, Dr. Etheridge says people shouldn't believe everything they hear on such self-help tapes. After all, the tapes are made for large audiences; not everything on each tape can possibly apply to you.

Weight-loss tapes, for instance, typically exhort people to "eat less and less and less . . . look nicer and nicer and nicer," Dr. Etheridge says. Good advice, right? Not for someone suffering from an eating disorder like anorexia nervosa, who feels she's overweight even when she's not. Many people who think they're too heavy actually need more to eat, not less.

"A lot of the people who make these tapes do not understand the human mind sufficiently to be wise in their word selection," Dr. Etheridge warns.

Self-help tapes probably won't hurt so long as you employ a reasonable amount of skepticism. The good tapes, however, really can help, she says. Most of us can benefit from extra reassurances, gentle nudges, and reminders that we can deal with our problems.

More and more therapists these days are using self-help tapes as adjuncts to conventional therapy. After all, few people are so rich—or so idle—that they can spend an hour or more a day in therapy. With shrinks shrunk to playback size, however, people can listen to their therapist whenever (and however often) they want. Unlike the doctor, the tape is always "in."

Self-help tapes are practically essential for some people. For instance, what would you do if you had agoraphobia, the fear of public places? Let's face it: People with agoraphobia often can't leave their homes by themselves, much less drive across town for a doctor's appointment.

Turn on the tape. Listen to your therapist . . . she's leading you, one step at a time . . . first down this street, then to the corner to the station. . . . Are you scared? It's okay—just listen.

Some people simply need to confront their problems by hearing about them over and over again. For instance, one therapist asked a client to record on tape the reasons for her obsessive fear of knives. Afterward, the woman listened to the tape ten times a day for more than two months. By then, she no longer was bothered by the idea of knives.

Not all self-help tapes seem to be equally helpful. Some experts feel that subliminal tapes—which supposedly deliver a subaudible message often masked by music—don't do much more than line the producers' pockets.

Dr. Etheridge says we routinely take in messages we're not aware of receiving. We stop at red lights, for instance, without thinking about why we're stopping. However, there's no evidence that subliminal audiotapes produce therapeutic results, she says.

People should only buy self-help tapes made by experts and distributed by reputable companies, Dr. Etheridge suggests. What's more, you shouldn't listen to them all day. For most people, two half-hour sessions a day is plenty, she says.

"You don't want to stay in a meditative state all the time," Dr. Etheridge says. "You want to apply what you learn to the real world."

self-help groups It took David a long time to admit that drugs and alcohol were—to put it bluntly—ruining his life. Money was tight because he spent it all on dope. He had trouble concentrating at work. And as for caring about his wife—all he really cared about was getting high.

David finally got smart enough to check into a private rehabilitation clinic, and therapists there eventually sent him to Alcoholics Anonymous— probably the nation's oldest self-help group.

"People told me if I didn't attend AA for the rest of my life, I'd either be in jail, or dead, or addicted," David remembers. Now 34, he's been sober more than four years.

His experience isn't unusual. Indeed, there may be half a million self-help groups in the United States, serving more than 17 million people.

There is a self-help group for just about every physical, social, and emotional problem. Alcoholics Anony-

mous, probably the largest of the self-help groups, is estimated to have more than 1.8 million members nationwide. Overeaters Anonymous and Gamblers Anonymous also have chapters in most large cities. There are self-help groups for senior citizens, for young parents, for teenagers.

In fact, you have a self-help group every time three (or three million) people get together to tackle common problems, says Ed Madara, director of American Self-Help Clearinghouse, a New Jersey–based organization that lists nearly 5,000 local and national self-help groups. The number is (201) 625-7101.

SHARED INSIGHTS

"When 20 people call us and there's no group for their problem, we ask them if they're interested in starting their own group," Madara says. By definition, self-help groups aren't run by therapists, Madara says—unless, of course, the therapists have the same problems as other people in the group.

There are exceptions, however. "We do not classify our groups—which are facilitated by licensed psychotherapists—as 'self-help' groups," says Harold H. Benjamin, Ph.D., founder of The Wellness Community, a nationwide program to help cancer patients become partners with their physicians in their fight for recovery. "However, the fundamentals are the same. The primary function of the facilitator is to help the participants in the groups share experiences, swap stories, and give emotional support. There is no better or more supportive way to decrease what are sometimes overwhelming burdens than to share your feelings with 12 other people who are going through the very same experiences."

How effective are self-help groups? At the University of Hamburg in Germany, researchers at the Institute for Medical Sociology asked 232 people if they felt better—experienced less fear, for example, or less emotional distress—after attending self-help groups. Eighty percent said they improved after attending the groups.

"You can go to a million lectures and be told you must not drink anymore," says a spokeswoman at the Alcoholics Anonymous general service office in New York. However, lectures don't work nearly as well as meeting people with the same problems, she says.

Self-help groups "become a lifelong process," says a spokesperson at the Overeaters Anonymous world service office. "Most people who come in find it becomes a way to cope with their life, deal with challenges, and make decisions."

Newcomers to self-help meetings always are a little nervous. Don't let that scare you. For one thing, everyone knows how you feel. Besides, people don't expect first-timers to talk much, anyway.

"A lot of people have been told you have to be a professional to start a self-help group, but this is not the case," Madara says. "Just a core group together—people who share your problem and your dream."

sex People have sex for many reasons. Starting a family is one reason. But sex is also a powerful physical drive: It demands satisfaction. It also satisfies our longings for romance and intimacy—what you might call our emotional drives.

Here's still another reason. Sex has some healing powers, too.

SUPPRESSES PAIN

If you have a little pain, for example, sex may help. Researchers report that sexual stimulation releases analgesic chemicals—endorphins, the body's "morphine," is one example— that raise pain thresholds and suppress sensory awareness. That's why you may not notice minor aches and pains during intercourse. You may not hear the doorbell, either.

Sex also stimulates the release of estrogen and progesterone. These hormones, like endorphins, also appear to make us less sensitive to pain.

Sexual intercourse may have other benefits as well. Vaginal atrophy, a decrease in the vagina's natural elasticity, occurs most often in postmenopausal women who rarely have intercourse. Conversely, vaginal atrophy is rare in sexually active women. The phrase "Use it or lose it," then, may have some validity.

Incidentally, just how active does one have to be to qualify as "sexually active"? In one study, researchers said sexually active women had intercourse at least three times a month for one consecutive year.

Some women claim that intercourse relieves painful menstrual cramping. How? During orgasm, the uterus contracts, sending blood coursing through the cervix. It's theorized that this may relieve the occasionally painful pressure of menstrual blood in the cervical canal.

A SLEEP INDUCER

Have you ever noticed that post-coital sleep—deep, satisfying, out-like-a-light sleep—seems darned near irresistible? No, it's not just you. Doctors say many people quickly fall asleep after sex.

Sex, however, isn't quite the same as a sleeping pill. When you feel your eyes pressing shut before you can say, "Good night, dear," it's merely the after-sex relaxation effect that's putting you out, says Timothy Roehrs, Ph.D., a scientist at the Henry Ford Hospital Sleep Disorders and Research Center in Detroit.

"When the sexual drive is satisfied, one is relaxed, and therefore sleep onset is very easy," Dr. Roehrs says. Don't count on sex to put you to sleep if you're not tired, he warns. It won't.

Some people insist they get their best sleep after sex. Sex may, in fact, promote deep sleep—but so does riding a bicycle or indulging in any sort of vigorous exercise, Dr. Roehrs says.

shiatsu. *See* **acupressure**

shoes, therapeutic Special feet require a special fit. That's the basis behind today's therapeutic shoes for adults, custom-made with certain goals in mind. Comfort is only one of them.

For the elderly who've lost most of the fat cushion beneath the soles of their feet, therapeutic shoes with soft inserts can prevent bone-grinding contact with the pavement.

For people with diabetes who have poor circulation and loss of sensation in their feet, therapeutic custom-made shoes may help distribute weight and relieve pressure in a way that prevents ulcers from developing, says Glenn Gastwirth, D.P.M., director of scientific affairs for the American Podiatric Medical Association.

Some people with severe arthritis can benefit from custom-made shoes that hold the feet in a position that alleviates pain, says Ellen Cohen-Sobel, D.P.M., Ph.D., assistant professor of orthopedics at the New York College of Podiatric Medicine in Manhattan. Therapeutic shoes may also offer an alternative to surgery for some cases of bunions, particularly in older patients, she says.

SHOPPING SMART

Some people opt for custom-fit therapeutic shoes for the sheer comfort of them. Of course, you don't have to go to that trouble—or expense—to find a pair of shoes that feel good and support your feet. You can get off to a good start by checking the one-page list of shoes given a "seal of acceptance" by the American Podiatric Medical Association. This is a voluntary list, so it only applies to shoes that manufacturers have submitted for review. The shoes have been judged for quality, construction, foot support, and shock absorption, Dr. Gastwirth says. You can obtain a copy by writing to the American Podiatric Medical Association, c/o Department of Public Affairs, 9312 Old Georgetown Road, Bethesda, MD 20814–1621.

When you're in the shoe store, keep these important guidelines in mind.

Make sure the back of the heel is fairly stiff, the midsole is rigid enough to be supportive, and the lower sole is flexible from the ball of the foot forward, says Richard Robinson, D.P.M., assistant clinical professor at the California College of Podiatric Medicine, Los Angeles.

Turn the shoe over. Look at the bottom of your foot and compare it with the curve of the shoe. Are the shapes similar, or will your foot be squeezed into an awkward position? Make sure the curves match. *See also* **orthoses**

skin grafts   We shouldn't, but we do. We take for granted one of our body's most vital organs, the skin. Although our birthday suit faithfully protects our insides from bumps, wounds, chemicals, bacteria, extreme temperatures, radiation, and water loss, we view it rather like an old, reliable shoe—it'll always be there when we need it.

But when it isn't there, when it has suffered real damage—in the case of a severe burn, for example, or the treatment of leg ulcers, or the removal of cancerous tumors—a surgical procedure called skin grafting can help.

A skin graft serves three purposes, says Gary Rogers, M.D., associate professor of dermatology and surgery at Boston University School of Medicine. First, it gives a slow-healing wound immediate protection from bacteria and germs by covering it up with another piece of skin. Otherwise, an infection and subsequent complications may occur.

Second, by covering up the wound with transplanted skin, new fragile skin will start growing underneath, protected by the graft. This new skin will eventually fill in that place left by the damaged skin.

Third, a graft stops the water in your body from seeping out through the exposed tissues of the wound, something that can cause dehydration, shock, and even death if the exposed area is large enough to allow substantial water loss.

SKIN DEEP

In a typical skin graft, says Dr. Rogers, the wound is first scraped clean of charred or dead tissue so that what remains is healthy underlying tissue that is rich with blood vessels, called vascularized or granulated skin. Then doctors cut off a new, healthy piece of skin from another part of the same patient's body, preferrably from a spot where the skin is similar to that surrounding the wound.

Doctors place the new skin on top of the wound and hold it in place with staples, stitches, and bandages.

In the meantime, the place from which the skin was removed, called the "donor site," is also bandaged. Usually donor sites heal well and new skin grows in and fills up the empty space without leaving unsightly marks or indentations.

If the graft is successful, the blood vessels and tissues in both the original wound and the new skin covering it will connect and grow together. Depending on the type of graft you need, it can take between 48 hours to a week for the new skin to start growing onto the healing skin, Dr. Rogers says.

Ideally, your own skin is used for grafts (a technique called autologous skin grafting), but in some cases this is not possible. For example, if a patient has severe burns over 80 percent of his body, there is not enough undamaged skin left to serve as a donor site. Because the biggest concern of doctors is to quickly cover up all exposed, damaged skin, temporary grafts using pig or human cadaver skin are done in such cases. Before long, the burns begin healing underneath the layer of temporary skin, and it is removed when healing is complete. (Ultimately, our bodies will always reject skin that isn't our own.)

THROUGH THICK AND THIN

To understand how the various kinds of skin grafts work, you need to understand exactly how skin is structured. The outer layer of skin, called the epidermis, is a very thin covering, only about $50/1000$ inch thick. This waterproof epidermis protects the skin's second layer, the dermis, which is meaty looking and rich with blood vessels. It is also where the hair follicles—something critical to the healing process—are located. The third layer, the hypodermis, contains loosely connected tissue and fat, and acts as insulation and padding. Think of it as our body's shock absorbers.

The depth and width of the wound determines the type of skin graft you will have. Here are the main types of grafts.

Full thickness graft. This is used on deeper wounds—such as those related to cancer, skin ulcers, and severe burns—where the top two layers of skin are damaged or missing. A full thickness graft provides the best functional results. It can only be used to cover limited areas, however.

After the damaged skin tissue has been removed, the remaining hole must be filled with fresh skin from the donor site—skin most likely to readily attach itself to the wound and grow. Ideally, the donor site would be located in a nearby area of the body where the skin is similar. For example, if you have a wound on your eyelid, then the best donor site would be the other eyelid. But if that isn't available, skin is often taken from the chest or behind the ear.

This type of graft takes about a week to heal, and it looks better cosmetically than other skin grafts.

Split thickness graft. This is typically used in cases such as extensive burns where large areas of skin have to be resurfaced. The immediate concern here is that because there is so much damaged, exposed tissue, infection or dehydration could occur.

In this case, doctors need to place a thin layer of epidermis with a tiny amount of blood-vesseled dermis onto the burn. It takes about 48 hours to begin attaching itself to the burn.

A split thickness graft is not as cosmetically attractive as a full thickness graft. But because of its lower metabolic demands, it has a better chance of surviving than a full thickness graft does in situations where there is poor blood supply, such as chronic leg ulcers.

Synthetic skin. One of the major problems with widespread burns is that doctors often can't find enough undamaged epidermis on the patient's body to cover the burn. But now they can actually grow large sheets of epidermis in incubators.

Physicians take a tiny piece of skin and place it into incubators filled with a liquid containing all the nutrients skin cells need to grow. Gases that skin cells would normally be exposed to are also pumped into the incubator. There is virtually no limit to the size of the sheet of skin that can be grown. Physicians report having treated about 100 patients with skin that was originally the size of a postage stamp. This cultured skin is laid on the burn patient's wounds without having to perform any surgery. The beauty of this is that a patient with extensive burns or large leg ulcers doesn't have to go through the trauma of having large portions of his healthy skin removed to cover the wounded areas.

slippery elm   They say music can soothe the savage breast. But how do you soothe savage sore throats, wounds, digestive upsets, or a mild case of hemorrhoids? Ask the Indians. Long before the Pilgrims invaded their shores, native Americans were using slippery elm for whatever irritated them (colonists not included).

Thanks in part to large elm forests that blanketed the East in those days, they had a steady supply of this all-purpose botanical. And the colonists picked up the habit in short order. It's probably no exaggeration to say that back then slippery elm was at the top of the nation's hit parade when it came to soothing home remedies.

MODERN USES

Even today, herbalists make good use of slippery elm. It's the mucilaginous inner bark that possesses the tree's healing properties. When powdered, it can easily be mixed with water. Herbal practitioners often recommend using the resulting mixture externally as a poultice to bandage wounds and to soothe irritated skin. And they use slippery elm tea as an expectorant and to aid in the treatment of sore throats, coughs, diarrhea, ulcers, and other digestive problems. Slippery elm has only a slight taste and a maplelike aroma.

One old-time remedy for colds and bronchitis is slippery elm lemonade: Mix 1 tablespoon of the powder with cold water to make a paste. Gradually stir in 1 pint of boiling water; add 2 tablespoons of lemon juice and honey to taste.

For a poultice to bandage wounds, gradually add enough water to make a paste and apply it to the affected area.

Herbalists also recommend sprinkling the power directly on the skin to soothe heat rashes and chafed skin.

Slippery elm is no longer as common or popular a remedy as it once was. Most people know it as a prime ingredient in old-fashioned lozenges sold in many health food stores for sore throats and colds.

The medical literature contains no reports of slippery elm causing harm, but as with all botanicals, allergic reactions are always possible.

soda crackers   For generations, queasy mothers-to-be have been nibbling on soda crackers to prevent morning sickness. So have hung-over drinkers and holiday overeaters with rumbling bellies, not to mention all those Thanksgiving Day overeaters who fairly stagger away from the table vowing never to eat again.

While there's no scientific proof that this bland little cracker can actually soothe an upset stomach, still there *are* some experts who insist this folk remedy deserves two thumbs-up for effectiveness.

When you are nauseated, your stomach needs some kind of food in it, explains Dudley Phillips, M.D., who has a family practice in Darington, Maryland. If you don't eat something, you're going to get even sicker from having *no* food.

And that's where soda crackers can come in real handy.

A soda cracker is very, very easy on the digestive system, according to Dr. Phillips. It's light and doesn't take much energy for the digestive system to handle it. So you're able to get food into your stomach without making your system work extra hard to digest it.

But there's an even more important reason why soda crackers help soothe the stomach. "Soda crackers eat up the acid in your stomach," Dr. Phillips explains. "A good part of what is in these crackers besides the flour is soda bicarbonate, which will neutralize stomach acid. A cracker or two just soaks it right up."

Dr. Phillips says salted crackers, graham crackers, or even the kind of wheat cracker used for hors d'oeuvres works almost as well as plain soda crackers. The latter, which are often called soup and oyster crackers, have very little sodium in them. "Any cracker that's been made with baking soda will probably do the trick."

Nibble Away

"I often tell my patients to eat a cracker or two if their stomach is in trouble," says Dr. Phillips. "If the reason you're feeling ill is because of something you ate—say, a big Thanksgiving dinner—my advice is to wait about 1 hour. That's about the time you have the most acid in your stomach. Eat a couple of crackers, wait another 2 hours, then have another one."

Dr. Phillips points out that soda crackers can work if the cause of the nausea is relatively minor and correctable. "But if your stomach upset is symptomatic of a serious disease or illness, obviously it's going to take more than a cracker to solve the problem." *See also* **antiemetics**

sore throat remedies Swallowing is normally as effortless as blinking your eyes. But this morning, your throat is so tender that when you've finished your cereal, you feel like you've just auditioned for a job as a sword swallower in the circus.

A sore throat is often the first sign that a cold virus has invaded your body. "You might not think of it this way, but your scarlet, swollen throat means that legions of infection-fighting white blood cells have mobilized and are waging war against enemy viral particles," says John Henderson, M.D., assistant clinical professor of ear, nose, and throat surgery at the University of California School of Medicine in San Diego.

Feel better yet? No? Well, there is something you can do besides wince each time you swallow. For starters, gargling with saltwater can be exquisitely soothing.

"When you add ½ teaspoon of salt to an 8-ounce glass of warm water, you create a saline solution that is very much like your body's own fluid," explains Dr. Henderson. "As long as it's weak, saltwater is less stimulating to sensitive nerve fibers than any other gargling liquid." What's more, the salt draws germs and fluids out of tissues and thus reduces swelling, he says. And when you gargle, the bubbling action is like a supersoft scrub brush, gently massaging away thick mucus that accumulates and irritates throat tissues.

SPRITZ AWAY PAIN

Gargling can only reach as far as the soft palate (that's the fleshy protuberance that hangs down like a stalactite in a cave). To reach a sore spot further down in your throat, try an anesthetic throat spray such as Chloraseptic. These sprays allow you to aim a pain-numbing jet stream of anesthetic directly at the irritated site and to direct the medication deeper in your throat.

But try not to get "trigger-happy" when using the spray. "The problem with anesthetic sprays is that the pain-killing effect is washed away with each swallow of saliva," says John Cormier, Pharm.D., associate professor and associate dean of the College of Pharmacy at the Medical University of South Carolina in Charleston. And when the anesthetic wears off, you may be tempted to spray your throat again immediately, instead of waiting the recommended 2 to 4 hours before your next spray. Soon you've created a vicious spray/pain/spray cycle.

Overuse of anesthetic throat sprays can make an angry, red throat worse, says Dr. Henderson. "The main ingredient in throat sprays is usually phenol, which is a harsh irritant. Used full strength, these sprays can cause a chemical burn on sensitive throat tissues."

MELT AWAY SORENESS

Throat lozenges have longer-lasting pain-relieving power than sprays simply because you hold them in your mouth for a longer period of time. But because the disk's painkilling effect lasts only 15 minutes after dissolving, you might be tempted to suck on another lozenge too soon afterward, to sustain the relief.

"If you use too much lozenge

medicine, you may irritate the mucous membranes of the mouth and throat," says Dr. Cormier. His advice? "Don't take lozenges more often than directed on the label."

Of course, you could simply swallow two ordinary pain-reliever tablets and be done with it, suggests Dr. Henderson. "Take two acetaminophen tablets, like Tylenol, for example, and in 20 minutes, the pain in your throat will be reduced."

Never chew or dissolve aspirin or aspirin-like pain relievers in your mouth, however. "Aspirin applied locally can eat into mucous membranes, resulting in painful ulcerations," says Dr. Cormier.

And don't rely on aspirin chewing-gum products for topical relief of sore throat pain, says Branton Lachman, Pharm.D., clinical assistant professor at the University of Southern California School of Pharmacy in Los Angeles: "Aspirin must be absorbed into your bloodstream in order for it to relieve pain."

Despite all your efforts, if your sore throat lingers beyond two days, see a doctor. See a doctor *first* if you have a fever over 102°F, your throat is swollen or covered with white patches, or you have difficulty swallowing or breathing. These symptoms may mean you have strep throat, a serious bacterial infection which can lead to pneumonia or rheumatic fever if not treated with antibiotics. *See also* **gargling; horehound; lozenges**

sphygmomanometer. *See* **blood pressure monitors**

spirulina (speer-YOO-lee-na) Ever since a popular national tabloid ran an article about the nutritional wonders of spirulina, this commercially grown blue-green algae (freeze-dried in the form of food supplements) has been touted as a superfood of the future. Supposedly, this "magic bullet" is capable of boosting your energy, lowering your cholesterol, reducing cancer, shrinking your waistline, and wiping out wrinkles.

Sound suspect? It is. It turns out that as far as nutrition goes, spirulina has no more to offer than many much more common foods. And in fact, by taking spirulina, you may be compromising your health instead of boosting it.

As far as the claim that it's the wonder food of the future, in truth, spirulina is a food from the past. Centuries ago, Africans would scoop the scum off lakes, dry it in the sun, grind it, mix it with flour, and eat it as a source of protein.

That made perfect sense for those people in that time and place, experts say. "Spirulina is almost three-quarters protein and has a superhigh iron content," says Elliot Shubert, Ph.D., professsor of biology at the University of North Dakota in Grand Forks. "It's also a good source of beta-carotene [which is converted to vitamin A in the body] and B vitamins."

But for modern Westerners, explains Dr. Shubert, spirulina has no more to offer nutritionally than protein sources such as chicken or eggs, or iron sources such as spinach, or beta-carotene sources such as carrots. "These foods are readily available, cheaper, and better tasting than algae," says Dr. Shubert. More important, these foods may be *safer* than spirulina.

A few years ago, Dr. Shubert and his colleagues were investigating spirulina for its iron bioavailability in a study sponsored by the U.S. Department of Agriculture. "We were intrigued to discover that the iron from this plant was readily retained by laboratory rats. That's unusual, since most biologically available iron comes from meat sources, not plant sources," he says.

But despite those positive findings, Dr. Shubert would not recommend that anyone take spirulina as an iron source. The reason? "In sample after sample, we found significant levels of mercury and lead—two elements that are highly toxic in the body if taken for prolonged periods," he says.

CLAIMS ARE UNPROVEN

Even if spirulina could be cultivated without these dangerous minerals, says Dr. Shubert, there is just no convincing scientific evidence that it can help you in any therapeutic way, as some manufacturers claim.

Take, for example, the claim that spirulina is a good diet pill. This is based on the algae's content of the amino acid phenylalanine, which supposedly affects the brain's appetite center, says Varro E. Tyler, Ph.D., professor of pharmacognosy at Purdue University. "But there is no evidence to support the claim that phenylalanine is especially effective in reducing the appe-

tite," says Dr. Tyler. "And even if it were, that amino acid is readily available from a wide variety of more economical protein sources." The Food And Drug Administration agrees with Dr. Tyler. They found that claims for spirulina as an appetite suppressant were unsubstantiated.

Okay, so it can't tame your appetite. But can it stop hungry cancer cells from eating up your life? If you're a hamster in an experiment, maybe. If you're a human, probably not.

In a study conducted by Joel Schwartz, D.M.D., D.M.Sc., associate professor of oral pathology at Harvard University School of Dental Health, a beta-carotene solution taken from purified extract of spirulina was applied to cancerous tumors in the mouths of hamsters. The solution inhibited, shrank, and destroyed cancer cells.

"This in no way suggests that the spirulina you buy in the health food store will help you fight cancer," cau-

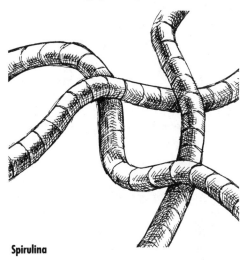

Spirulina

tions Dr. Schwartz. "There's a big difference between a purified extract and taking spirulina in a capsule."

What's more, he says, beta-carotene content can vary from sample to sample, depending on how the spirulina is grown.

Besides unknown potency, there is a question about the purity of spirulina. "Keep in mind that we're talking about bacteria [the other name for blue-green algae is cyanobacteria]," says Dr. Schwartz. "Bacteria like to grow in brackish ponds which can attract eggs of other organisms. Even though spirulina is now commercially cultivated in supposedly pristine ponds in California, you really have no guarantee of how pure it is."

Another point to consider: The Harvard researchers found that some components in spirulina appear to actually *promote* tumors.

"I would not recommend taking spirulina as a source of beta-carotene," says Dr. Schwartz. "You are better off eating a variety of fruits and vegetables rich in beta-carotene—such as broccoli, carrots, cauliflower, and papaya."

Dr. Shubert agrees. "There is no reason to take something that has no clear nutritional or therapeutic advantages over other readily available and safer food sources," he says.

On the other hand, spirulina might make a good supplemental food for astronauts some day. "NASA has been interested in spirulina because this lightweight algae can easily be grown in a test tube," says Dr. Shubert. Let's hope the scientists will come up with a way to cultivate spirulina that's both tasty and pure by the time we're ready to board the spaceship.

steroids   Most of us, when we think of steroids, probably imagine musclebound young men pumping iron at California's Muscle Beach. Well, athletes taking anabolic steroids certainly have received the lion's share of media attention. But all of us—athlete or bookworm—naturally churn out a variety of steroids. In fact, scientists have discovered more than 50 of them.

TWO BROAD CATEGORIES

Let's take a look at two major groups.

Corticosteroids. These include the steroid hormones naturally produced by our adrenal glands as well as synthetically derived copies. (Hydrocortisone, prednisone, and cortisone are a few examples of corticosteroids.)

Normally, corticosteroids help our bodies maintain healthy levels of blood sugars and mineral salts. Synthetic corticosteroids may be prescribed if your adrenal glands don't produce enough of the real thing. People with Addison's disease, for example, may take 20 to 30 milligrams of hydrocortisone a day to supply their needs. Taken in this way, the corticosteroids appear to be relatively safe.

Given in high doses, the corticosteroids are powerful anti-inflammatory drugs. Cortisone or prednisone may be injected into a joint to relieve the pain caused by rheumatoid arthritis, say, or the inflammation from an injury. Hydrocortisone, the active ingredient in many over-the-counter ointments, reduces the itching and inflammation of many skin diseases.

Doctors agree steroids do a fine job quelling inflammation. Like aspirin and other non-steroidal anti-inflammatory drugs, the corticosteroids inhibit your body's production of prostaglandins, compounds that kick off the inflammatory process. Steroids, injected into a swollen joint, permeate the lining and prevent additional inflammation-causing cells from getting in. They often give dramatic relief.

Corticosteroids fight all types of inflammation. Inhaled beclomethasone, for instance, often is used to help people with asthma get some extra breaths in. Also, doctors sometimes use large, intravenous doses of corticosteroids to defuse life-threatening asthma attacks.

Steroids, taken orally in small doses, may give long-term relief from rheumatoid arthritis pain. Hydrocortisone taken rectally is used to treat some forms of ulcerative colitis. Doctors also may use steroids to suppress your body's immune system. That helps reduce the risk of organ rejection following transplant operations. Steroids even have been found to reduce neurological damage when administered within the first 8 hours after spinal cord injuries.

Anabolic-androgenic steroids. Unlike the corticosteroids, the anabolic-androgenic steroids largely are produced in the testes. (Women produce small amounts in their adrenal glands.) The anabolic steroids that bodybuilders use simply are a synthetic variety of testosterone, the male sex hormone.

Athletes, of course, may use (and abuse) anabolic steroids to increase their muscle mass and endurance. But these benefits aren't free. Many people who take anabolic steroids, in fact, pay dearly.

What are the risks of taking anabolic steroids? Heart attack, liver cancer, stroke, and unfavorable blood cholesterol changes are major concerns. The drugs have also been linked with decreased sperm motility and testicular atrophy in men. In women, anabolic steroids have been linked with excessive and abnormal hairiness, decreased breast size, and menstrual irregularities.

THERAPY WITH RISKS

Although their use is often medically justified, the corticosteroids aren't much safer. The *Physicians' Desk Reference* lists this sampling of adverse reactions: hypertension, muscle weakness, osteoporosis, peptic ulcer, impaired wound healing, and pituitary unresponsiveness.

In fact, if you take large quantities of corticosteroids for a long time, your natural "factory" may simply shut down. You also may be prone to infections that take advantage of your steroid-depressed immune system. One doctor, in a letter published in the *Journal of the American Medical Association*, refers to the "treacherousness of corticosteroid therapy." It's a sentiment shared by many doctors.

This doesn't mean you should resist taking steroids if your doctor prescribes them. They are very useful, very powerful drugs—drugs that also require very careful medical supervision. *See also* **cortisone; hydrocortisone; prednisone**

stress management   Is stress bad for your health? Is the White House white? From acne to asthma, high blood pressure to herpes, ulcers to irregular menstruation, stress may often play a role. In fact, experts say your body's every organ can be negatively influenced by poorly handled stress.

So much for *why* you should manage your level of stress. Let's talk about *how*. To say the least, stress management is a broad term. It includes formal relaxation techniques like progressive relaxation, meditation, yoga, autogenic training, and deep breathing. But it also includes a walk in the park, a chat with a friend, a concert, a bike ride, a movie, a game of cards, a picnic, an evening of roller skating, a massage, or simply whistling "Yankee Doodle" in a hot shower.

STRESSBUSTERS AT WORK

The stress/disease connection works two ways. Those who succumb to stress get sick more often, while those who learn to manage their stress enjoy the benefits of greater health. Don't take our word for it. Look at the studies.

One study, published in the medical journal *Heart & Lung,* looked at 80 patients who had been admitted to a coronary care unit with symptoms of acute heart attack. While still under hospital care, a number were given three sessions a day of either progressive relaxation exercises (tensing and relaxing various muscle groups) or listening to soothing music. Both of these groups were able to reduce stress and lower their heart rates. Most importantly, they suffered fewer medical complications than did a third group that was not given any such sessions.

A 1990 study from the University of California at Los Angeles looked at a very different kind of stress management. The researchers wanted to see how often elderly Medicare patients made appointments to see their doctors, and whether this might be linked to how well they managed daily stress. The particular form of stress management the investigators chose to focus on was, of all things, pet ownership. The doctors' conclusion? Seniors who take time to snuggle with puppies, particularly during stressful times, needed fewer trips to see the doctor.

CHANT OR SHOOT HOOPS?

With all the different ways you can manage your stress, which should you try? Unfortunately, we can't tell you. "Relaxation is a very individual thing," says John E. Carr, Ph.D., professor of psychiatry and behavioral sciences and clinical psychologist at the University of Washington Medical School. "For some people the most beneficial kind of relaxation might be something akin to meditation. They may come home from work, flop down on the couch, put their feet up, and just flake out. For other people, relaxation means going to the gym and doing hard physical work," says Dr. Carr.

As a rough rule of thumb, you might look for optimum stress-management benefits in those things that provide contrast from your daily routine. For instance, if you labor all day swinging a hammer and lugging two-by-fours, you may not find working up a sweat at the gym as relaxing as does your friend the computer programmer.

Stress management is most effective when it becomes a part of your everyday lifestyle, rather than merely an added diversion, says Paul Rosch, M.D., president of the American Institute of Stress and a clinical professor of medicine and psychiatry at New York Medical College. Those who manage stress best, he says, are those who are doing things in life they enjoy and who feel that they are in control of their own lives.

Is there such a thing as an *ultimate* stress management strategy? You bet, says Dr. Rosch: "Do something you enjoy, something that utilizes your talents, and also benefits others." That, he says, is the secret of a relatively stress-free, healthy, and long life. *See also* **autogenic training; biofeedback; meditation; progressive relaxation**

stretching Human bodies, like paychecks, frequently need to be stretched.

Stretching is exercise that makes muscles and tendons more pliable "in hopes of achieving enhanced performance in a sport or activity, as well as to prevent injuries," says Robert P. Nirschl, M.D., medical director of Virginia Sportsmedicine Institute in Arlington. For some people—including those who have arthritis—stretching can be a form of therapy itself, as well as a way to reduce stress, he says.

Stretching alone is helpful, but for best results it should accompany whatever exercise program you do on a regular basis, says John W. Robertson, M.D., director of Seattle Sports Medicine. "Physical therapists and physicians prescribe both strengthening *and* stretching exercises for muscles," he notes.

A regular program of stretching leads to better flexibility, but all gains are only temporary and will be lost if you stop what you're doing. Stretching—like breathing and eating—"is a lifetime proposition," Dr. Nirschl says.

ARTHRITIS AID

Many physicians have observed that certain stretching exercises to promote flexibility "tend to diminish pain and enhance motion in arthritic or injured joints," says Dr. Nirschl. He says that arthritic pain and stiffness in muscles, tendons, ligaments, and joint linings are best relieved when stretching is combined with strengthening exercises.

Even patients whose x-rays show significant arthritic change within a joint "often do quite well if they're able to maintain good strength and flexibility in arthritic joints," says Dr. Nirschl. "There are patients I have observed who deferred surgery because they had embarked upon a successful stretching and strengthening program."

In addition to being used in some cases as therapy, stretching also can be of value to reduce stress—particularly when combined with regular aerobic activity, says Dr. Nirschl. "Anything which takes your mind off the stresses of the day and allows your brain to relax and refocus can be helpful," he says.

Just the simple act of stretching itself "unloads tight muscles and releases some stress," says D. W. Edington, Ph.D., director of the University of Michigan Fitness Research Center in Ann Arbor.

INJURY PREVENTION

Because muscles tend to tighten up after a tough workout, and because tight muscles are more injury-prone, "stretching can be very helpful" in preventing injuries, says Dr. Robertson.

Laboratory studies in which animals have been subjected to stretching demonstrate that "if tissue is made more pliable, it will accept more pressure before it tears," says Dr. Nirschl.

In other words, stretching may allow you to participate in exercise therapy until your muscles ripple—not rip. Stretching is essential for anyone just beginning an exercise program or returning to one after a long leave of absence, Dr. Robertson says. "In the first couple weeks you're going to be exercising those muscle groups in a fashion they're not used to," he adds.

Many people over 40 need to reeducate themselves about the proper way to stretch, says Dr. Nirschl. If you were an athlete in the distant or even not-too-distant past, you probably were taught to stretch *before* you worked out or competed—a concept that has since been found wrong, he says. Some experts now say that stretching should only be attempted after muscles are thoroughly warmed by exercise.

Serious stretching should always be done after warming up, says Dr. Edington. A five-part exercise regimen, for instance, should consist of a brief warm-up, light stretches, the main exercise, a cool-down, and then another series of stretches, he says. However, any time is appropriate for mild stretches—such as pulling back your shoulders to release stress at your desk.

SENSIBLE STRETCHING

When stretching, always use common sense. This isn't a donation to your favorite charity; you don't want a muscle to give until it hurts. If you feel pain, Dr. Robertson says, you're overdoing it. "There's a fine line between stretching an appropriate amount and overstretching until injuring a muscle," he says.

Stretching, like meditating, is best attempted alone in most cases, says Dr. Robertson. Although some people successfully stretch in pairs or groups, the concentration you need to stretch properly is sometimes lost if you're doing a stretch in tandem, he says.

"It isn't necessary for most people to stretch all muscle groups," says Janet Sobel, licensed physical therapist and director of rehabilitation at the Virginia Sportsmedicine Institute who works with elite athletes in a United States Tennis Association player development program. Sobel says that most young tennis players, for example, need to perform ten basic exercises to stretch all the muscle groups they use in their sport. Most people who walk for exercise can get by with stretching just four groups—the hamstrings (muscles on the reverse side of the knee), lower back, front of the hip, and shoulder. "However, the key is that each individual has her own specific needs based on her body type, lifestyle, and activities," says Sobel.

The proper way to stretch is to take a deep breath and to work the group as far as you can—then hold for 10 to 20 seconds, says Sobel. "Then take another breath and stretch a little farther," she says, noting that you should stop if you feel pain. Do each stretch three times.

Here is one example of a stretch you may want to call your own: a hamstring stretch. It's also good for the lower back because tight hamstrings

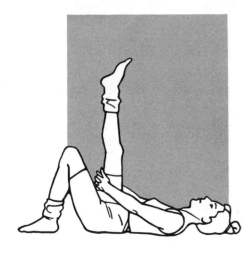

Hamstring stretch

may lead to lower back troubles, Sobel notes.

This stretch is for an area that is often injured or reinjured, says Sobel. "Because of our lifestyles, hamstrings in most people are tight," she says.

Lie on your back with your knees bent and feet flat. Raise and straighten one leg, bringing it toward your trunk. Bend your toes toward your face to stretch your calf. Straighten your leg as much as you can, but do not lock your knee. Hold 10 seconds. Repeat twice more. Then repeat the process with the other leg. *See also* **exercise therapy; yoga**

sugar   Although you may think of sugar as a natural sweetener that comes from sugar cane or sugar beets, some doctors think of it as a tool of medicine.

British studies indicate, for example, that a paste made of granulated sugar, powdered sugar, and hydrogen peroxide—the stuff that turns hair blonde—may do an even better job of stopping infection in wounds than more traditional antiseptics.

"All we have at this point are theories," says Bobby G. Spell, M.D., a surgeon at Methodist Rehabilitation Hospital in Jackson, Mississippi. It may be that sugar absorbs the moisture in a wound, which, in turn, dries out the wound bed and dehydrates the infection-causing bacteria. Or it may be that the bacteria feed so heavily on the sugar that they die from overeating.

But, theory aside, Dr. Spell has found in his practice that sugar paste works better than more conventional germ-killing ointments as a dressing for open and infected wounds, pressure sores, and the unhealed stumps of amputated limbs. The paste he uses combines sugar with the antiseptic povidine-iodine (Betadine), although plain sugar seems to work just as well.

"I like the sugar paste because it leaves the area so thoroughly clean of debris from the infection," says Dr. Spell. "When I change a dressing several hours later, the paste has already dissolved. I can basically wipe off the residual with a damp sponge. And it's safe and inexpensive."

Sugar can also be used to fill a deep wound, adds Dr. Spell, although he cautions that anything deeper than a scratch should always be checked by a physician.

HYDRATION HELPER

Sugar is also used by doctors to help the body absorb nutrient-dense fluids and prevent the dehydrating effects of prolonged vomiting or diarrhea.

How? Sugar actually enables the body to absorb salt, explains gastroenterologist Margaret Khouri, M.D., assistant professor of medicine at Hahnemann University Hospital in Philadelphia. And when given in multinutrient rehydration formulas, sugar enables the salt to literally pull life-giving nutrients and fluids into the cells.

Although these formulas are primarily used with people who are seriously dehydrated from diseases that cause prolonged vomiting or diarrhea, anyone who experiences such symptoms for even a day or two—from the flu or an intestinal virus, for example—is generally advised to sip a similar substance, says Dr. Khouri.

The magic elixir? Generally fruit juice or Gatorade, says Dr. Khouri. Both work the same way as rehydration formulas to replenish cellular fluids.

THE QUICK FIX

Sugar can also provide a quick fix for people with insulin-dependent diabetes whose blood sugar levels have dipped dangerously low, says Marion Franz, R.D., vice-president of nutrition at the International Diabetes Center, Minneapolis.

That's why people with this disease often carry plain sugar cubes as insurance against the times they've taken too much insulin, skipped a meal, or exercised too hard or too long. A few cubes can counteract the low blood sugar that these activities can cause and prevent an insulin reaction.

The advantage of carrying a few sugar cubes instead of a candy or piece of pastry, experts say, is that people may not be as tempted to eat the sugar cubes when they don't need them.

sunlight Pity ol' Sol. Once we proudly basked in his glowing warmth for hours, eager to have him toast our milky skin; now we are advised to trowel on the sunscreen just to pick up the mail. Once Mom shoved us outside the moment he peeked through the clouds in an effort to keep us "healthy" (and her sane); now our doctor keeps us inside with warnings about premature wrinkles.

And wrinkles are just the beginning. From headache to heat exhaustion, from cataracts to cancer, the sun and his nasty ultraviolet (UV) rays get the blame for a host of ills. And each year, the forecast gets gloomier.

Sure, get too much sun—without the proper sunblock—and that mighty force 93 million miles away can do some up-close-and-very-personal damage, especially to your skin. But before you paint your windows black or move to Seattle, check out what else is in those rays.

BONE PROTECTION

The elderly might note that sunlight can help prevent one of their most common and serious threats—hip fractures, which are often caused by bone-weakening adult rickets.

Yes, rickets. Before you dismiss this ailment as a quaint blast from the past, understand that rickets is very much a modern-day problem—particularly among the elderly. "We found that in the Boston area, between 60 and 80 percent of the nursing home population was vitamin D-deficient, which can cause osteomalacia [adult rickets]," says Michael F. Holick, Ph.D., M.D., director of the Clinical Research Center at Boston University Medical School and head of its vitamin D laboratory. "Most vitamin D for the elderly comes in the form of sunlight, so regular exposure to sunlight can help them prevent rickets." Vitamin D helps the body absorb calcium, essential for maintaining strong bones.

That's why it's especially needed by the elderly. "There is evidence that in the United States and Europe, between 30 and 40 percent of people with hip fractures are vitamin D-deficient," adds Dr. Holick.

To prevent deficiency, he recommends you get between 10 and 15 minutes of sunlight on your face, arms, and hands two to three times weekly; those who are extremely fair-skinned or sunlight-sensitive should limit their exposure to about 5 minutes in the morning or late afternoon. In addition, and especially during winter months, he advises a daily supplement with 400 I.U. of vitamin D, or three to four glasses of skim milk a day.

Besides the elderly, the sun may help bring some relief to those with psoriasis. "There are no set rules for treating psoriasis with the sun," says Al Lane, M.D., associate professor of dermatology and pediatrics at Stanford University Medical Center. "Just being exposed to sunlight usually helps people with this annoying skin condition, however."

Meanwhile, travelers might note that sunlight helps beat jet lag by keeping our internal body clocks stimulated. "The general rule of thumb is when you are traveling east to west, through six or fewer times zones, you want to be outdoors at the end of the afternoon for 1 to 2 hours for the first two or three days after you arrive at your new destination," says Alfred Lewy, M.D., Ph.D., professor of psychiatry at Oregon Health Sciences Center University in Portland. "When you travel west to east, be outdoors in the morning. That's because the evening sun shifts your body rhythms later, while the morning sun shifts your rhythms earlier. And if you're going through more than six time zones, be outdoors in the middle of the afternoon, avoiding morning light when traveling east and avoiding late afternoon light when traveling west."

For traveler and nontraveler alike, though, that strong midday sun can spell danger—especially to children.

"It turns out that about 80 percent of the dangerous UV exposure we get occurs *before* age 18," says Dr. Lane. "If kids—actually, those up to age 20—would regularly use sunscreen with an SPF [sun protection factor] of at least 15, we could probably decrease skin cancers by between 75 and 80 percent."

His advice for raising skin-healthy kids (who are less likely to get wrinkles or skin cancer as adults): "Basically, avoid the noonday sun. When your shadow is shorter than you are, find some shade. And *always* wear sunscreen." *See also* **light therapy**

syrup of ipecac.   *See* **emetics**

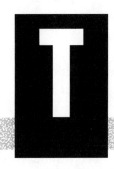

t'ai chi. *See* **exercise therapy**

tea One of the oldest beverages in the world is becoming one of the newest subjects of study in the medical laboratory.

For thousands of years, tea has been revered mystically by the Chinese for its curative powers; and the British, who popularized its use in much of the rest of the world, were so enraptured with the stimulant effect of the herb that they based its English name on the Greek word for "goddess," *thea.*

The mystic and mythic cape that cloaks the folklore, though, is being broken down into its component fibers as scientists identify and test the various chemicals in tea.

While many herbs can be brewed and steeped into a liquid called tea, what we commonly refer to today as tea comes from *Camellia sinensis,* a plant indigenous to the Far East. The way in which its leaves are processed determines not only the flavor of the brewed drink but the healthful properties it contains, according to John H. Weisburger, M.D., Ph.D., a senior member

of the American Health Foundation in Valhalla, New York.

The three kinds of tea available—green, oolong, and black—represent increasing degrees of leaf fermentation. The less fermented the leaves, the more chemicals retained to be transferred into a steaming cup of tea.

TANNINS ARE THE KEY

Tannins, derived from polyphenols in the tea, are the chemicals linked to tea's medicinal qualities. Black tea has been used for many of the folklore remedies favored in the West, researchers say, but green tea contains higher concentrations of the polyphenols and is the subject of most of the current laboratory study.

"Tannins have antibacterial, antiasthmatic, and anticariogenic [anticavity] properties," according to Daniel Mowrey, Ph.D., director of the American Phytotherapy Research Laboratory in Salt Lake City who specializes in studying the ways plants affect health.

Theophylline in tea helps to ease respiratory problems and the symptoms of bronchial asthma, Dr. Mowrey says. Other tannin agents, particularly those in green tea, can protect against tooth decay.

Tea also contains an astringent property that helps stop bleeding. Because of that, it has been thought helpful in treating diarrhea and hemorrhoids, although Dr. Mowrey believes "that's stretching it a bit." He also cautions that the detrimental effects of the caffeine in tea may outweigh any benefits for healthy people.

The astringency of tea has been used to cure canker sores in the mouth and to lessen foot perspiration and odor. Jerome Z. Litt, M.D., assistant clinical professor of dermatology at Case Western Reserve University School of Medicine in Cleveland, Ohio, recommends boiling two tea bags in a pint of water for 15 or 20 minutes, then adding the brew to 2 quarts of cool water, in which the feet should soak for about 30 minutes a day for the first week. Then repeat two to three times a week until odor and sweat are significantly reduced, then weekly or monthly as needed.

"It will literally tan the hide" of your feet, Dr. Litt says, but the brownish coloration will go away, as should the sweat and odor. Treatments then can be reduced to once a week or once a month as needed. The procedure also is effective in reducing excessively sweaty palms, he says.

Holding a wet tea bag on a canker sore can bring "almost instantaneous relief" in many cases, Dr. Litt says. And if you bite your tongue, a wet tea bag can stop the bleeding.

CANCER FIGHTER?

An increasing number of studies indicate that green tea may play a crucial role in the prevention and reduction of cancer, Dr. Weisburger says. Drinking green tea "may reduce heart diseases and several types of cancer, including cancer of the breast, colon, lung, bladder, stomach, and kidney among others," he says. It also may "reduce the carcinogenic effect of some chemicals, including those in cigarette smoke, and can lower cholesterol and triglycerides in the blood."

The green tea chemical primarily responsible for the anticancer claims is called epigallocatechin gallate, or EGCG. Studies have shown that green tea or EGCG extract suppressed or reduced sarcoma tumors in mice, decreased the number of lung tumors in mice exposed to tobacco carcinogens, and significantly lessened the size of skin tumors in mice exposed to ultraviolet-B light, a cancer-causing component of sunlight.

In addition, Dr. Mowrey says other studies indicate EGCG may play a role in protecting the body against cancer in the esophagus, stomach, and colon.

The polyphenol prevents oxidation of the cells, helping to stop the kind of tissue damage that may lead to cancer, according to Chi-Tang Ho, Ph.D., a professor in the Department of Food Science at Rutgers University who has studied green tea.

While green tea can act to prevent cells from mutating, according to Hasan Mukhtar, Ph.D., a professor in the Department of Dermatology at Case Western Reserve University in Cleveland, "whether it has the ability to stop the conversion of benign lesions to malignancy is not known."

Even though the active green tea agents "substantially lowered tumor prevalence in animals exposed to a variety of carcinogens," Dr. Mukhtar says, it will not be known if humans can benefit until "far into the future."

Nonetheless, population studies in Japan indicate that people who drink green tea regularly have a lower cancer mortality rate. Since green tea's constituent chemicals are nontoxic and have shown remarkable beneficial effects, Dr. Mukhtar says, there is an advantage in consuming tea as a beverage.

The green variety is the easiest to test in the laboratory, adds Dr. Ho, but the "little bit of study done so far" on black tea indicates it may be equally effective in promoting health and guarding against the onset of cancer.

tears, artificial Face the wind. Don't blink, don't squint. Feel the dry burn, the sandy irritation in the eyes, and know the pain and discomfort of dry-eye syndrome. For those afflicted, no matter how much they blink, their eyes don't have it—the ability to coat the cornea with a thin, protective layer of tears.

Millions of people suffer from dry-eye syndrome—known clinically as keratoconjunctivitis sicca—and doctors say anyone at any age can get it, although women of menopausal age and older are the most likely candidates.

Symptoms range from an overall feeling of dryness or the sense that some foreign matter is in the eye to severe burning or irritation.

Lack of vitamin A in the diet, certain skin diseases, arthritis, allergies, and use of antihistamines or diuretics all can cause the tear wells to run dry.

Barring surgery to correct any underlying eye abnormalities, there is no cure for dry eyes, experts say. The main treatment is frequent use of artificial tears, special solutions that add a soothing layer of moisture to the surface of the eye and the inside of the eyelid.

Originally, all artificial tear preparations contained cellulose derivatives, which are natural substances, says Mitchell Friedlaender, M.D., of the Scripps Clinic and Research Foundation's division of ophthalmology in LaJolla, California. While effective in moistening the eyes, Dr. Friedlaender says, these thick solutions often blurred vision. Even today, they still tend to form a crust on eyelids.

In the 1960s, tears made of polyvinyl alcohol were developed. They aren't as viscous and vision blurring as cellulose-based formulas. And later advances in the 1970s brought other polymeric solutions that are not gooey at all.

Most artificial tear preparations are sold over the counter. They are applied from a bottle or a single-dose vial. There are also pellets, available by prescription, that slowly release the lubricant. These must be inserted inside the lower eyelids.

PRESERVATIVE PROBLEMS

To destroy bacteria and extend shelf life, many artificial tear solutions contain chemical preservatives. Though harmless with only occasional, temporary use, Dr. Friedlaender and other ophthalmologists say that long-term exposure to preservative-laden brands can produce allergic and toxic reactions and even damage the cornea, the blood vessels in the eye, and the membranes that coat the surface of the eye and inner eyelids. People who use artificial tears several times a day might be better off using the preservative-free types, doctors suggest.

Preservatives offer cause for concern, Dr. Friedlaender says, because of the very nature of dry-eye syndrome: Sufferers have insufficient natural tears to dilute and wash away the additives.

One of the most common preservatives found in artificial tears, benzalkonium chloride, has caused corneal damage in laboratory test rabbits in concentrations just slightly higher than the 0.013 percent permitted in the solutions. Other preservatives to watch out for on the labels of artificial tear products are edetic acid formulations and thimerosal, both of which can cause allergic reactions or inflame the cornea and eyelids. Studies have discovered no major toxic complications with the use of another preservative, chlorobutanol, although it has been found to concentrate in soft contact lenses, causing some mild inflammation.

Doctors recommend the use of artificial tears about four times a day in mild cases of dry-eye syndrome. Those with severe cases, though, should consult a physician. They may need to apply the solution as often as every hour or even every 15 minutes.

tea tree oil   It almost sounds too good to be true. The oil of the tea tree is said to chase away acne, boils, and athlete's foot. It purportedly wipes out candida, mouth ulcers, and ringworm. According to some folks, it can even rid your pooch of that packload of fleas.

But in *this* case, what's "too good" might indeed be true. This pine-scented oil, which comes from the crushed leaves of the Australian *Melaleuca alternifolia* (or tea tree), is a healing gift from nature—a safe, natural antibiotic that can wipe out a battalion of bacteria with just a few drops.

Of course, this is no surprise to Australians, who have used it for centuries to treat infected wounds. As recently as World War II, physicians and dentists in Australia used it extensively as a topical solution to combat germs and a variety of fungal infections.

Numerous studies back up the effectiveness of tea tree oil, including one by the National Institute of Phytotherapy that found the majority of patients with yeast infections successfully eliminated the problem after being treated with tea tree oil.

"Basically, the essential oil that comes from tea tree leaves has an active ingredient called terpinen-4-ol," explains psychopharmacologist and phytotherapist Daniel Mowrey, Ph.D, director of American Phytotherapy

Research Laboratory in Salt Lake City. "This compound and other ingredients in the oil have the ability to either kill bacteria or stop it from spreading. But because there is little acid in it, the surrounding skin tissues are not damaged."

Dr. Mowrey says that because tea tree oil is highly concentrated, you don't need to use much.

"Apply just a few drops directly onto the infected area and very lightly massage it in," he recommends. "If you have sore gums, place the drops on your finger first, and rub it into the swollen area.

"The concentrated oil can work," says Dr. Mowrey, but adds: "Be wary of products advertising tea tree oil in them, like shampoos, toothpastes, even dish detergents. The quantities of tea tree oil in them are so small that it is unlikely that they would have any effect."

tender loving care.   *See* **TLC**

tetracycline   Two generations of acne sufferers have reason to be grateful for this reliable but less-than-perfect antibiotic. Tetracycline has lost some ground to newer prescription drugs since its introduction in 1953, but it's still an old standby for acne and is considered the treatment of choice for several other diseases, too.

How does it work? Unlike penicillin, tetracycline usually doesn't actually *kill* germs, says John Connors, Pharm.D., assistant professor of clinical pharmacy at Philadelphia College of Pharmacy and Science. Instead, it interferes with the ability of certain bacteria and protozoa to grow and multiply. "It's not the antibiotic that cures people," Dr. Connors explains. "Your body heals you. These drugs just help your body get the infection under control."

That's how tetracycline combats serious infections like pneumonia or syphilis. But no one really knows why tetracycline has been so effective with acne. "It's thought to inhibit bacterial growth on the skin," says Dr. Connors. Tetracyclines may also reduce the formation of trouble-making fatty acids in sebum, the oil in your skin.

Tetracycline taken orally can help bring acne under control in one to three months. It won't cure acne, however. (Acne isn't considered curable.) Once the problem clears, you'll probably remain on a lower maintenance dose to prevent new pimples. Just be aware that in rare instances, prolonged use can cause problems with the liver, kidneys, or bone marrow. Talk to your doctor about periodic blood tests if you've been on tetracycline for a few years.

Tetracycline is available in a form that can be applied directly to the skin, but it's not as popular with dermatologists as clindamycin and erythromycin, the two top-selling topical antibiotics for acne sufferers. One problem unique to topical tetracycline is that it can temporarily make the skin yellowish.

INFECTION FIGHTER

What else is tetracycline used to treat? The drug is useful for people with chronic bronchitis. Some doctors recommend it to control or prevent chest infections.

Tetracycline is considered the treatment of choice in adults for Rocky Mountain spotted fever and Lyme disease, and chlamydia, a common sexually transmitted disease that often accompanies gonorrhea. Doctors who treat gonorrhea with seftriaxone will usually add a seven-day course of tetracycline to knock out the chlamydia, says Dr. Connors.

While tetracycline is useful, it's far from perfect. For one thing, it may make your skin hypersensitive to sun and sun lamps. And like almost any antibiotic, it can cause a suprainfection. This happens when certain harmful microorganisms that aren't susceptible to tetracycline flourish in place of those reduced by the drug. Yeast organisms, the kind that cause vaginal infections, are common suprainfection culprits. Tetracycline can also hamper the effectiveness of oral contraceptives.

Some people develop diarrhea, nausea, and vomiting from the drug. If that happens to you, stop the tetracycline and call your doctor.

Children under the age of eight aren't good candidates for tetracycline therapy, because it can permanently stain developing teeth. Pregnant women and nursing mothers should also avoid the drug.

Keep in mind that tetracycline doesn't mix well with certain drugs and foods. Antacids and calcium can block its absorption. Iron can zap its effectiveness. That means that if you've just eaten a meal, you should wait 2 hours to take the tetracycline. Or take the tetracycline first, and wait 1 hour before you eat.

The beneficial effects of tetracycline may not kick in for up to three days. Once it does start working, it may do its job so well, you'll be tempted to stop taking it before you've finished your prescription. Don't! Doctors warn that the original infection can recur with a vengeance if you stop the treatment too soon. *See also* **antibiotics**

theophylline. *See* **bronchodilators**

therapeutic touch Practitioners of therapeutic touch believe in a life energy that permeates every cell. This energy extends beyond the body's surface, they claim, creating a bioelectric field. Using their hands, they sense and assess what they call weaknesses or congestion in the field. Then they direct energy into the field to balance it. Sometimes, practitioners actually touch the skin. Most prefer to work a few inches above it. The whole process takes 15 to 20 minutes.

When New York University offered its first class on therapeutic touch to nurses in 1975, techniques that claimed to work by directing the "universal life energy" were considered unorthodox, to say the least. Today, however, therapeutic touch is more widely accepted. That's because many of its practitioners are traditionally trained nurses and because university research shows there really *is* something to therapeutic touch.

Studies have found that therapeutic touch increases hemoglobin levels in the blood, induces physical relaxation, and decreases anxiety, says Janet Quinn, R.N., Ph.D., former associate professor and department director of medical-surgical nursing at the University of South Carolina. A University of Missouri study found that the procedure could reduce headache pain by up to 70 percent in most of the people tested.

FASTER HEALING

Janet Macrae, R.N., Ph.D., an instructor of therapeutic touch at New York University, says she has observed how the technique can speed wound healing and reduce the amount of time patients need to be on pain medication.

"I think that's significant," she says. "Therapeutic touch won't block the experience of pain as well as painkillers do. But the fact that people who have such treatments don't need the pain medicine for long shows that therapeutic touch does facilitate healing. I think it's a very effective complement to orthodox medicine."

In her book *Therapeutic Touch: A Practical Guide,* Dr. Macrae says she has used the method with varying degrees of success on children suffering from acute asthma attacks. One boy stopped wheezing immediately, one kept wheezing but found it easier to breathe, and a third didn't respond at all, she says. In another case, eight months of weekly treatments brought rather dramatic improvement to a woman with emphysema, she reports. The proven relaxation benefits of therapeutic touch also make it helpful for people with high blood pressure, ulcers,

and those in the midst of an emotional crisis, she says.

Therapeutic touch can be a pleasant experience. You simply sit in a chair or lie down and relax while the therapist sweeps her hands along the contours of your body, keeping her palms a few inches away from the body itself. Some say they feel warmth emanating from the therapist's hands; others report tingling in the areas where she's working.

Practitioners begin by establishing their intent to heal, perhaps by saying a prayer. Then they use their hands to scan the body's field to see where the problems lie. Next they use the hands to clear away energy in areas where it seems too dense, or to bring more energy to places where it seems to be depleted. What they're after is a feeling that the body's energy is evenly balanced.

Dr. Macrae has taught the technique to nurses, psychotherapists, and massage practitioners around the country. Chances are there's a therapeutic touch practitioner in your community, perhaps at a local hospital. You can also teach yourself how to do therapeutic touch with Dr. Macrae's book.

"It's a skill that everybody can learn," she says. "It's not just for nurses. I think it would be great in families. Once you learn, you can develop your skills through practice."

thyme Long popular as a seasoning, thyme has also been a staple in the herbalist's bag of tricks since ancient times. Used mostly as an antiseptic, cough remedy, and digestive aid, thyme extract is found even today in some mouthwashes and decongestants.

Through the ages, thyme was used to combat diverse ailments such as leprosy, sciatica, headaches, and shortness of breath. It was even regarded as a remedy for nightmares, which may explain the popularity of thyme-stuffed pillows. As late as World War I, thyme oil was employed as an antiseptic and even used on the battlefield.

A MUSCLE RELAXANT

Modern herbalists recommend thyme tea as a sweat-inducing weapon against the common cold. And they say the tea eases flatulence and soothes the digestive system. That may be because of thyme's antispasmodic properties. In other words, it helps relax the smooth muscles of the stomach. One recipe for tea to combat indigestion, according to Michael Weiner, Ph.D., author of *Weiner's Herbal,* calls for steeping ½ ounce or 3 tablespoons of dried thyme in 2 cups of boiling water. Strain before drinking.

Used externally, thyme baths are often recommended to ease rheumatic pains. And the oil is sometimes found in liniments and massage oils.

It's even said that thyme's antiseptic properties extend to fighting dandruff. A noted hair stylist recommends a thyme rinse made by boiling 4 heaping tablespoons of dried thyme in 2 cups of water for 10 minutes. He says to strain and cool the mixture before pouring it over clean, damp hair, making sure the liquid covers the scalp.

A few cautions: As a culinary herb, thyme is perfectly safe; the concentrated essential oil, however, can be toxic. Taken in pure form, even small doses can cause headache, nausea, weakness, and dizziness. Even applied externally, the oil may cause irritation if you have sensitive skin.

thyroid. *See* **glandulars**

TLC Henrietta was having a rough day. Blind, arthritic, suffering from Alzheimer's disease, and strapped into a wheelchair in her room at a northern Idaho nursing home, she was struggling to eat a bowl of ice cream. Most of it wound up on the floor or on her dressing gown.

An acquaintance who had been visiting a relative at the home happened to walk by and saw Henrietta's plight. The woman touched Henrietta on the arm and gently took the spoon out of her hand. Then the woman fed Henrietta and talked to her for a few moments in a soothing voice. As the woman left, she heard Henrietta cry out, "Love you, love you."

Bestowing a gentle touch or a meaningful hug, sharing a good joke or a timely kiss, wiping away tears, or listening attentively are just a few of the hundreds of ways that we can show tender loving care, or TLC. Yet the importance of those gestures of kindness as a healing therapy are often overlooked by medical professionals and laypeople alike.

"Tender loving care is the last thing that many medical students and faculty are aware of. They're often focusing on the latest treatments and drugs," says Judith Alexander Brice, M.D., a psychiatrist in Pittsburgh, Pennsylvania. "I think that's a big mistake. I think 80 percent of patients would do better if someone just took time to listen to them."

Dr. Brice should know because she has been a patient, too. A few years ago, she suffered from ulcerative colitis, a chronic inflammation of the colon, and had to undergo surgery. Later, she also had to have surgery to repair her hips, which were damaged by the steroid drugs she had been taking to control her colitis. She says nurses and doctors treated her poorly after both surgeries: "Frequently, when [my surgeon] came to see me, he would not look at me. His gaze would often avoid mine to wander toward the window or the television. I yearned for him to sit for a minute, hold my hand, give me some reassurance. He never did."

Other patients recall similar experiences.

PATIENTS ARE PEOPLE

"Doctors tend to transform you into a statistic when you're seriously ill. Well, I'm not a statistic, I'm a person," says Kari Fedorchak, a 25-year-old Tempe, Arizona, woman whose acute myeloblastic leukemia has been in remission for four years. "I know they have to prepare you for all the things that could happen. But, hey, I wish they would loosen up a bit, and let you know that it is possible to lick this thing."

"Treatment is a human activity that goes well beyond the medical procedures involved," agrees Robert Dozor, M.D., who treats acquired immune deficiency syndrome patients at Community Hospital in Santa Rosa, California.

He encourages his patients to take an active role in their treatment. "We advocate asking patients the explicit question, 'How do you want me to work with you?' [This] allows the physician to know when he or she is needed as a fighter, teacher, parent, technician, or covenanter," Dr. Dozor says. "We need to listen to determine when the disease is perceived as a spiritual challenge or as a brutal enemy, as an invasion of chaos or opportunity for growth and resolution."

But friends and family members also can be insensitive to the importance of TLC. Within days of her diagnosis, for example, Fedorchak's boyfriend left her.

"I didn't know if I was going to live or die. That weekend, he went out partying. Then he borrowed my car to impress a date. I loved him, but he didn't want anything to do with me. It was just another kick in the side that I didn't need right then," Fedorchak recalls.

Many of her friends didn't offer much more support. "They didn't know what to say to me. They didn't know how to treat me so they just stayed away," she says.

HOW TO GIVE TLC

So what *can* you say, what *can* you do to show the ill person that you care? First, remember that communication is a form of love, says Dr. Dozor.

"Physicians and families are forced to look at and see the reality of different human lives in circumstances that involve compassion that transcends old chasms of communication," he says. "The miracle of unconditional love flourishes best in the face of adverse circumstances."

But avoid being a cheerleader. Instead, listen to the feelings that the sick person is expressing. "Few ever really listened to me. People really need to sit there and let you pour out your feelings," Fedorchak says.

Thomas Kirk, director of patient and family services for the Alzheimer's Disease and Related Disorders Association, agrees. "People with Alzheimer's, for example, still have feelings. We need to listen to them express their feelings and let them know that we understand," he says.

Even if they can't communicate with you, don't assume that they don't understand what you're saying. Avoid talking about them in their presence as if they weren't there. "Instead of talking about them, talk with them," he says.

Learn to use your nonverbal communication skills, too. "We still can communicate with them by hugging, kissing, patting on the back, holding hands, and looking them in the eyes," Kirk says.

Finally, remember that TLC also means encouraging people to do as much as they can for themselves. "We need to assure people and encourage them to use their remaining skills to the best of their ability," Kirk says. "Our jobs as caring, concerned people is to treat them with dignity and help them when they need help. But we shouldn't overdo things for them or discount their abilities." *See also* **touch therapy**

touch therapy Touch is back in vogue among health professionals. It's back in hospital nurseries, where daily massage is used to stimulate neurological development and weight gain in premature babies. It's visible in the bedside manner of the best nurses, who know that a reassuring touch can help speed healing. And it's being recognized by a growing number of psychotherapists and bodywork practitioners as a way to harmonize the physical and mental components of well-being.

While strict taboos against touch are still in place in traditional psychoanalysis and other therapeutic quarters, that wisdom is challenged by a spate of new research. Touch, it seems, is vital to well-being.

New research suggests that the need for touch is brain-based. Studies of animals at Duke University have shown that depriving infants of maternal contact apparently causes their brains to release a chemical that interferes with weight gain and growth. Studies of infant monkeys at the University of Wisconsin suggest that those separated from their mothers may even suffer long-range immunological consequences.

BIGGER, BRIGHTER BABIES

For ethical reasons, researchers don't do separation studies on human infants, but they have found that newborns thrive better when given *extra* touch. In a University of Miami study, premature babies were all held, rocked, and given the usual amount of human stimulation. But some babies were also caressed and massaged for 15 minutes three times a day for ten days. This group gained weight 47 percent faster than other preemies left to nap in their incubators.

"The massaged infants showed signs of faster neurological development and became more active and responsive than the other babies," says University of Miami Medical School psychologist Tiffany Field, Ph.D. Researchers theorize that certain biochemicals released by touching—or others released in the absence of touch—may be the underlying factor.

And reviewing the available research, Theodore D. Wachs, Ph.D., of Purdue University, concluded that babies who are held more in the first six months of life were likely to have an advantage in mental development over babies held less.

Of course, touch isn't just for babies. Adults have as plentiful a supply of nerve endings in the skin and chemicals in the body that register the pleasure of touch—all of which makes touch therapeutic at any age, says Norman Shealy, M.D., Ph.D., director of the Shealy Institute For Comprehensive Health Care in Springfield, Missouri.

Dr. Shealy is a firm believer in the "prescription" Virginia Satir, the prominent family therapist, often gave to her patients. Satir considered four hugs a day from loved ones the minimum daily requirement for emotional well-being. *See also* **massage; therapeutic touch; TLC**

tranquilizers Prescription tranquilizers can induce calm in as little as 30 minutes. They're typically prescribed for three reasons: to reduce general anxiety, to overcome insomnia, and to quell the anxiety that sometimes sets in following the loss of a job, the breakup of a marriage, or the death of a loved one.

They are sometimes used to treat ailments made worse by anxiety, like peptic ulcers. Tranquilizers are often prescribed after a heart attack, too, to prevent anxiety from triggering a second attack.

The most widely prescribed tranquilizers in the United States today belong to a chemical family known as benzodiazepine compounds. One of these, Valium, is among the all-time best-selling medications. Since Valium also relaxes the muscles, it's sometimes prescribed for people with back problems.

One of the problems with Valium is that it tends to cause drowsiness, although this side effect often disappears over time. The drug is always dangerous in combination with alcohol. In rare cases, it can lower a person's inhibitions. But the biggest concern with Valium is that it is potentially habit forming and can lead to dependency problems.

Another benzodiazepine, Librium, is similiar to Valium in almost every respect. Even its side effects are similar, including withdrawal symptoms when the drug is stopped.

QUIETING THE HUBBUB

Benzodiazepines like Valium and Librium work by promoting the action of a chemical, gamma-aminobutyric acid (GABA). GABA attaches to the brain cells, blocking the transmission of electrical impulses. This reduces the excessive communication between brain cells that is thought to cause anxiety.

Valium and Librium remain effective for about 8 hours, but small amounts of these drugs can stay in the body for days. New benzodiazepines are completely eliminated from the body after several hours, preventing dangerous buildup.

The newest of this new breed of Valium-type tranquilizers is Xanax. It is just as powerful as Valium but considered safe because it is short-acting; its effects last 8 to 12 hours. Xanax recently overtook Valium as the largest-selling prescription drug in the United States. The drawback with Xanax and other short-acting tranquilizers is that they tend to produce rebound anxiety and insomnia after a few weeks of constant use. Ativan and Halcion, two other drugs in this category, can also produce episodes of amnesia.

The benzodiazepines have become so popular, they've eclipsed long-standing tranquilizers like barbiturates and meprobamate (marketed as Seconal and Miltown.) On occasion, a psychiatrist will still prescribe Equanil or Miltown for someone who doesn't respond to the benzodiazepines.

Beta blockers, another type of calming drug, are used to minimize physical signs of anxiety: shaking, sweating, and heart palpitations. They're helpful for people who experience excessive anxiety in specific situations, like job interviews or public appearances.

Ideally, medical experts say tranquilizers should be reserved for short-term relief of incapacitating anxiety. They can work well to relieve panic reactions, muscle tension, and insomnia for a couple of days or weeks, but they won't resolve the emotional conflict that continues to generate these symptoms. *See also* **antianxiety drugs; sedatives**

Tylenol. *See* **acetaminophen**

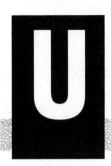

ulcer drugs Not so long ago, people tried to soothe their ulcers by drinking a tall, cool, creamy glass of milk. Milk, it was thought, coated their insides and protected the stomach's delicate lining from corrosive gastric acids.

Milk may feel good going down, but doctors now know it won't do a thing for your ulcer—except possibly make it *worse*, since milk actually *stimulates* the secretion of ulcer-causing stomach acids. People watching their cholesterol, of course, have additional reasons for drinking less milk.

Fortunately, there are anti-ulcer drugs that *do* work. Antacids, as the name suggests, simply neutralize stomach acid. Acid inhibitors inhibit the production of gastric acid, and mucosal defenders help protect the delicate linings of the stomach and duodenum (the first part of the small intestine) from acid onslaughts.

When trouble occurs, *any* form of help is welcome. "The normal mucosa [the protective lining] in your stomach looks pink and healthy," says Sacramento, California, internist Joshua Hoffman, M.D. "But if you get an ulcer, the mucosa looks sore, it looks angry. There's a good chance it will bleed. If it bleeds *and* perforates, that's a surgical emergency."

NEUTRALIZE THE ACID

Until recently, antacids were *the* treatment for stomach and duodenal ulcers. Still recommended for easing ulcer pain, over-the-counter antacids such as Tums, Maalox, and Mylanta also help prevent ulcers from coming back.

Antacids have the disadvantage of being short-acting—people often have to take them several times a day. By contrast, some modern ulcer drugs only have to be taken once a day. Another possible problem with antacids is they sometimes contain considerable amounts of sugar or sodium, a concern for people with diabetes or high blood pressure.

"You can definitely relieve ulcers with antacids, but there are other drugs that do a better job and are certainly more convenient," says Dr. Hoffman.

REDUCE THE FLOW

Left to itself, the stomach sometimes produces too much acid for its own good. A class of drugs called H_2-blockers can help prevent that. (H_2 is shorthand for the type of histamine receptor responsible for ordering yet *more* acid.)

Today, the H_2-blockers generally are considered the ulcer drugs of choice. Perhaps the best-known is cimetidine (Tagamet), although famotidine, nizatidine, and ranitidine also are widely used.

Convenience is one reason for their popularity. Cimetidine, for example, may be taken once a day. They also work quickly, often reducing ulcer pain in as little as one week. (Complete healing may take one to two months.) Doctors sometimes recommend cimetidine *and* an antacid for quicker relief.

There are two new drugs that are rapidly gaining acceptance, Dr. Hoffman says. Omeprazole, currently approved by the Food and Drug Administration for esophageal reflux, is said to profoundly inhibit acid secretions that may lead to ulcers. Misoprostol, prescribed to protect the stomach from ulcers caused by non-steroidal anti-inflammatory drugs, such as ibuprofen, both inhibits acid secretions *and* strengthens the gastric mucosa.

STRENGTHEN THE LINING

Unlike most ulcer drugs, sucralfate (Carafate) does little to reduce acid production or its potency. Rather, sucralfate forms a pasty, protective barrier over the ulcer, protecting it from further acidic assaults.

Sucralfate generally is prescribed for the short-term treatment (up to two months) of duodenal ulcers. "I will add Carafate if the H_2-blockers haven't been completely effective," Dr. Hoffman says. For hospitalized people who are prone to stress ulcers, however, Carafate may work better than the H_2-blockers, he adds.

FINALLY, RELAX

Doctors don't know for sure if stress actually *causes* ulcers, but it almost certainly triggers ulcer *symptoms.* That's why ulcers tend to flare when people are stressed and go away when they're relaxed. A little R&R isn't a drug, exactly, but it may help.

Sometimes a week on the beach isn't enough. If you do need drugs to treat an ulcer, which of the alternatives above is likely to be most helpful?

Most ulcer drugs are safe and effective, Dr. Hoffman says. However, it may take some trial and error before your doctor can determine the best regimen for you. *See also* **antacids**

ultrasound   Ultrasound refers to vibrations that are of the same physical nature as sound, but with frequencies higher than the range of human hearing. Imagine those sound waves stripping a wound clean of bacteria—painlessly, quickly, without leaving a mark. Or picture them penetrating the pores of the eye, to relieve the fluid buildup of glaucoma. This is ultrasound at work as a healer.

Most of us are more familiar with ultrasound, the diagnostician. The waves have a number of useful properties that make them especially useful for non-invasive snooping inside the body. They can bounce off organs and other structures, discriminate between soft-tissue densities, and echo back their findings. The information is then electronically transformed into a picture.

Obstetricians rely on ultrasound when they suspect birth defects. Cardiologists call on it to confirm their suspicions of heart disease. It is also used to determine the severity of atherosclerosis.

As a healer, however, ultrasound is just coming into its own.

In tests with animals, Larry Nichter, M.D., of the University of Southern California, found that immersing the injured area in a sterile bath and passing ultrasonic waves through the water shakes loose bacteria and other contaminants without damaging healthy tissue.

If tests on people are successful, Dr. Nichter predicts that ultrasonic cleaning may become standard practice in emergency rooms and doctors' offices.

With prostate cancer, ultrasound is used to help direct the placement of cancer-killing radioactive seeds. This new treatment reduces the risk of nerve damage and impaired sexual function associated with prostate surgery.

TREATS GLAUCOMA

Because ultrasound can penetrate such small spaces, it's also useful in the treatment of glaucoma, an eye disease characterized by high pressure within the eyeball. The Food and Drug Administration has approved a new ultrasound device for glaucoma.

It works like this: A probe placed over the eye releases pulses of high-intensity sound waves. The waves do two things: They create small pores in the whites of the eyes, releasing the built-up fluid that has been causing the pressure. And they decrease the eye's production of fluid.

The procedure is painless—a local anesthetic is used. The usual side effect is temporary inflammation of the treated eye.

Ultrasound treatment is not for every glaucoma patient, though. Michael E. Yablonski, M.D., former chief of the glaucoma service at Cornell University Medical Center, thinks that patients who can't be treated with drugs should next turn to laser surgery. If that fails, ultrasound is the next step. (In certain cases, where surgery is

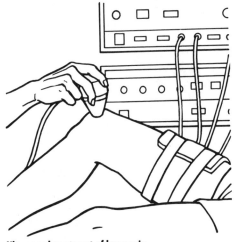

Ultrasound treatment of knee pain

known to have a low success rate, ultrasound may be used first.) Dr. Yablonski believes that the new treatment can correct 70 to 75 percent of the glaucoma cases that surgery can't.

Ultrasound devices are also used by physical therapists to treat sprains, bursitis, tendinitis, and other painful conditions. The sound waves heat injured tissue and increase blood circulation, says Mel Strapmeyer, Ph.D., chief of the Health Sciences Branch at the Food and Drug Administration's center for devices. He says ultrasound energy is absorbed by muscle so it gets to where it's needed. Ultrasound devices have also been used for cleaning teeth, he says.

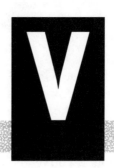

V

valerian (vah-LEH-ree-an) We might as well give it to you straight: Valerian has an odor only a rat could love. In fact, legend has it that the Pied Piper used this very herb—more so than his hypnotic music—to lure the rodents from Hamelin. But if you can get past valerian's unpleasant aroma, say herbalists, you might find that its natural tranquilizing properties have the power to lure your cares away.

For at least 1,000 years, valerian has been valued by herbalists as a tranquilizer, calmative, and sedative. At various times it was also recommended for epilepsy, chest congestion, convulsions, sores, wounds, digestive problems, menstrual discomforts, and the plague. Valerian seemed to have so many uses that the early European herbalists nicknamed it "all-heal." In true cure-all fashion, valerian was said to be both a sedative for agitated people and a stimulant for those who are tired.

HELPED INSOMNIACS

Today in Europe, where herbal medicine is more widely practiced than in America, valerian is the active in-gredient in scores of over-the-counter tranquilizers and sleep aids. In at least one study, researchers found that insomniacs who took valerian root extract showed significantly greater improvement in sleep quality than those taking a look-alike pill. And unlike prescription drugs such as Valium, valerian is not potentially addictive. Nor does it react dangerously with alcohol and barbiturates as Valium can.

Valerian's main drawback, says Varro E. Tyler, Ph.D., professor of

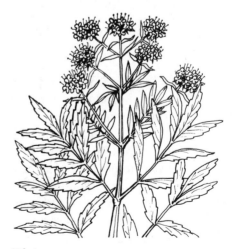

Valerian

485

pharmacognosy at Purdue University, is that some of its components tend to be unstable. That means you can't be sure—even with homegrown and dried valerian root—how much of the healing compound you're getting. Dr. Tyler is convinced that valerian tea or capsules are effective as minor tranquilizers, but is not sure to what extent. He writes in *The New Honest Herbal:* "The fact that [valerian] is very widely employed and has long been popular in Europe would seem to indicate a considerable degree of practical application."

If you'd like to be your own judge and give valerian a try, herbalists often recommend steeping 2 teaspoons of powdered root in 1 cup of water. Drink before bed. To help disguise valerian's distinctive taste, sweeten the tea with honey or sugar and flavor it with lemon. But don't get carried away with your home dose: Large amounts of valerian may cause headaches, blurred vision, nausea, and morning grogginess.

Valium. *See* **antianxiety drugs; tranquilizers**

vaporizers These steam humidifiers that boil water to produce a fine mist may help you breathe easier.

If your nose is clogged and you must breathe through your mouth, inhaling heated moist air could help you breathe more comfortably and keep your throat from drying out. If your child has the barking cough of croup—a condition resulting from airway obstruction—running a steam vaporizer might help ease breathing.

But don't expect a steam vaporizer to cure or halt a common cold, experts say. "The major benefit of using a steam vaporizer is to help you feel more comfortable when you're feeling lousy," says Michael Macknin, M.D., head of general pediatrics at the Cleveland Clinic. "Comfort is often the only relief we can offer cold sufferers."

So if your nose is stuffy, your throat sore, and your chest congested, go ahead and get steamed. But use extreme caution when operating a steam vaporizer around kids and pets. The most serious drawback of these units is that they could cause severe scalding if they tip over.

A safe alternative to using steam machines is to create your own steam tent. Fill a basin with boiling water, drape a towel over your head, lean over the basin, and sniff the steamy vapors. *See also* **humidifiers**

vegetarian diet When Bob Finnell went on a vegetarian diet, six of his eight coronary arteries became less blocked. When Werner Hebenstreit switched to the same diet, his angina disappeared.

Bob and Werner are 2 of 18 people who reversed their heart disease following a nondrug treatment program, including a very-low-fat vegetarian diet, devised by Dean Ornish, M.D., assistant clinical professor of medicine at the University of California, San Francisco.

RISKS REDUCED

Studies have long shown that vegetarian diets—that is, diets that omit meat, fish, poultry, and sometimes eggs and dairy products—are associated with a lower risk of developing heart disease. But Dr. Ornish's study goes further, showing that a plant-based diet can help *reverse* atherosclerosis (blocked arteries leading to the heart) once the disease has taken hold.

Vegetarians also may be at lower risk than nonvegetarians for a number of other diseases, including noninsulin-dependent diabetes, high blood pressure, kidney stones, gallstones, diverticular disease, arthritis, and breast, prostate, and colon cancer. Researchers suspect a vegetarian diet is healthier because it's lower in saturated fat, which can raise cholesterol levels and help block arteries, and higher in fiber, which may protect against certain other conditions.

In Dr. Ornish's program, people on the vegetarian diet experienced more dramatic results than others who followed the standard American Heart Association diet, which limits fat but allows meat and dairy products. And the more severe their blockages, the more noticeable was their improvement, Dr. Ornish reported.

Other studies have shown that adopting a vegetarian diet can help lower blood pressure, relieve constipation, and soothe painful joints in people with rheumatoid arthritis. It can also help you lose weight, even if you don't eat less, according to a study at Purdue University. And a study at Loma Linda University showed that vegetarian diets, because of their high carbohydrate content, can help double or triple endurance in athletes.

PLANNING THE DIET

Over the past two decades, vegetarian diets have been studied extensively, and vegetarians are no longer considered outside the mainstream. But experts caution that a vegetarian diet takes more planning than an unrestricted diet to avoid nutritional deficiencies. The American Dietetic Association advises vegetarians to choose from a variety of foods, including fresh fruits, vegetables, whole grain breads and cereals, nuts and seeds, legumes, and fortified soy substitutes. If you eat eggs or dairy products, limit yolks to two or three a week and choose low-fat milk, cheese, and yogurt.

You don't necessarily have to mix grains, legumes, seeds, and nuts together at one meal to benefit from the partially complete proteins they contain, as was previously believed. Eating various kinds of plant-based protein over the course of a day is okay.

Getting enough iron on a vegetarian diet is more of a concern than getting enough protein. While some plant foods contain considerable amounts of iron, it's less easily absorbed than iron in meat. So vegetarians should include a good source of vitamin C, like peppers or orange juice, with meals to enhance iron absorption. Also, total vegetarians, who abstain from all animal products, would do well to supplement their diet with vitamins B$_{12}$ and D, which plant foods lack. Dietitians also caution vegetarians against eating too many sweets, fats, and other empty-calorie foods, which can cancel out many of the benefits of a meatless diet. *See also* **macrobiotic diet**

vision therapy   Sometimes called vision training, this treatment consists of a variety of eye exercises designed to retrain your eyes and improve your vision. While programs are tailor-made for each particular patient, most regimens prescribe specific eye movements or manipulate vision with corrective lenses of varying strengths.

"Vision therapy is very valuable for certain eye conditions," says Irwin Suchoff, O.D., professor of optometry at the State College of Optometry at the State University of New York and editor of the *Journal of Behavioral Optometry.* He cites studies showing that vision therapy works for amblyopia (also called lazy eye) and vision discomfort due to problems with convergence (keeping both eyes properly aligned), fixation, and accommodation (focusing).

Vision therapy seems to help some people with a type of myopia (nearsightedness) that develops when their eye muscles either become too tense to focus properly or become rigidly focused on close objects. To perform one typical exercise prescribed for myopia, patients use a wall calendar. Taking off their glasses, patients stand far enough away so some numbers are clear. They rock forward on their feet until all the numbers are clear. Then they rock back until the numbers blur. With practice, the eye muscles supposedly learn to relax enough to focus sharply from the far position. Improvement may take anywhere from 10 minutes to three weeks, according to practitioners.

MANY SKEPTICS

Despite the improvement reported by people who have tried eye exercises, vision therapy is controversial. Optometrists (trained to treat vision only) tend to be more enthusiastic about its potential than ophthalmologists (medical doctors who treat eye disease with medicine or surgery). There are exceptions, however. Some ophthalmologists, for example, prescribe eye exercises before and after surgery for strabismus, or cross-eye.

"Vision therapy is pretty much

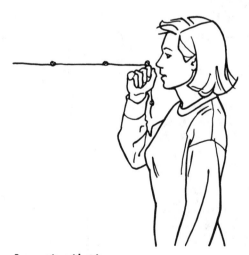

Eye exercise with string

optometry's 'baby,' and always has been," says Dr. Suchoff. "Ophthalmologists tend to pooh-pooh nonmedical, nonsurgical interventions like vision therapy." But many now recognize its value, and vision therapy is becoming more accepted than in the past.

Vision therapy isn't appropriate for eye diseases like cataracts or glaucoma. And Dr. Suchoff says vision therapy doesn't work for presbyopia, a condition in which people have difficulty seeing print at normal reading distance. This normally occurs around age 40 as the lens of the eye grows less elastic.

Some vision therapists teach tennis players and other athletes eye exercises to improve performance. Critics say that, strictly speaking, athletes aren't really improving their vision, but merely increasing the speed and accuracy with which eye muscles focus, thereby improving their ability to track moving objects. Of course, if you can keep your eye on the ball, you'll probably play better.

For vision therapy to work, practitioners say you have to stick with it. ("It's not like taking a pill," quips Dr. Suchoff.) To locate an eye care practitioner trained in vision therapy, contact either the College of Optometrists in Vision Development, P.O. Box 285, Chula Vista, CA 92012–0285, or the Optometric Extension Program Foundation, 2912 South Daimler Street, Santa Ana, CA 92705.

visualization. *See* **imagery**

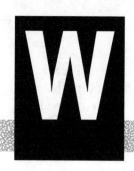

walking. *See* **exercise therapy**

water Vitamins, minerals, protein . . . you name it — as important as they are, they are *all* out-glimmered by the nutritional importance of water. "Water is *the* most vital nutrient — without it, you couldn't live for more than three or four days," says Kathleen M. Zelman, R.D., spokeswoman for the American Dietetic Association and dietetic internship director at Ochsner Medical Institutions in New Orleans.

You *are* one-half to four-fifths water, says Zelman. That water gurgles in every cell of your body. It lubricates your joints, cools your skin, washes wastes from your digestive tract, cushions your organs, and allows you to salivate. In short, water keeps you from turning into an overgrown beef jerky with arms.

At certain times your body will need more water than usual, such as when you're racing about town on a hot July afternoon, laboring in a dry air-conditioned office, or dancing fervently till beads of sweat run down your chest. If you ever find yourself with kidney stones, a urinary tract infection, the flu, or any ailment that brings fever, vomiting, or diarrhea, don't be surprised if the very first thing your doctor gushes is "drink more water."

WATER, WATER EVERYWHERE

But wait a minute. If water is so essential, how can it be that there are some people who seem to never touch the stuff? And how is it that almost no one drinks anywhere *near* the 10 cups of water a day that many experts insist our body needs? The answer to these mysteries is clear, says Zelman. "Your body is capable of extracting the water it needs from other fluids you drink and foods you eat."

All fluids, including juice, tea, soda, milk, eggnogs, and Shirley Temples, are mostly water. Even most "solid" foods are awash in water. Veal, for instance, is 60 percent water, and roast turkey is 68 percent. Most fruits and vegetables contain even more. Some foods — like lettuce, cantaloupe, watermelon, and gelatin — are well over 90 percent water.

On average, we only need to drink from six to eight glasses of our daily water needs. The remainder, we "eat." Fortunately, nature gave us a nifty little mechanism that tells us automatically if our bodies are not getting enough water. It's called thirst. Most often, you can think of your thirst as a close and dear friend—trust it implicitly. There are times, however, when your friend may let you down.

PASS THE GLASS

If you engage in heavy, sustained exercise, for instance, you may easily fall short on water. The problem is that through heavy sweating you may lose so much water so fast that your thirst mechanism simply can't keep up, says Zelman.

The solution? Consume about 8 ounces of water 30 minutes before you exercise, says Hinda Greene, D.O., a staff internist with the Cleveland Clinic Florida in Fort Lauderdale. While you're exercising, continue to drink—"take small amounts every 15 to 20 minutes," says Dr. Greene. Keeping well hydrated can help prevent painful stitches and cramps.

Likewise, vomiting, diarrhea, or fever due to illness of any kind may result in the rapid loss of water from your body. You should therefore make a conscious effort to replace it, says Dr. Greene.

If you are suffering from a urinary infection, the very first thing your doctor may recommend along with antibiotics is to drink more water. The trick here is to keep drinking and urinating, drinking and urinating, drinking and . . . "You need to increase your fluid intake during urinary tract infections to replace excess water loss that occurs from fever and your increased urination," says Dr. Greene. "So keep drinking as long as you're awake—put a couple of extra quarts in you throughout the day."

Similarly, if you have a kidney stone, your doctors may recommend turning your gullet into a funnel for lots and lots of water. The more water you pass, the better your chances of waving goodbye to your stone. "If you can pass the stone, then perhaps you can avoid surgery," says Dr. Greene. "I'd recommend an extra 2 liters [a little more than 2 quarts] of water a day," she says.

Late in life, as some of us know too well, our senses sometimes start to falter. Our sense of thirst is no exception. "Up around 'Medicare age' your thirst mechanism is not as responsive," says Dr. Greene. The change is as gradual as the tide and can long go unnoticed. To avoid dehydration, be on guard to make sure you're drinking a sufficient quanitity of water and eating foods with high water content. You may notice that your mouth and skin are dry, you're urinating less, or your urine is a darker color, says Dr. Greene. But these are not infallible signs. They may indicate dehydration but could also be the effects of medication.

Whether young, old, or in between, drink water in moderate amounts throughout the day. "It's important not to drink all your water at one sitting, but to space it out," says Zelman. "Drink six to eight glasses at once, and you'll just urinate it out. Your body won't be able to use it." *See also* **fluids; hydrotherapy**

weight loss Big may be beautiful, but—don't kid yourself—it isn't healthy.

"What one person considers beautiful or sexy is purely a subjective matter. But where health is concerned, there's nothing subjective about it—the numbers don't lie. If you're overweight and you lose weight, you'll likely live longer and improve the quality of your life," says Peter D. Vash, M.D., assistant clinical professor of medicine at the University of California in Los Angeles and president of the American Society of Bariatric Physicians (doctors who treat obesity).

Slimming down may improve the quality and duration of your life by preventing a number of health problems and actually *reversing* others. For instance, weight loss is often the treatment of choice—typically chosen *before* medications or any other therapies—for high blood pressure and most diabetes. And for America's top killers, heart disease and cancer, weight loss may make you less susceptible. But the story doesn't end there. The size of your waistline may at least partly determine whether you'll have a number of other health problems, like joint aches, varicose veins, heartburn, or gallstones.

HEFTY BENEFITS

Lose weight, lower your blood pressure. Nothing could be more clear—except perhaps the connection between high blood pressure and stroke. "Weight loss should be the first line of attack against high blood pressure," says Dr. Vash. In a study published in the *Archives of Internal Medicine,* doctors went on the attack. Fifty overweight people with high blood pressure were encouraged to shed an average of 23 pounds over 16 weeks. They did, and they saw their blood pressure plummet—the average systolic reading (the top number) fell 16 points, and the diastolic reading, 14 points.

Similarly, there's no question that the most common form of diabetes, Type II or noninsulin-dependent diabetes, is closely related to body weight. Excess mass (which many diabetics have plenty of) directly affects the body's ability to balance blood sugar. So it stands to reason: "Removing the excess weight can be curative, and is certainly the first line of treatment for approaching the Type II diabetic," says Dr. Vash. An overweight diabetic who loses weight "will usually be able to reduce or stop his need for insulin injections within the first month," he says.

Backaches, knee pain, and other sorrows of the bones and muscles are often related to heft as well. The more weight you carry, the heavier the load on your frame. One study at the University of Toronto looked at over 100 severely overweight people (overweight by at least 100 pounds), most of whom reported daily torment in their backs, knees, ankles, and other body parts. After doffing their handicap, the great majority experienced relief of pain in one or more joints.

SLIM YOUR ODDS

Other diseases may not be so easily treated by weight loss, but their progress could be slowed—or they might even be prevented. Take coronary heart disease. "You may lose weight and still develop heart disease, but you'll probably get it when you're 75 years old rather than 55," says Dr. Vash.

Flabbiness affects your heart in a number of wicked ways, says Artemis P. Simopoulos, M.D., president of the Center for Genetics, Nutrition, and Health in Washington, D.C., and former head of the Nutrition Coordinating Committee of the National Institutes of Health. As we've seen, overweight contributes to high blood pressure, which puts strain on the heart. Overweight is associated with lower levels of HDL, the good kind of cholesterol that helps keep your arteries clean, whereas weight loss is associated with higher HDL levels. And excess weight *also* changes the chemistry of the blood, making it clot more easily, so increasing the chances of heart attack.

Cancer can't be cured by losing weight, but perhaps it may be prevented, says Dr. Simopoulos. From a number of large population studies, doctors know that cancers of the uterus and breast are higher among overweight women after menopause. Some studies show that women who have had breast cancer and lose weight slim their odds of developing new tumors. In men, various cancers also seem to attack the overweight disproportionately—foremost are cancers of the prostate and colon.

But the connection between overweight and disease doesn't end there. "Women over 40 who are obese have a much higher incidence of gallstones—in medical school you're taught that from the very beginning," says Dr. Simopoulos. The stout are also more likely to suffer from heartburn, or acid reflux, because body fat exerts pressure on the stomach, which tends to force digestive juices upward. Even accidents, such as falling down stairs, may strike the overweight more often. "People who are obese generally have more difficulty maintaining balance," says Dr. Simopoulos.

Finally, the effects of flab go beyond the physical. "Being overweight often affects the overall attitude a person has about life," says Dr. Simopoulos. "An obese person often feels discriminated against—even if he's not discriminated against."

TAKE THIS TEST

Before we talk about how to lose weight, you should determine if you really need to. There's no simple formula that will give you a definite answer. But with a tape measure you can get a rough idea, says Dr. Vash. Measure around your waist where it is most narrow, then measure your hips where they are widest. Divide the number of inches in your waist by the number of inches in your hips to get a ratio. Men: If your ratio is below 1.0, you're probably all right. Women: A ratio below 0.8 is desirable. (This test reflects the most recent medical evidence that flab around the middle is worse for your health than flab down below.)

The more you're above your ideal weight (the higher your waist to hip ratio), the more your health is at risk, says Dr. Vash.

Over 30 percent of all Americans surpass their ideal weight. If you're among them, here's how to take those pounds off.

START SMART

No, losing weight is *not* easy, nor should it be too rapid. In fact, the first sign of a *bad* diet plan is one that makes promises such as "*You can lose 10 pounds in one week!!*" Yes, 10 pounds in one week is sometimes possible—but it's going to be mostly water weight that you'll quickly regain, says Kelly Brownell, Ph.D., professor of psychology at Yale University and a well-known expert on weight loss.

So what's the very best weight-loss program around? "There is no such thing," says Dr. Brownell. "Weight Watchers is very effective for some people, not so effective for others. Overeaters Anonymous is a similar case. It depends on who you are. One program isn't necessarily better than another—they're just different from one another," he says.

And these differences can be enormous. "Some plans are completely do-it-yourself, like buying a diet book. Others are low-cost, self-help type groups, like Overeaters Anonymous. There are commercial programs, like Weight Watchers. There are diet centers, like Optifast . . . specialty university clinics . . . and special spas and resorts," says Dr. Brownell.

How do you choose from so many options? "Shop around. Talk to friends. Comb the newspapers. Make calls. Ask a few places to send literature. Go and visit and find out how each meets your needs," says Dr. Brownell. But, he adds, "you must make sure that certain minimum criteria are met by any program."

Among these criteria, sensible weight-loss programs usually aim for a loss of about 1 pound a week, sometimes 3 or 4, but *never* 10. "Any program that makes dramatic claims for the speed and amount of weight loss should be suspect," says Dr. Brownell. A diet that advocates less than 1,500 calories per day for a man or under 1,200 for a woman should only be followed under medical supervision.

Sensible weight-loss programs are also built on a sound nutritional framework. They advocate a diet that includes all the basic food groups—not just one or two foods. And they advocate exercise. "Diet and exercise work better than either alone," says Dr. Brownell. Any weight-loss program—if it's going to be successful—*must* deal with changing both your long-term dieting *and* exercise habits, he says.

What about diet pills? "Those you can buy over the counter are likely to have a trivial effect on your weight," says Dr. Brownell. Your doctor may prescribe something that's a bit more effective (often with side effects). But in the end, says Dr. Brownell, "it's your behavior that's going to make a difference—not any pill." *See also* **exercise therapy; fasting; low-fat diet**

weight training.   *See* **exercise therapy**

Wellbutrin.   *See* **antidepressants**

whirlpool bath.   *See* **hydrotherapy**

willow bark   When your back hurts, your head is pounding, and you've got the flu, it might be a good time to pop a couple aspirin and jump into bed.

You're out of aspirin? No problem. You might find some pain relief if you go out on a limb—a willow limb, that is. The inner bark of willow trees contains salicin, a chemical relative of acetylsalicylic acid, better known as aspirin.

Long before pharmacists were pressing powders into pills, native Americans were brewing willow tea and chewing willow bark, says James A. Duke, Ph.D., a botanist and toxicology specialist with the U.S. Department of Agriculture in Beltsville, Maryland.

"I think a lot of people out in the boonies still use willow bark," Dr. Duke says. "I've chewed up a small twig and put it near a toothache, and that seemed to help. If I thought I had something like rheumatism or arthritis, I would boil it up in a tea."

Willow bark has a distinctly bitter taste, Dr. Duke says. That may explain why it's more often drunk as a tea than chewed fresh off the tree.

How does willow bark compare to aspirin? Dr. Duke estimates that a third of an ounce of bark might contain a gram of salicin—about the equivalent of three aspirin. Bark brewed as a tea, of course, would be quite a bit weaker.

Many herb stores stock willow bark extracts, says Mark Blumenthal, executive director of the American Botanical Council in Austin, Texas. The bark may be sold in bulk, like tea. It also may be packed into capsules, for easy consumption.

A HEALING REPUTATION

Willow bark is reputed to reduce inflammation, cool fevers, and relieve the aches and pains of colds and flus. Drunk regularly, it's theorized it might help prevent some strokes and heart attacks by inhibiting the formation of clots in the bloodstream. In short, willow bark is thought to do many of the same things that aspirin does.

Unlike aspirin, however, willow bark isn't standardized. There's no telling how strong—or weak—a given dose will be.

Experts agree willow bark has earned a place in the annals of folk medicine. That doesn't mean, however, that they all use it themselves.

"I'm not going to chew willow bark if I have a headache—that's silly," says David Spoerke, pharmacist and director of the Denver-based POIS-INDEX Information System, a toxicology computer network. "If I have a headache, I'll take an aspirin."

Dr. Duke, on the other hand, makes occasional raids on nearby willow trees. "If I started sneezing, I would go home right away and brew a tea by boiling some honeysuckle and forsythia—both seem to contain virucides [agents that destroy viruses]—and I'd just strip some willow bark and throw it in," he says. "Whatever I was sick with, I'd be throwing a double whammy at it." *See also* **aspirin**

wintergreen. *See* **oil of wintergreen**

witch hazel You might call witch hazel the "baking soda" of skin care: It's a simple, all-purpose, old-fashioned product that's been used for generations. When distilled and combined with alcohol, the aromatic oil extracted from the bark of the witch hazel shrub makes a soothing and mildly astringent lotion. Its clean, fresh fragrance dissipates quickly after being applied to the skin, a characteristic which appeals to many. And with only 14 percent alcohol, the lotion is nondrying and hypoallergenic—two added bonuses.

"The active ingredient in witch hazel is a tannic acid derivative called catechol tannin, much like the tannins present in tea," says Richard Kirpas, senior vice-president and technical director for The E. E. Dickinson Company, manufacturers of Dickinson's Witch Hazel. "Tannins are vasoconstrictors—they constrict the tiny capillaries and venules [junctions between veins and capillaries] below the skin surface. So witch hazel lotion reduces minor swelling and irritation caused by insect bites, bruises, sunburn, windburn, sprains, scratches, and abrasions."

In the 1920s and 1930s, barbers used witch hazel lotion as an after-shave and hair tonic. Even today, Kirpas says, Dickinson gets hundreds of letters from customers who say they splash on witch hazel as an after-shave.

Perhaps the leading use of witch hazel, though, is to cleanse the skin and remove makeup. And although witch hazel isn't sold as an acne fighter, many teens report that it reduces the swelling of minor pimples and blemishes.

Also, when incorporated into pads and ointments with other ingredients like glycerin, witch hazel is said to help shrink external hemorrhoids.

Witch hazel lotion is sold at most pharmacies and supermarkets.

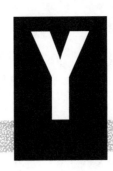

yoga The woman stands absolutely still, feet apart, arms at her sides, eyes straight ahead. Slowly she slides her hands up to her waist and rests them on her hips. She takes a deep breath, then slowly leans over backward until you half-expect her to topple over. But she doesn't. She balances perfectly, hair falling down her back, eyes closed, sensing the gentle stretching of her body.

It can be a bit startling to actually see someone assuming a yoga posture—an *asana*—for the first time. Surely, you think, the human body wasn't meant to stretch that far or in that particular direction. But it was and—with a little practice—it can.

Yoga is actually derived from a 4,000-year-old Indian tradition. The word *yoga,* which literally means "union," refers to a number of specific disciplines. One discipline emphasizes the use of postures or stretches, another stresses study of yoga's ancient literature and history, yet another emphasizes service to others.

A TOTAL BODY BOOST

Most Westerners are familiar with the discipline that emphasizes stretches and poses—called *Hatha* yoga—because they've seen examples of it in television programs, exercise videos, or even classes at a local YWCA/YMCA.

Why is it so popular? Studies indicate that this particular type of yoga may reduce mental fatigue, increase your ability to think and remember, and improve breathing capacity, reaction time, and metabolism. And, most yoga practitioners will tell you that it helps them relax and respond in a healthier, more productive manner to stressful situations than they did before they began yoga.

Orthopedists and sports medicine doctors particularly like yoga's ability to relax muscles. As Allentown, Pennsylvania, physiatrist Charles Norelli, M.D., points out, "If your back hurts because you've got a muscular problem, than there's a good chance yoga can help."

He also considers yoga beneficial for chronic headaches caused by muscle tension, and for fibromyalgia, a condition characterized by widespread aches and pains, insomnia, and morning stiffness. "People who have fibromyalgia need to relax the muscles as they're stretching them," says Dr. Norelli. And yoga does exactly that.

THE THREEFOLD HELPER

Another physician impressed with the benefits of yoga is Mary Pullig Schatz, M.D., a Nashville pathologist who also practices physical medicine. Because yoga did such a good job of healing her own bad back, she now prescribes it for many of her patients.

Basically, any disease or condition that can be helped with relaxation can be helped with yoga, says Dr. Schatz. Muscular strains and sprains, anxiety, high blood pressure, colitis, asthma, and other respiratory diseases all fit into that category.

Yoga works on three levels, she explains. It boosts circulation, triggers the body's relaxation mechanisms, and helps to correct bad habits of posture that have gotten "locked" into the body. "Slouched posture, for example, can lead to neck, shoulder, and upper back pain. Yoga can help correct that."

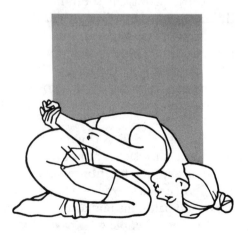

Yoga asana: the Moon

Want to give yoga a try? The Moon asana described here is said to be a particularly calming yoga posture. (Note: This exercise should be avoided if you have high blood pressure.) Kneel on a flat surface and sit on your heels. Grasp your right wrist with your left hand behind your back. Inhale, and as you exhale, bend forward slowly from the hips until your forehead is on the ground—or as close to the ground as you can get it. If your forehead won't reach the ground, rest your forehead on a folded towel or blanket. Let go of your wrist and allow your arms to rest on the floor on either side of you. Hold this position for a moment or two, then, as you slowly inhale, lift yourself back up until you are once again upright in a kneeling position. *See also* **Relaxation Response**

yogurt The sour, custardy food we know as yogurt comes from the marriage of milk and certain bacteria that cause the milk to ferment. *Lactobacillus bulgaricus* and *Streptococcus thermophilus* are the bacteria cultures used to make yogurt. When you eat them in their live, active state, these bacteria multiply in your gastrointestinal tract and supplement the friendly bacteria normally present there.

The bacterial fermentation process makes the protein in yogurt easier to digest than the protein in milk. That fact, combined with its high calcium content, makes yogurt a nutritiously worthy addition to just about anyone's diet.

But if you are looking to yogurt

for benefits beyond good nutrition, know this: There is no solid, scientific evidence for any health claims made about yogurt, says Sherwood L. Gorbach, M.D., a Tufts University researcher whose special area of interest is lactobacilli and human health.

DIARRHEA PREVENTED

There is some evidence, however, that yogurt may have even more to offer. Studies suggest that eating yogurt with active cultures can prevent the diarrhea that so often develops when a person is taking antibiotics.

In a study at the University of Lille in France, nine out of ten volunteers on erythromycin therapy remained diarrhea free while eating three servings of yogurt a day, despite the antibiotic's reputation for causing bowel upset. Yogurt without the beneficial bacteria didn't have the same protective effect.

Yogurt may be of benefit against other intestinal disorders, too. In one study, mice who were fed yogurt successfully fought off the type of salmonella poisoning people get from eating contaminated poultry. The researchers discovered that the yogurt-fed mice had a more plentiful supply of immune cells in their blood, liver, and spleen than mice who were fed the usual diet. The yogurt-fed mice also had fewer salmonella organisms sticking onto their intestinal walls. This effect has not been demonstrated in humans.

Yogurt bacteria may even exert a protective effect against cancer. In one laboratory study, *L. bulgaricus* was shown to possess potent antitumor activity in the test tube. In another, yogurt consumption brought about a 28 to 35 percent reduction in tumor cells in mice, compared to a control group fed milk. The researchers involved in these cancer studies stress that there is no proof that yogurt—or yogurt bacteria—can prevent cancer in humans.

"In general, yogurt is a very good product," says Khem M. Shahani, Ph.D., an expert at the University of Nebraska–Lincoln who has done numerous cancer/yogurt studies himself. "But it should not be used as a medicine to treat cancer."

If you want to take advantage of the best yogurt has to offer, follow this simple rule: Choose only live-culture products. Most brands you find on the grocer's shelf contain active beneficial bacteria. In such cases, the product label often says "contains active yogurt cultures." But check before you buy. If the label says "heat-treated after culturing," that means the active bacteria probably have been killed. Keep in mind, too, that while frozen yogurt typically does contain live cultures, there may be significantly fewer than in regular yogurt. *See also* **acidophilus**

Z

zinc.   *See* **cold remedies**